Study Guide

Pharmacology

A Patient-Centered Nursing Process Approach

8th Edition

Joyce LeFever Kee, MS, RN
Associate Professor Emerita
School of Nursing
College of Health Sciences
University of Delaware
Newark, Delaware

Evelyn R. Hayes, PhD, MPH, FNP-BC
Professor
School of Nursing
College of Health Sciences
University of Delaware
Newark, Delaware

Linda E. McCuistion, PhD, RN, ANP, CNS
Professor
South University
Richmond Campus
Richmond, Virginia

Study Guide prepared by

Lisa A. Hollett, BSN, RN, MA, MICN, CFN
Trauma Program Manager
Department of Trauma Services
St. John Medical Center
Tulsa, Oklahoma

ELSEVIER
SAUNDERS

ELSEVIER
SAUNDERS

3251 Riverport Lane
St. Louis, Missouri 63043

STUDY GUIDE FOR PHARMACOLOGY:
A PATIENT-CENTERED NURSING PROCESS APPROACH ISBN: 978-1-455-77053-3

International Standard Book Number 978-1-455-77053-3

Executive Content Strategist: Lee Henderson
Content Manager: Jennifer Ehlers
Content Development Specialist: Jacqueline Twomey
Publishing Services Manager: Jeffrey Patterson
Project Manager: Clay S. Broeker
Publishing Services: Lisa Hernandez

Printed in the United States of America

Last digit is the print number: 9 8 7 6 5 4 3 2 1

Preface

This comprehensive *Study Guide* is designed to provide the learner with clinically based situation practice problems and questions. This book accompanies the text *Pharmacology: A Patient-Centered Nursing Process Approach*, Eighth Edition, and may also be used independently of the text.

Opportunities abound for the enhancement of critical thinking and decision-making abilities. Hundreds of study questions and answers are presented on nursing responsibilities in therapeutic pharmacology. For example, Chapter 14 is composed of six sections, each devoted to a specific area of medications and calculations. Multiple practice opportunities are provided in the areas of measurement, methods of drug calculations, calculation of oral and injectable dosages (including pediatrics), and calculation of intravenous fluids. Each chapter follows a format that includes study questions (including multiple choice, matching, word searches, crossword puzzles, and completion exercises), NCLEX review questions (including alternate-item format questions), and case studies.

There are more than 160 drug calculation problems and questions, many relating to actual patient care situations and enhanced with real drug labels. The learner is also expected to recognize safe dosage parameters for the situation. The combination of the instructional material in the text and the multiplicity of a variety of practice problems in this *Study Guide* preclude the need for an additional drug dosage calculation book.

The nursing process is used throughout the patient situation–based questions and case studies. Chapters have questions that relate to assessment data, including laboratory data and side effects, planning and implementing care, patient/family teaching, cultural and nutritional considerations, and effectiveness of the drug therapy regimen.

Because of the ever-expanding number of drugs available, pharmacology can be an overwhelming subject. To help students grasp essential content without becoming overwhelmed, chapters have been divided into multiple smaller sections. The result is a layout that is user-friendly.

To underscore the importance of the nurse's role in patient safety, a new safety icon has been added to call attention to questions concerning safe patient care. As one of the six core competencies of the Quality and Safety Education for Nurses (QSEN) initiative, patient safety has never been more at the forefront of nursing education.

Answers to all questions are presented in the Answer Key to make studying easier. New to this edition are rationales for selected application-level questions and case study questions.

The *Study Guide* is part of a comprehensive pharmacology package, including the textbook and Instructor and Student Resources available on the companion Evolve website. This package and each of its components were designed to promote critical thinking and learning. We are excited about this edition of the *Study Guide* because it offers the learner a variety of modalities for mastering the content.

Contents

1 Drug Action: Pharmaceutic, Pharmacokinetic, and Pharmacodynamic Phases

Study Questions

Crossword puzzle: Use the definition to determine the pharmacologic term.

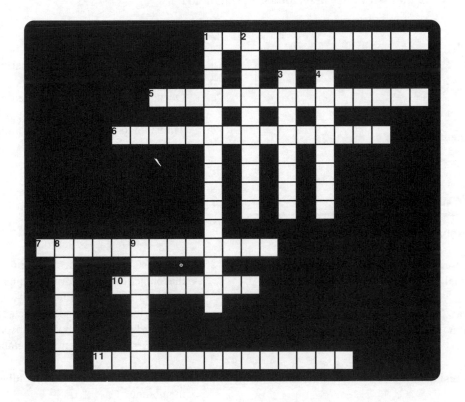

Across

1. Dissolution of the drug
5. Effect of drug action because of hereditary influence
6. Four processes of drug movement to achieve drug action
7. Drug tolerance to repeated administration of a drug
10. One-half of the drug concentration to be eliminated
11. Drug bound to protein

Down

1. Effect of drug action on cells
2. Drug that blocks a response
3. Toxic effect as a result of drug dose or therapy
4. Located on a cell membrane to enhance drug action
8. Drug that produces a response
9. Psychologic benefit from a compound that may not have the chemical structure of a drug effect

Match the terms in Column I with their descriptions in Column II.

Column I

_____ 12.   Protein-bound drug

_____ 13.   Unbound drug

_____ 14.   Hepatic first pass

_____ 15.   Dissolution

_____ 16.   Passive absorption

_____ 17.   Nonselective receptors

Column II

a.   Breakdown of a drug into smaller particles

b.   Proceeds directly from intestine to the liver

c.   Drugs that affect various receptors

d.   Free active drug causing a pharmacologic response

e.   Causes inactive drug action/response

f.   Drug absorbed by diffusion

g.   Drug requiring a carrier for absorption

Match the terms in Column I with their descriptions in Column II.

Column I

_____ 18.   Onset

_____ 19.   Peak action

_____ 20.   Duration of action

_____ 21.   Therapeutic index

Column II

a.   Length of time a drug has a pharmacologic effect

b.   The margin of safety of a drug

c.   Occurs when a drug has reached its highest plasma concentration

d.   Time it takes a drug to reach minimum effective concentration

NCLEX Review Questions

Select the best response.

22.   Which drug form is most rapidly absorbed from the gastrointestinal (GI) tract?
   a. Capsule
   b. Sublingual
   c. Suspension
   d. Tablet

23.   Where does disintegration of enteric-coated tablets occur?
   a. Colon
   b. Liver
   c. Small intestine
   d. Stomach

24.   Usually food has what effect on dissolution and absorption of medication?
   a. Accelerates
   b. Decelerates
   c. Has no effect
   d. Prevents

25.   Which statement places the four processes of pharmacokinetics in the correct sequence?
   a. Absorption, metabolism, distribution, excretion
   b. Distribution, absorption, metabolism, excretion
   c. Distribution, metabolism, absorption, excretion
   d. Absorption, distribution, metabolism, excretion

26.   Which type of drug passes rapidly through the GI membrane?
   a. Lipid-soluble and ionized
   b. Lipid-soluble and nonionized
   c. Water-soluble and ionized
   d. Water-soluble and nonionized

27.   Which factor(s) most commonly affect(s) a drug's absorption? *(Select all that apply.)*
   a. Body mass index
   b. Hypotension
   c. Pain
   d. Sleep
   e. Stress

28. The patient is taking diazepam (Valium) for anxiety. Two days later she is started on dicloxacillin for an infection. What does the nurse know will happen to the diazepam in the patient's body?
    a. The diazepam remains highly protein bound.
    b. The diazepam is deactivated.
    c. Most of the diazepam is released, and it becomes more active.
    d. The diazepam is excreted in the urine unchanged.

29. Which body organ is the major site of drug metabolism?
    a. Kidney
    b. Liver
    c. Lung
    d. Skin

30. What route of drug absorption has the greatest bioavailability?
    a. Intramuscular
    b. Intravenous
    c. Oral
    d. Subcutaneous

31. Which is the best description of a drug's serum half-life?
    a. The time required for half of a drug dose to be absorbed
    b. The time required after absorption for half of the drug to be eliminated
    c. The time required for a drug to be totally effective
    d. The time required for half of the drug dose to be completely distributed

32. The patient is taking a drug that has a half-life of 24 to 30 hours. In preparing discharge teaching, what is the dosing schedule the nurse anticipates will be prescribed for this medication?
    a. Daily
    b. Every other day
    c. Twice per day
    d. Three times per day

33. Which type of drug can be eliminated through the kidneys?
    a. Enteric-coated
    b. Lipid-soluble
    c. Protein-bound
    d. Water-soluble

34. The older adult patient has a creatinine clearance of 30 mL/min. He has been prescribed trimethoprim (Proloprim) for a urinary tract infection. If the normal dose is 200 mg per day, what does the nurse anticipate will occur with the dosing regimen?
    a. The dose will double.
    b. The dose will decrease by one-half.
    c. The dose will stay the same.
    d. The dose will increase to three times per day.

35. Which is the best determinant of the biologic activity of a drug?
    a. The fit of the drug at the receptor site
    b. The misfit of the drug at the receptor site
    c. Inability of the drug to bind to a specific receptor
    d. Ability of the drug to be rapidly excreted

36. Which type of drug prevents or inhibits a cellular response?
    a. Agonist
    b. Antagonist
    c. Cholinergics
    d. Nonspecific drug

37. A receptor located in different parts of the body may initiate a variety of responses depending on the anatomic site. Which type of receptor responds in this manner?
    a. Ligand-gated
    b. Nonselective
    c. Nonspecific
    d. Placebo

38. Which indicator measures the margin of safety of a drug?
    a. Therapeutic range
    b. Therapeutic index
    c. Duration of action
    d. Biologic half-life

39. The nurse has just given the patient her prescribed antibiotic. Which measurement checks for the highest plasma/serum concentration of the drug?
    a. Peak level
    b. Minimal effective concentration
    c. Half-life
    d. Trough level

40. Before administering a medication, the nurse checks a drug reference book or pamphlet to obtain pertinent data. Which data should the nurse note? *(Select all that apply.)*
    a. Contraindications
    b. Half-life
    c. Maximum effective concentration
    d. Protein-binding effect
    e. Therapeutic range

41. Which type of physiologic effect is not related to the desired effect(s) and are predictable or associated with the use of a specific drug?
    a. Severe adverse reactions
    b. Side effects
    c. Synergistic effects
    d. Toxic effects

42. The nurse is giving a large initial dose of a drug to rapidly achieve minimum effective concentration in the plasma. What is this type of dosage called?
    a. Therapeutic dose
    b. Toxic dose
    c. Loading dose
    d. Peak dose

43. A time-response curve evaluates parameters of a drug's action. Which parameter(s) is/are part of the time-response curve? *(Select all that apply.)*
    a. Duration of action
    b. Onset of action
    c. Peak action
    d. Therapeutic range
    e. Minimum effective concentration

44. Which intervention(s) regarding drug therapy should the nurse implement? *(Select all that apply.)*
    a. Assess for side effects, with a focus on undesirable side effects
    b. Check reference books or drug inserts before administering the medication
    c. Teach the patient to wait one week after appearance of side effects to see if they disappear
    d. Check the patient's serum therapeutic range of drugs that have a narrow therapeutic range
    e. Evaluate peak and trough levels prior to administering the medication

Case Study

Read the scenario and answer the following questions on a separate sheet of paper.

M.E. has been prescribed verapamil (Calan) for angina. The nurse knows that this medication is part of the ligand-gated ion channel receptor family.

1. Explain the receptor theory and the four receptor families. What class of medication is verapamil, and how does it work?

2. What key teaching points will the nurse provide to M.E. regarding this medication?

2 The Drug Approval Process

Study Questions

Crossword puzzle: Use the definition to determine the pharmacologic term.

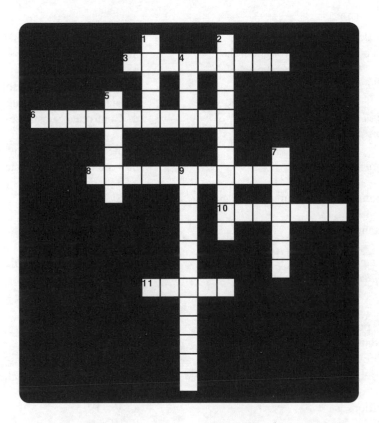

Across

3. Derived from the foxglove plant
6. A drug dose that results in the patient's death
8. Omitting a drug dose that results in the patient's death
10. Schedule II drug—American
11. Name owned by the manufacturer

Down

1. Approval seal of reputable online pharmacies
2. Giving the right drug by the wrong route that results in the patient's death
4. Toxic to children in large doses
5. Schedule I drug—Canadian
7. Nonproprietary name
9. Schedule III drugs—Canadian

Match the act or amendment in Column I with the description in Column II.

Column I

_____ 12.   Kefauver-Harris Amendment

_____ 13.   Food, Drug, and Cosmetic Act

_____ 14.   The Orphan Drug Act

_____ 15.   Durham-Humphrey Amendment

Column II

a.   Determines which drugs can be sold with or without a prescription

b.   Tightened controls on drug safety and testing

c.   Promotes the development of drugs used to treat rare illnesses

d.   Empowered the FDA to monitor and regulate the manufacture and marketing of drugs

NCLEX Review Questions

Select the best response.

16.   What resource provides the basis for standards in drug strength and composition throughout the world?
    a.   *United States Pharmacopeia/National Formulary*
    b.   *American Hospital Formulary Service (AHFS) Drug Information*
    c.   *MedlinePlus*
    d.   *International Pharmacopeia*

17.   What is the current authoritative source for drug standards?
    a.   Controlled Substances Act
    b.   *MedlinePlus*
    c.   The *Medical Letter*
    d.   *United States Pharmacopeia/National Formulary*

18.   What is the primary purpose of federal legislation related to drug standards?
    a.   Provide consistency
    b.   Establish cost controls
    c.   Ensure safety
    d.   Promote competition

19.   Which legislation identified those drugs that require a new prescription for a refill?
    a.   Controlled Substances Act
    b.   Durham-Humphrey Amendment
    c.   Food, Drug, and Cosmetic Act of 1938
    d.   Kefauver-Harris Amendment

20.   The Kefauver-Harris Amendment was passed to improve safety by requiring which information to be included in the drug's literature?
    a.   Recommended dose
    b.   Pregnancy category
    c.   Side effects and contraindications
    d.   Adverse reactions and contraindications

21.   What state law controls drug administration by nurses?
    a.   Nurse practice act
    b.   Food, Drug, and Cosmetic Act
    c.   State board of nursing
    d.   Controlled Substances Act

22.   In the United States, how many categories/schedules are controlled substances grouped into?
    a.   3
    b.   5
    c.   7
    d.   9

23.   Drugs on which schedule have accepted medical use?
    a.   I through IV
    b.   I through V
    c.   II through V
    d.   III through V

24.   What is correct about schedule drugs' potential for abuse?
    a.   V > IV
    b.   III > I
    c.   I > III
    d.   V > III

25.   The patient presents to the emergency department with hallucinations. The patient's friends state he has been using lysergic acid diethylamide (LSD) and mescaline. To which schedule do these drugs belong?
    a.   Schedule IV
    b.   Schedule III
    c.   Schedule II
    d.   Schedule I

26. In which schedule would the nurse find codeine, which is included in cough syrup?
    a. II
    b. III
    c. IV
    d. V

27. Where must controlled substances be stored in an institution/agency?
    a. Double-wrapped and labeled
    b. In the patient's medicine bin
    c. Near the nurse's station
    d. In a locked, secured area

28. In Canada, on what drug schedule is morphine?
    a. I
    b. II
    c. III
    d. IV

29. In Canada, over-the-counter preparations are administered by which group of the respective provinces?
    a. Pharmacy Acts
    b. Canadian Food and Drug Act
    c. 1961 Narcotic Control Act
    d. Health Protection Act

30. Which legislation decreased the time for approval of drugs so they could be developed and marketed to the public more rapidly?
    a. Patient Protection and Affordable Care Act
    b. Drug Regulation Reform Act of 1978
    c. Durham-Humphrey Amendment
    d. Kefauver-Harris Amendment

31. Which drug reference is published annually and updated monthly?
    a. *United States Pharmacopeia/National Formulary*
    b. *Prescriber's Letter*
    c. *American Hospital Formulary Service (AHFS) Drug Information*
    d. The *Medical Letter*

32. The nurse must be alert for counterfeit prescription drugs. What is/are clue(s) to identification of counterfeit products? *(Select all that apply.)*
    a. Different color
    b. Different dose
    c. Different taste
    d. Different labeling
    e. Different shape

Case Study

Read the scenario and answer the following question on a separate sheet of paper.

L.L. has received a prescription for a medication to treat bronchitis and is preparing for discharge from the emergency department. He says to the nurse, "I don't understand all of this paperwork that I have to sign. I sign this same form every time. What is HIPAA, and why should I even care?"

1. How will the nurse explain HIPAA to the patient as it pertains to his medications?

3 Cultural and Pharmacogenetic Considerations

Study Questions

Match the term in Column I with its definition in Column II.

Column I

_____ 1. Assimilation

_____ 2. Complementary health practices

_____ 3. Pharmacogenetics

_____ 4. Ethnopharmacology

_____ 5. Traditional health practices

_____ 6. Alternative health care

Column II

a. Study of drug responses unique to an individual due to social, cultural, and biological phenomena

b. The effect of a drug varies from the predicted response due to genetic factors

c. The use of new therapies in place of mainstream therapies to treat an illness

d. Includes the use of teas, herbs, spices, and special foods

e. Occurs when a less powerful group changes its ways and practices to blend in with the dominant group

f. Combines traditional beliefs with mainstream practices

NCLEX Review Questions

Select the best response.

7. Which statement reflects the physiologic response of African-American individuals to medications?
    a. They are less responsive to beta blockers than are European Americans and Hispanics.
    b. They are more responsive to beta blockers than are European Americans and Hispanics.
    c. They experience fewer toxic side effects with psychotropic medications than do European Americans.
    d. They experience fewer toxic side effects with antidepressant medications than do European Americans.

8. Which ethnic or cultural group may experience increased problems with lactose intolerance?
    a. African descent
    b. Asian descent
    c. Latin American descent
    d. Native American descent

9. What communication style is characteristic of people of European descent?
    a. Comfortable with periods of silence
    b. Maintenance of eye contact
    c. Use a soft voice
    d. Utilize few words

10. The patient, who is Jamaican, is currently 4 months pregnant and informs the nurse during a prenatal visit that she eats red clay to provide nutrients to the fetus. She states that this is a practice her grandmother told her would ensure a healthy pregnancy. What is the best action by the nurse?
    a. Contact Child Protective Services.
    b. Insist that she stop the practice immediately.
    c. Determine the amount of clay she eats daily.
    d. Discuss the research about dietary intake of clay.

11. The older adult patient is newly diagnosed with diabetes and has been started on metformin. The patient's healer has recommended that the patient drink sabila tea three times per day to improve nutrition and help control blood sugar. What is the nurse's best action?
    a. Encourage the patient to drink it four times per day instead.
    b. Discourage the practice because sabila tea potentiates metformin.
    c. Tell him he must stop the tea immediately.
    d. Advise him he can continue to drink the tea, but he also needs to continue his medications.

12. Which factor(s) may affect a patient's physiologic responses to medications? *(Select all that apply.)*
    a. Age
    b. Diet
    c. Genetics
    d. Language
    e. Values

13. Which factor(s) may affect a patient's adherence to medication regimens? *(Select all that apply.)*
    a. Access to health care
    b. Heredity
    c. Poverty
    d. Trust in provider
    e. Use of same language

Case Study

Read the scenario and answer the following questions on a separate sheet of paper.

A Chinese couple brings their 4-year-old, 19-kg daughter to the emergency department (ED). She was seen in the same ED 2 days earlier and was diagnosed with a pulmonary infection. During her previous visit, she was prescribed erythromycin 200 mg, 1 teaspoon every 6 hours for 10 days. The parents are concerned that their daughter is not well yet. They bring the bottle of liquid erythromycin with them in a plastic bag, along with a porcelain soup spoon that is the size of a tablespoon. The bottle is almost half empty.

1. What is the nurse's first concern?

2. How will the nurse approach the family and child to provide culturally competent care?

4 Drug Interactions and Over-the-Counter Drugs

Study Questions

Crossword puzzle: Use the definition to determine the pharmacologic term.

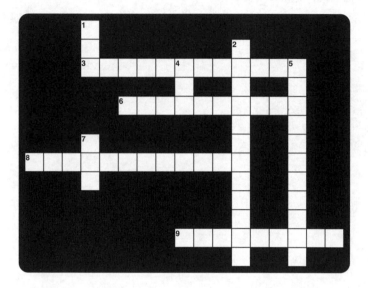

Across

3. No longer found in over-the-counter (OTC) weight-control drugs
6. Movement of a drug from the site of administration into body fluids
8. How a drug becomes available to body fluids and body tissues
9. Elimination of a drug from the body

Down

1. Monitors safety of drugs
2. To break down a drug
4. Category of OTC drugs considered to be ineffective (spell out)
5. When two drugs are given together, one can potentiate the other
7. Drugs obtainable without a prescription (abbreviation)

Match the terms in Column I with the letter of the definition in Column II.

Column I

_____ 10. Drug interaction

_____ 11. Drug incompatibility

_____ 12. Adverse drug reaction

_____ 13. Pharmacokinetic interaction

_____ 14. Pharmacodynamic interaction

Column II

a. Undesirable drug effect

b. Changes that occur in the absorption, distribution, metabolism, or excretion of one or more drugs

c. Altered effect of a drug as a result of interaction with other drugs

d. A chemical or physical reaction that happens between two or more drugs in vitro

e. Interaction that results in additive, synergistic, or antagonistic drug effects

Match the agents in Column I with the letter of the action in Column II. Each agent may have multiple actions. Select all that apply.

Column I

_____ 15. Laxatives

_____ 16. Aspirin

_____ 17. Antacids

_____ 18. Food

_____ 19. Opioids

Column II

a. Decrease drug absorption

b. Increase drug absorption

c. Block drug absorption

d. Change urine pH to alkaline

e. Change urine pH to acid

f. Increase drug excretion

NCLEX Review Questions

Select the best response.

20. The 6-year-old patient is complaining of a sore throat, productive cough, and bilateral knee pain, and the health care provider has started the child on an antibiotic. The child's parent is about to administer several OTC medications. What will concern the nurse about a child taking multiple OTC medications? *(Select all that apply.)*
    a. The OTC medications may interact with one another.
    b. The OTC medications may interact with the prescription medication.
    c. OTC medications must be taken with food.
    d. OTC medications can never be taken with prescription medications.
    e. OTC and prescription medications should not be taken without consulting a provider.
    f. This child is too young for OTC medications.

21. The patient is taking carbamazepine (Tegretol) for seizures. She is also taking warfarin (Coumadin) because she has a history of deep venous thrombosis (DVT). What will concern the nurse about the interaction of this drug and warfarin?
    a. A larger dose of warfarin may be needed.
    b. A smaller dose of warfarin may be needed.
    c. These medications cannot be taken together.
    d. An alternative to carbamazepine must be utilized.

22. The older adult patient is a vegetarian and has a history of atrial fibrillation. The patient is taking warfarin and states that his favorite vegetables are spinach, broccoli, and Brussels sprouts. What will concern the nurse about the patient's diet and the type of anticoagulant he is taking?
    a. The green vegetables are high in vitamin K, which increases the effects of warfarin.
    b. The green vegetables are low in vitamin K, which increases the effects of warfarin.
    c. The green vegetables are high in vitamin K, which decreases the effects of warfarin.
    d. The green vegetables are low in vitamin K, which decreases the effects of warfarin.

23. The patient is taking digitalis for atrial fibrillation. The patient complains to the nurse that she has problems with constipation so she takes a laxative three to four times per week. What concerns the nurse about the frequency of laxative use?
    a. Laxatives slow down gastric emptying, which increases drug absorption.
    b. Laxatives increase gastric emptying, which decreases drug absorption.
    c. Laxatives impact the liver's metabolism of medications, thereby increasing their effects.
    d. Laxatives impact the liver's metabolism of medications, thereby decreasing their effects.

24. The patient is taking ciprofloxacin (Cipro) for an infection. When completing the discharge teaching, what foods will the nurse advise the patient to avoid while taking the medication?
    a. Cheese
    b. Grapes
    c. Hamburger
    d. Oatmeal

25. Which drug group is primarily absorbed by the small intestine?
    a. Anticonvulsants
    b. Barbiturates
    c. Salicylates
    d. Xanthine derivatives

26. The patient has been injured playing football and has been prescribed two different analgesics for pain relief. Two drugs with similar action are administered to achieve which effects?
    a. Additive
    b. Antagonistic
    c. Combined
    d. Synergistic

27. The patient had surgery yesterday for hernia repair. He was discharged home and has been prescribed two medications to be taken at the same time, a narcotic and an antihistamine. The administration of these drugs together will produce which type of effect?
    a. Additive
    b. Antagonistic
    c. Combined
    d. Synergistic

28. The patient presents to the emergency department unresponsive. The patient's friend states the patient was "shooting heroin" and stopped breathing. The nurse is preparing to administer naloxone (Narcan) to reverse the effects of the narcotic. This drug will be administered to produce which type of drug effect?
    a. Additive
    b. Antagonistic
    c. Combined
    d. Synergistic

29. A major drug-food interaction occurs between monoamine oxidase inhibitors and foods rich in what component?
    a. Acetylcholine
    b. Caffeine
    c. Fiber
    d. Tyramine

30. The patient has a history of hypertension and congestive heart failure. The patient is taking digoxin and furosemide. What statement by the patient indicates an understanding of a potentially dangerous drug-drug interaction?
    a. "I only have to take the furosemide when I feel short of breath."
    b. "I need to make sure I eat plenty of foods rich in potassium."
    c. "I cannot take my medicines with cranberry juice."
    d. "I must be sure to not go outside during the day for too long."

31. How are most drugs excreted from the body?
    a. Feces
    b. Lungs
    c. Saliva
    d. Urine

32. Based on review by the Food and Drug Administration, OTC medications are assigned to one of how many categories?
    a. Two
    b. Three
    c. Four
    d. Five

33. Which statement by the patient indicates an understanding of how to prevent a potential drug-induced photosensitivity reaction?
    a. "I must only go out after dark."
    b. "I need to increase my vitamin C intake."
    c. "I should wear sunscreen when I am outside."
    d. "I must stop taking my medication before going on vacation."

34. The patient has a history of hypertension and impaired renal function. The patient is not on dialysis. Which medication(s) should be avoided? *(Select all that apply.)*
    a. Acetaminophen
    b. Aspirin
    c. Ibuprofen
    d. Quinidine
    e. Valproic acid

35. Absorption of which medication is impaired by altered gastrointestinal flora?
    a. Angiotensin-converting enzyme (ACE) inhibitors
    b. Antipsychotics
    c. Phenytoin
    d. Oral contraceptives

36. The patient has a history of angina and migraines. The patient takes a calcium channel blocker for angina, and the health care provider wants to start preventive medication for migraines. Which medication will raise a concern with the nurse?
    a. Acetaminophen
    b. Propranolol
    c. Levetiracetam
    d. Butalbital

5 Drugs of Abuse

Study Questions

Crossword puzzle: Use the definition to determine the pharmacologic term.

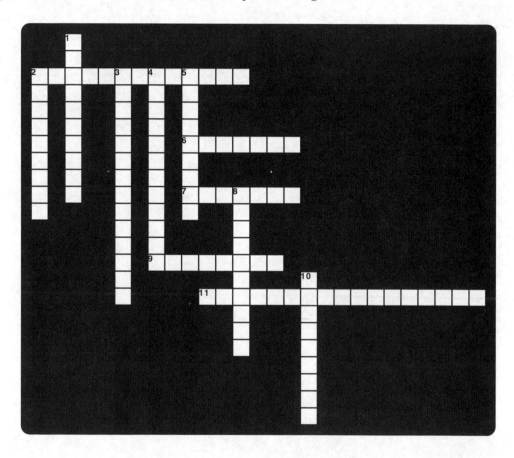

Across

2. Uncontrolled craving for a substance (2 words)
6. Return to drug use after a period of non-use
7. Most potent of the abused stimulants
9. Addictive agent in tobacco
11. A common cause of relapse (3 words)

Down

1. Recreational use of a chemical substance (2 words)
2. Overindulgence in a chemical substance resulting in negative functioning (2 words)
3. Treating an intoxicated patient to remove drugs from the body
4. Under the influence or being affected by a drug
5. Need for larger doses of a drug to obtain original euphoria
8. Sustained avoidance of substance use
10. Antidepressant used to treat nicotine addiction

Match the term in Column I with the definition in Column II.

Column I

_____ 12. Korsakoff's psychosis

_____ 13. Wernicke's encephalopathy

_____ 14. Cross-tolerance

_____ 15. Withdrawal syndrome

Column II

a. Inflammation of the brain from deficit of thiamine
b. Short-term memory loss and inability to learn
c. Can include gross tremors, seizures, and hallucinations
d. Tolerance to one drug causes tolerance to another in the same category

NCLEX Review Questions

Select the best response.

16. The patient presents to the emergency department (ED) under the custody of local law enforcement. The patient reportedly swallowed a small balloon full of cocaine. What clinical manifestations would the nurse expect to see if the balloon ruptured?
    a. Dilated pupils and diaphoresis
    b. Hypotension and tachycardia
    c. Insomnia and fine tremors
    d. Respiratory depression and pinpoint pupils

17. A patient is taking a tricyclic antidepressant as a prophylactic medicine for migraines. She also abuses cocaine. What effect may result from the interaction between these two substances?
    a. Bradycardia
    b. Dysrhythmias
    c. No interaction
    d. Reflex tachycardia

18. Which medication can be given to aid a patient with opioid withdrawal?
    a. Disulfiram (Antabuse)
    b. Lorazepam (Ativan)
    c. Methadone (Dolophine)
    d. Naloxone (Narcan)

19. Which drug contains the only Food and Drug Administration–approved cannabis preparation?
    a. Dronabinol (Marinol)
    b. Lorazepam (Ativan)
    c. Methadone (Dolophine)
    d. Naloxone (Narcan)

20. The patient has decided to quit smoking. What key point(s) must the nurse include in the teaching plan? *(Select all that apply.)*
    a. Assess that the patient is motivated to quit.
    b. Set a quit date of one month.
    c. Help the patient identify triggers or high-risk situations.
    d. Advise the patient he may use chewing tobacco as a substitute.
    e. Provide the patient with a list of over-the-counter and prescription options for smoking cessation aids.
    f. Advise that the patient must use an aid to quit.

21. What percentage of nurses abuse drugs and demonstrate impaired practice due to that abuse?
    a. 1%-2%
    b. 3%-6%
    c. 7%-10%
    d. 11%-15%

22. A mother brings her 13-year-old daughter to the ED because she is "acting strange." The mother states she found a package of "bath salts" in her daughter's bedroom. "Bath salts" are classified as which type of drug?
    a. Amphetamine
    b. Benzodiazepine
    c. Hallucinogenic
    d. Synthetic stimulant

Case Study

Read the scenario and answer the following questions on a separate sheet of paper.

C.L., 57 years old, presents to the ED. He is unresponsive to verbal and painful stimuli and smells strongly of intoxicants. Vital signs include temperature 36.2° C, heart rate 104 beats/minute, respiratory rate 8 breaths/minute, and blood pressure 92/70 mm Hg. Oxygen saturation is 90%.

1.   What is the initial treatment for C.L.?

2.   What is the difference between alcohol withdrawal and Wernicke's encephalopathy? How would each be treated?

6 Herbal Therapies

Study Questions

Crossword puzzle: Use the definitions to determine the correct terms.

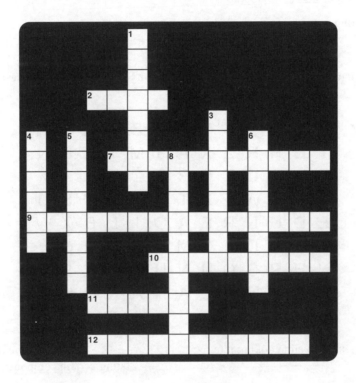

Across

2. Dries up mother's milk
7. Thought to decrease prostate size (2 words)
9. Natural estrogen promoter (2 words)
10. Helps prevent urinary tract infections
11. Increases immune function
12. Its extract may help to prevent liver damage (2 words)

Down

1. Used to treat menstrual cramps (2 words)
3. "Herbal Valium"
4. Decreases nausea in pregnancy
5. May promote healthy vision
6. Used to relieve migraine headaches
8. Increases bile flow

Match the description in Column I with the letter of the reference in Column II.

Column I

_____ 13. "Reasonable certainty" reported on specific herbal remedy

_____ 14. The authoritative source for therapeutic substances

_____ 15. Supports study of alternative therapies

_____ 16. Reviews global literature on herbal studies by clinicians and researchers

_____ 17. Plant-based remedies

_____ 18. Two primary types of herbal monographs

_____ 19. Clarified marketing regulations for herbal remedies

Column II

a. *United States Pharmacopeia*

b. Natural Standard Research Collaboration

c. Phytomedicine

d. German Commission E

e. Office of Alternative Medicine

f. Dietary Supplement Health and Education Act of 1994

g. Therapeutic and qualitative

Complete the following word search. Clues are given in questions 20-25. Circle your responses.

```
P U R Y S T P J B W Q S A
I E H R Z X A J M I Y B N
T I N C T U R E Z P I I X
D A T W E X T R A C T S U
L D U E R E A O I L B X W
W V F D A O M T Y R N O L
N H R S Q U N U E Q P P I
W K L M P Z A H A R C U R
```

20. Adding a sweetener to an herb and cooking it results in a(n) _____.

21. Soaking dried or fresh herbs in boiling water makes a(n) _____.

22. A(n) _____ is derived from soaking fresh or dried herbs in a solvent.

23. _____ have more reliable dosing by isolating certain components.

24. Soaking dried herbs in oil and heating for a long time results in a(n) _____.

25. Enzyme activity may cause fresh _____ to decay in a few days.

Match the herb in Column I with the letter of its description in Column II.

Column I

_____ 26. *Ginkgo biloba*

_____ 27. Peppermint oil

_____ 28. Yarrow

_____ 29. Saw palmetto

_____ 30. Kava

_____ 31. Goldenseal

_____ 32. Psyllium

_____ 33. Echinacea

_____ 34. Ginger

_____ 35. St. John's wort

Column II

a. Provides muscle relaxation

b. Widely used as laxative and with Crohn's disease

c. Immune enhancer

d. May be helpful in Raynaud's and Alzheimer's diseases

e. Relief from stiffness and pain of osteoarthritis and rheumatoid arthritis

f. Tonic, astringent, and relieves congestion of the common cold

g. May be effective treatment for tension headache

h. May decrease International Normalized Ratio (INR)

i. "Herbal Prozac"

j. "Plant catheter"

NCLEX Review Questions

Select the best response.

36. Which herb is commonly used for external treatment of insect bites and minor burns?
    a. *Aloe vera*
    b. Feverfew
    c. Licorice
    d. Yarrow

37. The patient presents to the clinic with complaints of abdominal discomfort and nausea. When obtaining the health history, the nurse inquires about herbal preparations. Which herb would the nurse recognize as one that provides relief of digestive and gastrointestinal distress?
    a. Chamomile
    b. Kava
    c. Licorice
    d. St. John's wort

38. What is the most commonly prescribed herbal remedy worldwide?
    a. Echinacea
    b. Ginger
    c. *Ginkgo biloba*
    d. Peppermint

39. The pregnant patient has been complaining of a sore in her mouth. Her grandmother suggested she try "something natural" due to her pregnancy. Which preparation does the nurse recognize as unsafe due to causing uterine irritability?
    a. Feverfew
    b. Ginger
    c. Goldenseal
    d. Psyllium

40. The patient drinks three to four alcoholic beverages per day and reports that he takes a variety of herbal preparations. Which herb does the nurse recognize as dangerous for this patient given his history?
    a. Kava
    b. Licorice
    c. Milk thistle
    d. Peppermint

41. The patient has just started taking warfarin (Coumadin) for atrial fibrillation. Health teaching for this patient would include information on which herbal product(s)? *(Select all that apply.)*
    a. Evening primrose
    b. Garlic
    c. Ginseng
    d. Hawthorn
    e. Sage

42. The nurse is concerned that a patient may be abusing ginseng. What will the nurse assess in a patient with ginseng abuse syndrome? *(Select all that apply.)*
    a. Edema
    b. Heart tones
    c. Bowel sounds
    d. Reflexes
    e. Pupillary response

43. Which statement(s) by the patient reflect(s) prudent use of herbs? *(Select all that apply.)*
    a. "Herbs are fine to use when breastfeeding."
    b. "Do not take a large quantity of any one herbal product."
    c. "Give the herb time to work for a persistent symptom before seeking care from a health care provider."
    d. "Do not give herbs to infants or young children."
    e. "Brands of herbal products are interchangeable."

44. The nurse is caring for a patient who takes a variety of herbal products and is starting a prescription antidiabetic medication. Which herb(s) will change the effect of the antidiabetic drug? *(Select all that apply.)*
    a. Cocoa
    b. Dandelion
    c. Evening primrose
    d. Feverfew
    e. Garlic

45. The patient tells the nurse he is taking ginkgo. Which medication(s) has/have negative interactions with ginkgo? *(Select all that apply.)*
    a. Antiplatelet agents
    b. Nifedipine (Procardia)
    c. Omeprazole (Prilosec)
    d. Flumazenil (Romazicon)
    e. Carbamazepine (Tegretol)

46. The patient has a history of hypertension, atrial fibrillation, chronic obstructive pulmonary disease, and insomnia. She tells the nurse at discharge, "I really love the taste of licorice. It motivates me to walk every day." What medication alteration(s) is/are seen when given in combination with licorice? *(Select all that apply.)*
    a. Antihypertensive medication effects are decreased.
    b. Corticosteroid effects are increased.
    c. CNS depressant medication effects are decreased.
    d. Digoxin effects are increased.
    e. Rifampin effects are decreased.

Case Study

Read the scenario and answer the following questions on a separate sheet of paper.

K.E., 21 years old, has a history of nausea and vomiting and severe migraine headaches. She has started missing classes and tells the nurse, "I really can't stand feeling terrible all the time." K.E. tells the nurse she has started trying "a bunch" of herbal remedies to attempt to get her symptoms under control. She does not know the names of any of them. She has presented to the student health clinic with a headache.

1. Which medications would the nurse suspect this patient is taking for these symptoms, and what is their presumed mechanism of action?

2. What medications do these herbals interact with?

3. What health teaching will the nurse provide for K.E. regarding the use of herbal preparations?

7 Pediatric Pharmacology

Study Questions

Complete the following.

1. Infants have _____ protein sites than adults, so _____ dosages of medications are needed.

2. The degree and rate of absorption of medications in a pediatric patient are based on _____, _____, _____, and _____.

3. Gastric pH does not reach adult acidity until between _____ and _____ year(s) of age.

4. Distribution of a medication throughout the body is affected by _____, _____, _____, and effectiveness of various barriers to medication transport.

5. Until about the age of _____, the pediatric patient requires a(n) _____ dose of water-soluble medications to achieve therapeutic levels.

Match the child's age group in Column I with a cognitive element to consider when administering medications in Column II.

Column I

_____ 6. Infant

_____ 7. Toddler

_____ 8. Preschool

_____ 9. School-age

_____ 10. Adolescent

Column II

a. Allow some choice
b. Involvement in administration process
c. Contract regarding plan of care
d. Simple explanation
e. Use minimum restraint necessary

NCLEX Review Questions

Select the best response.

11. The nurse is administering an oral medication with a low pH to the 2-week-old infant. What is the impact of the patient's age on the absorption of this medication?
    a. Absorption may be slower in this patient.
    b. Absorption may be quicker in this patient.
    c. This medicine will be absorbed at the same rate as an older patient.
    d. Oral medications should not be administered to this age group.

12. The 18-month-old child has been prescribed an oral medication that is water-soluble. Based on the nurse's knowledge of medication distribution, how may the dosage need to be modified for the patient in order to reach therapeutic levels?
    a. Alternate route
    b. Decreased
    c. Increased
    d. No change

13. The blood-brain barrier in infants is immature. Which outcome is more likely in infants?
    a. Increased effect of medication
    b. More side effects from medication
    c. Quicker results of medication
    d. Toxicity risk is higher

14. The 3-year-old patient requires a topical medication. What does the nurse know about the rate of absorption for topical medications in this age group?
    a. The medication will absorb faster.
    b. The medication will absorb slower.
    c. There will be no difference.
    d. It depends on the sex of the child.

15. What are the components of pharmacokinetics? *(Select all that apply.)*
    a. Absorption
    b. Distribution
    c. Excretion
    d. Metabolism
    e. Onset

16. The 12-year-old patient has been admitted for nausea, vomiting, and diarrhea, and the health care provider has prescribed several medications. What concern(s) will the nurse have regarding medication administration? *(Select all that apply.)*
    a. Renal tubular function is decreased.
    b. Dehydration may lead to toxicity.
    c. The medications should not be administered by the oral route.
    d. Rectal administration will promote quick absorption.
    e. Developmental levels must be considered.

17. The nurse is teaching a group of parents how to administer medications to their children. Which element(s) of medication administration will be included in the teaching? *(Select all that apply.)*
    a. Allow the child to determine the time of medication administration.
    b. Lightly restrain the child as needed.
    c. Praise the child after successful administration.
    d. Never threaten the child into taking the medication.
    e. Never tell the child what to expect, just give the medication.
    f. Herbal preparations should not, in general, be given to children.

Case Study

Read the scenario and answer the following questions on a separate sheet of paper.

A.M., 4 years old, fell from a tree branch and fractured her forearm. An IV needs to be established and analgesia administered.

1. What strategies may the nurse implement to provide developmentally appropriate care for this patient?

2. Discuss the utilization of topical anesthetics prior to IV starts.

3. How may the caregiver be involved in the patient's care while the IV is established?

Study Questions

Crossword puzzle: Use the definition to determine the correct term.

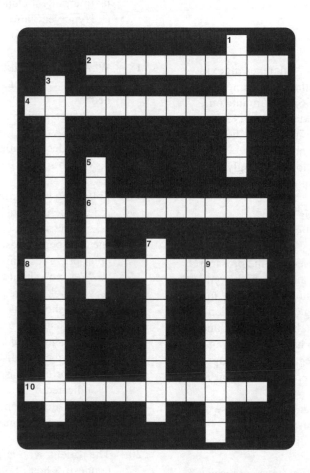

Across

2. Affected by alkaline gastrointestinal pH found in older persons
4. Affected by loss of binding proteins
6. Type of drugs usually prescribed for heart failure or hypertension
8. Taking multiple medications together
10. Not taking medications as prescription indicates

Down

1. Long-term use of this drug must be monitored due to its narrow therapeutic range
3. Drug metabolism that occurs in the liver and contributes to clearance of drugs
5. Major organ involved in drug excretion
7. 75% of nursing home residents take this type of drug
9. Taking medications as prescribed

NCLEX Review Questions

Select the best response.

11. What is an indicator of the glomerular filtration rate and the normal value for an adult?
    a. Creatinine clearance: 80-130 mL/min
    b. SGOT: 4-12 mL/min
    c. Troponin: 80-120 mL/min
    d. Urea: 1.2-4.5

12. The safest antihypertensive agents for older adults have a low incidence of what side effect?
    a. Constipation
    b. Electrolyte imbalance
    c. Loss of appetite
    d. Vision disturbances

13. The patient, who is 84 years old, takes digoxin (Lanoxin) for atrial fibrillation. The home health nurse finds a heart rate of 46 beats/minute on assessment, and the patient tells the nurse that he has been nauseous and vomiting since the last visit. Why does this concern the nurse?
    a. This could be an indication of hypoglycemia.
    b. This is an indication of possible digoxin toxicity.
    c. This patient probably has the flu.
    d. This patient may be malnourished.

14. The older adult patient presents to the provider's office for a follow-up visit and also with complaints of sneezing, runny nose, headache, and scratchy eyes after working out in the garden. The patient states he takes digitalis, fluoxetine, and a multivitamin regularly and has started taking diphenhydramine since he began having symptoms. What statement by the patient indicates that further teaching is needed?
    a. "I cannot work outside anymore because of the digitalis."
    b. "I think I need to find a different allergy medicine to take."
    c. "I take fluoxetine because I have depression."
    d. "I should not take my wife's headache medicine."

15. Which medication would have fewer adverse and toxic effects?
    a. Fat-soluble, half-life of 50 hours
    b. Fat-soluble, 90% protein bound
    c. Half-life of 4 hours, 50% protein bound
    d. Fat-soluble, 60% protein bound

16. Which specific lab value(s) should be monitored in a geriatric patient to assess kidney function? *(Select all that apply.)*
    a. BUN
    b. Creatinine clearance
    c. CBC
    d. Lipase
    e. Triglycerides

17. The patient, who is 75 years old, reports feeling dizzy every morning when he gets outs of bed. What effect does the nurse recognize the patient is probably experiencing?
    a. Bradycardia
    b. Intermittent claudication
    c. Hyperventilation
    d. Orthostatic hypotension

18. What changes will the nurse recommend to a patient who experiences dizziness when arising from bed?
    a. Change positions slowly.
    b. Move a chair close to the bed.
    c. Take deep breaths.
    d. Take his pulse before standing.

19. Following hospitalization, the older adult patient receives a home visit from the nurse. The patient asks if she should continue to take the medications she took before hospitalization. What is the most appropriate response?
    a. "Yes, you should continue to take the drugs that you took before going to the hospital."
    b. "You should take one-half the dosage of each drug that you took prior to hospitalization."
    c. "You should take only the drugs that have been prescribed on discharge and not drugs that you took prior to hospitalization unless otherwise indicated."
    d. "You should continue to take those drugs that have been helpful to you."

20. The patient, who is 73 years old, has a history of congestive heart failure and has recently been hospitalized due to complications. She tells the nurse that before this hospitalization, she was taking digoxin 0.125 mg/day. The new prescription is for digoxin 0.25 mg/day. The patient asks the nurse what she should do. What is the nurse's best response?
    a. "You should take digoxin 0.125 mg/day."
    b. "You should take digoxin 0.25 mg/day."
    c. "You need to check with a pharmacist first."
    d. "You must take digoxin 0.125 mg in the morning and 0.25 mg at bedtime."

21. The older adult patient states he has difficulties opening his bottle of celecoxib (Celebrex). What is the nurse's best response?
    a. "Please ask your pharmacist to place your medication in a bottle with a non-childproof cap."
    b. "You can keep your medication in a glass cup in the medicine cabinet."
    c. "You could place your medicine in an envelope."
    d. "A family member could help you with your daily medication regimen."

22. An older adult patient is to take newly prescribed drugs at different times. The patient has vision problems. What will the nurse suggest so that the patient can comply with the medication regimen?
    a. "Line up the bottles of medications on a table and take them in that order."
    b. "Obtain a daily (preferably) or weekly pill container from the drugstore and fill the container the day or week before with the drugs."
    c. "Ask a neighbor to give the daily medications."
    d. "Write down the drugs that you have taken each day."

23. The patient, who is 80 years old, has been started on a tricyclic antidepressant. Which clinical manifestation(s) suggest(s) that she is experiencing side effects of this class of drug? *(Select all that apply.)*
    a. Bradycardia
    b. Constipation
    c. Hypertension
    d. Nausea
    e. Urinary retention

24. In older adults, drug dosages are adjusted based on which factor(s)? *(Select all that apply.)*
    a. Amount of adipose tissue
    b. Height
    c. Nutritional status
    d. Laboratory results
    e. Response to medication

25. Before administering drugs to the older adult, what should the nurse know? *(Select all that apply.)*
    a. Whether the drug is highly protein bound
    b. Half-life of the drug
    c. Patient's last bowel movement
    d. Serum levels of drugs with narrow therapeutic range
    e. Baseline vital signs

Case Study

Read the scenario and answer the following questions on a separate sheet of paper.

M.Z., 80 years old, presents to her health care provider for her annual checkup. She has a medical history of diabetes, insomnia, and hypertension. Vital signs are temperature 37.2° C, heart rate 83 beats/minute, respiratory rate 16 breaths/minute, blood pressure 142/90 mm Hg, and blood glucose 96. During the health history, M.Z. complains of having trouble falling asleep and staying asleep, and having to get up several times per night to go to the bathroom. M.Z. says her current medications include hydrochlorothiazide (HCTZ), triazolam (Halcion), and chamomile tea. "I try to remember to take my medications, and sometimes I take an extra one, just in case I forgot one," she says.

1. What laboratory tests would the nurse anticipate for this patient?

2. What suggestions can the nurse make to help with M.Z.'s sleeping difficulties?

3. What further teaching will the nurse provide to the patient about her medication regimen?

9 Collaboration in Community Settings

Study Questions

Complete the following word search. Clues are given in questions 1-7. Circle your responses.

```
R C U L T U R A L C O N S I D E R A T I O N S J O A J V S V L Z
C E N Z E S B X A E F H R X U H S T E B S I D X E V S N E Y J R
G Q G W G W F E N O O L I V Z U Z X R I G L E U E O V S L U R Z
K V Q U T C S E L E Z E B K L I D K D A J I N Y Q I L U F H J T
S R I L L F H K I A Z E X J X O U E D U D N Y K Q D E X A N R O
G D X N N A L T K L P S M Q R F E E D K R I V J J B T C D Y C F
Q C L I D S T T K F E T O N U F L H C Y S Q T A E G T R M U O F
R L I E P I W O C H O B O X F E Z U P E C T H I X B N O I K E P
I L A E G V E B R W Y W L E B B G X Z U P H E G O X I F N U C G
U W S V M A W T B Y O X C A K X Z K T Q Z X M E G N P Z I J D U
R G R E U V L V I B F T L U N F K Z I U F X Z D M X A S S H X C
F E G J N T L B B J S L L E H O S M C G I B E I R U A L T C U J
S Z N E R X W O R G A R E C G C S H D Z A C X B F F W B R Y E O
I K B U N X H O I N R X J Z U F I R Z L J Y F M E W Z H A P R M
L W I E I E Q Y I S K O L V B L O N E A Y R E T Z Q V V T W J P
S X X D G D R G E F O H A G D C L M I P L I Y H V W G O I K Q C
B C V Q I U I A L T I E W S O N O W I I Q N X W E B Z I O F G S
T T P X U R Z B L J V O A I K H R B Q C K G D K C B K A N H H W
L H Y H O M W T R R A F L D D P R O F E S S I O N A L R R I F N
X B X B U F P D S Q E B O W V N L Z J W G W S F R E H T Y Q A V
```

1. Medication administration in any community setting must be consistent with _____, _____, and _____ requirements.

2. Communication and tracking are required to _____ untoward responses and medication errors.

3. The five areas of suggested patient teaching are _____, _____, _____, _____, and _____.

4. In all aspects of medication administration, patient _____ is of primary concern.

5. Two necessary qualities related to the storage of medications are _____ containers; with _____ caps, as necessary.

6. As part of the cultural assessment, the nurse initially assesses the patient's _____.

7. Nurses may demonstrate respect for cultural diversity by including _____ and _____ practices in the health care plan.

NCLEX Review Questions

Select the best response.

8. The patient will be administering his own medication via a subcutaneous route at home. What statement by the patient indicates the need for more teaching?
   a. "I must throw away my needles in a special sharps container."
   b. "I should never administer my medications in the dark."
   c. "If I have a question, I should wait until my next appointment."
   d. "I need to notify my health care provider if I have any side effects."

9. The nurse is teaching a patient about medications and appropriate diet during medication therapy. Which statement made by the patient indicates a need for more education?
   a. "I can take all of my medications together first thing in the morning with breakfast."
   b. "When taking my monoamine oxidase (MAO) inhibitor, I should not eat any cheese products."
   c. "I should not drink any form of alcohol while taking my pain medication."
   d. "I will eat a banana every day while taking my potassium-wasting diuretic."

10. The nurse is teaching a patient about medication side effects. What is the purpose of this teaching? *(Select all that apply.)*
    a. To help the patient understand what to monitor for when taking the medication
    b. To help the patient understand that some side effects are expected
    c. To inform the patient what clinical manifestations should be reported to the health care provider
    d. To help the patient understand the importance of taking the medication
    e. To allow the patient to ask questions about what can be expected

11. What suggestion will the nurse give the patient who is allergic to a medication?
    a. "Avoid all antibiotics."
    b. "Receive an annual flu shot."
    c. "Take extra vitamin C."
    d. "Wear Medic-Alert identification."

12. Which standard ultimately regulates administration of medication?
    a. ANA guidelines
    b. Local laws
    c. State nurse's association
    d. State's nurse practice act

13. A nurse at the work site may be responsible for identifying self-care centers for specific conditions. Which conditions are best suited for this level of service?
    a. Abdominal pain and low-grade fever
    b. Common cold and chest pain
    c. Common cold and minor cuts
    d. Headache and numbness in arm

14. The older adult patient lives alone on a fixed income. She has a complicated medical history and takes medications for angina, hypertension, diabetes, and asthma. The patient tells the nurse, "I don't know what I'm going to do anymore. My rent just went up, and I can't afford all of my pills. I guess I will stop taking some of them." The nurse will suggest which option to assist with obtaining prescription medications?
    a. American Red Cross
    b. Patient assistance programs (PAPs)
    c. March of Dimes
    d. Salvation Army

15. The patient has just been prescribed an antibiotic for pneumonia and a cough suppressant. What will the nurse include in the dietary teaching for this patient? *(Select all that apply.)*
    a. Instructions on alcohol use
    b. Drug-food interactions
    c. Foods to avoid
    d. Foods high in fiber
    e. Importance of fluid intake

Case Study

Read the scenario and answer the following questions on a separate sheet of paper.

The nurse is providing new student orientation to parents at the beginning of a school year. As part of the orientation, the nurse is covering medication administration and what is required for the students to receive medication from the school nurse. The school is located in a predominantly Asian neighborhood and serves over 700 middle school students.

1. Which medications does the nurse anticipate will be frequently administered at school?

2. What is required for the school nurse to administer medications to a student, and what needs to be in place to assure the safety of the medication administration?

3. Are there any cultural considerations the nurse needs to keep in mind for this population to provide culturally competent care?

10 The Role of the Nurse in Drug Research

Study Questions

Match the phrase in Column I to the applicable description in Column II.

Column I

_____ 1. Placebo

_____ 2. Quasi-experimental design

_____ 3. Intervening variables

_____ 4. Probability sampling

_____ 5. Crossover design

_____ 6. Matched pair design

_____ 7. Double- and triple-blind design

_____ 8. Independent variable

_____ 9. Control group

_____ 10. Experimental group

_____ 11. Dependent variable

Column II

a. Comparison of effectiveness of two antibiotics using two groups: patients receiving antibiotic A and patients receiving antibiotic B

b. Subjects randomly selected from the population

c. Subject serves as his or her own control

d. Pharmacologically inert substance

e. Preferred for drug research

f. Subjects matched on intervening variables and randomly assigned to experimental or control group

g. May include disease and state of severity, age, and weight

h. Participant receives treatment

i. The drug itself

j. Provides a baseline to measure the effects

k. Subjects' clinical reactions

Match the terms in Column I with the definitions in Column II.

Column I

_____ 12. Risk-to-benefit ratio

_____ 13. Respect for person

_____ 14. Beneficence

_____ 15. Justice

_____ 16. Informed consent

_____ 17. Veracity

_____ 18. Autonomy

Column II

a. Individual should be treated as capable of making decisions in his/her own best interest

b. Right to self-determination

c. Telling the whole truth, even bad news

d. The patient has the right to be informed and make decisions without coercion

e. Weighing the risk versus the benefit to the patient

f. All people should be treated fairly

g. Duty to do good

NCLEX Review Questions

Select the best response.

19. What is an integral component of respect for persons regarding nurses involved in research?
    a. Autonomy
    b. Beneficence
    c. Justice
    d. Risk

20. Which principle includes the objective allocation of social benefits and burdens?
    a. Autonomy
    b. Beneficence
    c. Justice
    d. Risk

21. For every 5,000-10,000 new compounds that are screened as potential new medications, how many are actually entered into clinical trials on average?
    a. 5
    b. 50
    c. 250
    d. 500

22. The new research nurse is working with the health care provider to write a proposal. What does the nurse know is a purpose of a phase I clinical trial?
    a. To determine the cost of creating the medication
    b. To discover the feasibility of a national study
    c. To determine the pharmacokinetics of the medication
    d. To study the drug in an animal population

23. The nurse is helping to enroll patients in a study about a potential new chemotherapeutic agent for ovarian cancer. Which type of person would the nurse anticipate to be in phase II of this study?
    a. Healthy adults
    b. Patients with ovarian cancer
    c. Pediatric patients
    d. Only female patients

24. Drug "X" is now in phase IV of a drug study. The nurse knows that one of the purposes of phase IV studies is to determine the long-term data for chronic usage and what other purpose?
    a. Carcinogenic properties of the drug
    b. Use in pregnant and lactating women
    c. New indications for the approved drug
    d. Implications of generic compared to trade version

25. What is the standard for the many aspects of clinical trials?
    a. Declaration of Helsinki
    b. FDA Modernization Act
    c. Good Clinical Practice (GCP)
    d. Institutional review boards (IRBs)

26. What is required in an appropriate experimental study design? *(Select all that apply.)*
    a. Alternate treatment methods
    b. Control groups
    c. Double-blinded subjects
    d. Random assignment
    e. Institutional review board approval

27. The nurse is working with a patient in a clinical drug trial. Which intervention(s) is/are required for the nurse to provide to the patient? *(Select all that apply.)*
    a. Answers to questions regarding the study
    b. A copy of the signed consent
    c. Financial compensation
    d. Permission to withdraw from the study at any time
    e. The IRB proposal
    f. Results from the study

Case Study

Read the scenario and answer the following questions on a separate sheet of paper.

The nurse is working with a drug company that is in phase II of a double-blind clinical trial. The drug has been shown to have several minor side effects, but it has been approved to move to phase III.

1. What is involved in a double-blind trial?

2. What might prevent a drug from moving forward into phase IV?

11 The Nursing Process in Patient-Centered Pharmacotherapy

Study Questions

Match the step of the nursing process in Column II with the phrases in Column I.

Column I

_____ 1. Noncompliance related to forgetfulness

_____ 2. Current health history

_____ 3. Goal setting

_____ 4. Patient's environment

_____ 5. Action to accomplish goals

_____ 6. Drug allergies and reactions

_____ 7. Referral

_____ 8. Patient/significant other education

_____ 9. Use of teaching drug cards

_____ 10. Laboratory test results

_____ 11. Effectiveness of health teaching and drug therapy

Column II

a. Assessment
b. Nursing diagnosis
c. Planning
d. Implementation/intervention
e. Evaluation

Match the clinical manifestations in Column I with the data type in Column II.

Column I

_____ 12. Productive cough

_____ 13. Pain in left ear

_____ 14. Lab values

_____ 15. Nausea

_____ 16. Heart rate

_____ 17. Patient perception of drug's effectiveness

_____ 18. Reported allergies

Column II

a. Subjective
b. Objective

NCLEX Review Questions

Select the best response.

19. *Risk for injury* would be included in which phase of the nursing process for a patient who is taking a sedative-hypnotic?
    a. Assessment
    b. Implementation
    c. Planning
    d. Nursing diagnosis

20. The patient has congestive heart failure and has been prescribed a diuretic. *Obtain patient's weight to be used for future comparison* is included in which phase of the nursing process?
    a. Assessment
    b. Evaluation
    c. Planning
    d. Nursing diagnosis

21. *The patient will receive adequate nutritional support through enteral feedings* is included in which phase of the nursing process?
    a. Assessment
    b. Implementation
    c. Planning
    d. Nursing diagnosis

22. *The patient will be free from hyperactivity* is included in which phase of the nursing process?
    a. Assessment
    b. Evaluation
    c. Planning
    d. Nursing diagnosis

23. The patient has been diagnosed with angina and hypertension and has been started on medication. *Instruct patient to avoid caffeine-containing beverages* is included in which phase of the nursing process?
    a. Evaluation
    b. Implementation
    c. Nursing diagnosis
    d. Planning

24. Revision of goals is included in which phase of the nursing process?
    a. Assessment
    b. Evaluation
    c. Implementation
    d. Planning

25. The patient has been prescribed a diuretic to treat hypertension and is currently taking an over-the-counter allergy medication. *Sleep pattern disturbance* is included in which phase of the nursing process?
    a. Assessment
    b. Evaluation
    c. Implementation
    d. Nursing diagnosis

26. The pediatric patient has been started on antibiotics for strep throat. *Advise patient to report adverse reactions such as nausea and vomiting to the health care provider* is included in which phase of the nursing process?
    a. Assessment
    b. Implementation
    c. Planning
    d. Potential nursing diagnosis

27. The patient has been prescribed an opioid pain medication after hip surgery. *Acute confusion* is included in which phase of the nursing process?
    a. Implementation
    b. Evaluation
    c. Nursing diagnosis
    d. Planning

28. *Instruct patient not to discontinue medications abruptly* is included in which part of the nursing process for a patient with epilepsy who is taking phenytoin (Dilantin)?
    a. Assessment
    b. Evaluation
    c. Implementation
    d. Planning

Case Study

Read the scenario and answer the following question on a separate sheet of paper.

O.Y., 53 years old, has been diagnosed with diabetes and has been prescribed insulin. In speaking to the nurse, O.Y. says, "I don't think I can give myself shots. I can't stick myself with a needle."

1. Utilizing the nursing process, how will the nurse develop a teaching plan for O.Y.?

12 Safety and Quality in Pharmacotherapy

Study Questions

Match the statement in Column I with the nursing implication of drug administration in Column II.

Column I

_____ 1. Right route

_____ 2. Right patient

_____ 3. Right time

_____ 4. Right documentation

_____ 5. Right assessment

_____ 6. Right drug

_____ 7. Right dose

_____ 8. Right to education

_____ 9. Right to refuse

_____ 10. Right evaluation

Column II

a. Measurement of a patient's apical pulse

b. Amount of medication given as prescribed

c. Medication given IM as prescribed

d. Teaching a patient about possible side effects of the medication

e. The patient refuses to take medication

f. Verification of patient ID

g. Nurse charts that patient pain was decreased after drug administration

h. Patient receives the prescribed medication

i. Nurse checks blood pressure following blood pressure medication administration

j. Drug given at the time prescribed

Match the instructions in Column II with the situation in Column I.

Column I

_____ 11. Drugs poured by others

_____ 12. Patient states that drug is different than usual

_____ 13. Bad-tasting drugs first, then pleasant-tasting drugs

_____ 14. Drugs transferred from one container to another

_____ 15. Drugs with date and time opened and your initials on label

_____ 16. Medications left with visitors

Column II

a. Do not administer

b. Do administer

Match the pregnancy category with the correct definition.

Categories

_____ 17. A

_____ 18. B

_____ 19. C

_____ 20. D

_____ 21. X

Definitions

a. Animal studies indicate a risk to the fetus. Risk versus benefit of the drug must be determined.

b. A risk to the human fetus has been proven. Risk outweighs the benefit, and drug should be avoided during pregnancy.

c. No risk to fetus. Studies have not shown evidence of fetal harm.

d. No risk in animal studies, and well-controlled studies in pregnant women are not available. It is assumed there is little to no risk to pregnant women.

e. A risk to the human fetus has been proven. Risk versus benefit of the drug must be determined. It could be used in life-threatening situations.

NCLEX Review Questions

Select the best response.

22. The patient has been prescribed antibiotics that are scheduled for every 8 hours. What statement by the patient indicates the need for more teaching by the nurse regarding the drug regimen?
   a. "I take this medicine every 8 hours around the clock."
   b. "I have to take the medicine even if I feel better."
   c. "I just spread out the three doses while I'm awake."
   d. "I cannot take it more often even if I don't feel better."

23. The patient has been prescribed a medication to be taken a.c. and h.s. What instructions should the nurse give the patient?
   a. "Take this medicine every 6 hours."
   b. "Take this medicine before meals and at bedtime."
   c. "Take this medication after meals and first thing in the morning."
   d. "Take this medication after meals and as needed."

24. What is the purpose of the "tall man" letters?
   a. To assist with medication reconciliation
   b. To aid in labeling medication allergies
   c. To promote safety between drugs with similar names
   d. To label differences in dosage strength of the same medication

25. The nurse is calculating an opioid dose for the patient. The dose seems "large." What is the best initial action for the nurse to take?
   a. Check the patient's name band and administer the medication.
   b. Call the health care provider.
   c. Recalculate the dose.
   d. Withhold the medication and document as not given.

26. The nurse working in a clinic will be administering flu shots from a multidose vial. What is/are the correct piece(s) of information that the nurse must use to label the bottle? *(Select all that apply.)*
   a. Address of the clinic
   b. Nurse's full name
   c. Date vial opened
   d. Prescribing provider
   e. Time vial opened
   f. Expiration date

27. The older adult patient tells the nurse, "I'm not taking that pill. I don't want it, and I won't take it!" What is the nurse's first action?
   a. Document the patient's refusal.
   b. Force the patient to take the medication.
   c. Educate the patient on the importance of the medication.
   d. Call the health care provider.

28. What abbreviation(s) is/are not allowed by the Joint Commission? *(Select all that apply.)*
    a. IM
    b. U
    c. IU
    d. q.d.
    e. MS

29. The "right to education" includes which action(s)? *(Select all that apply.)*
    a. Drug trial information collected before administration of the drug
    b. Education about the medication and why it has been prescribed
    c. Evaluation of the patient's response
    d. Laboratory monitoring of baseline values
    e. Possible side effects

13 Medication Administration

Study Questions

Complete the following.

1. _____ and _____ capsules must be swallowed whole to be effective.

2. Handheld nebulizers deliver a very _____ spray of medication.

3. When giving a patient a medication via handheld nebulizer, the patient should be placed in _____ position.

4. A nasogastric tube should be flushed with _____ mL of water (or the prescribed amount) following medication administration.

5. Following insertion of a rectal suppository, the patient should remain in a side-lying position for _____ minutes.

Match the route in Column I with the correct length of needle in Column II.

Column I

_____ 6. Subcutaneous (SQ)

_____ 7. Intradermal

_____ 8. Intramuscular (IM)

Column II

a. $\frac{3}{8}$ to $\frac{5}{8}$ inch in length
b. 1 to 1½ inches in length
c. ½ to $\frac{5}{8}$ inch in length

Complete the following.

9. The injection site that is well-defined by bony anatomic landmarks is _____.

10. The preferred site for intramuscular injections for infants and children is _____.

11. The site that is easily accessible but is suitable for only small-volume doses is _____.

12. The preferred site for the Z-track technique is _____.

13. The site (not visible to the patient) that has the danger of injury if incorrect technique is used is _____.

NCLEX Review Questions

Select the best response.

14. The patient is vomiting and has been prescribed an antiemetic. Which route does the nurse know is contraindicated for this patient?
    a. Intradermal
    b. Intravenous
    c. Oral
    d. Rectal suppository

15. The 2-year-old patient has been prescribed antibiotic ear drops. The nurse is providing education to the parents. Which is the correct direction in which to pull the auricle?
    a. Down and back
    b. Forward and back
    c. Forward and up
    d. Up and back

16. The patient has been prescribed an intramuscular injection. The medication is thick and must be administered deep IM. Which does the nurse choose for the injection site?
    a. Deltoid
    b. Dorsolateral
    c. Vastus lateralis
    d. Ventrogluteal

17. What is the preferred site for an IM injection for an 8-week-old infant?
    a. Deltoid
    b. Dorsogluteal
    c. Vastus lateralis
    d. Ventrogluteal

18. The patient is being discharged on new medications. Which statement made by the patient would indicate that more teaching is required?
    a. "I can take any over-the-counter medication or herbal preparation that I think would be helpful."
    b. "I need to make sure I keep appointments with my health care provider."
    c. "I need to report any side effects to my health care provider."
    d. "I will contact my pharmacy if I am going out of town to ensure that I have enough medication."

19. The patient has been started on a new oral prescription. What information will the nurse include in the patient teaching? *(Select all that apply.)*
    a. Desired effect of the medication
    b. Dietary considerations
    c. Storage of all medication in the refrigerator
    d. Research testing and development
    e. Written instructions on how to administer the medication

20. The patient has been prescribed a steroid metered-dose inhaler (MDI) for asthma. What statement by the patient indicates understanding of how to use this medication?
    a. "I can use it as often as I need it."
    b. "I need to rinse out my mouth after I use it."
    c. "I should put my mouth tightly over the end."
    d. "I can administer multiple puffs at one time."

21. The nurse is administering a medication via the Z-track method. Which site(s) is/are acceptable for administration by this method? *(Select all that apply.)*
    a. Deltoid
    b. Dorsogluteal
    c. Vastus lateralis
    d. Ventrogluteal
    e. Forearm

14 Medications and Calculations

Introduction

The medications and calculations chapter in this Study Guide is subdivided into six sections: (14A) Systems of Measurement with Conversion; (14B) Methods for Calculation; (14C) Calculations of Oral Dosages; (14D) Calculations of Injectable Dosages; (14E) Calculations of Intravenous Fluids; and (14F) Pediatric Drug Calculations.

Numerous drug labels appear in the drug calculation problems. The purpose is to familiarize the user with reading drug labels and calculating drug dosages from the information provided on the drug labels.

Drug calculation practice problems in each of the six sections provide an opportunity for the user to gain skill and competence in collecting and organizing the required data. Practice problems have examples of the administration of medications via a variety of routes, including both oral and parenteral (subcutaneous, intramuscular, and intravenous).

It is recommended that the user first read the practice problem and estimate an answer. The user should select one of the four methods (basic formula, ratio and proportion, fractional equation, or dimensional analysis) for drug calculations that are presented in the textbook. After completing the required calculations, the user can compare the estimate with the calculated answer. In the event of a discrepancy, the user should review both the thought process used in answering the problem and the actual mathematical calculation. It may be necessary to review the related section in Chapter 14 of the textbook. Practice problems provide reinforcement for the user to gain expertise in the process of actually calculating drug dosages.

Section 14A—Systems of Measurement with Conversion

Metric and Household Systems

Match the term in Column I with the appropriate abbreviation in Column II.

Column I

_____ 1. Gram

_____ 2. Milligram

_____ 3. Liter

_____ 4. Milliliter

_____ 5. Kilogram

_____ 6. Microgram

_____ 7. Nanogram

_____ 8. Meter

_____ 9. Grain

_____ 10. Fluid ounce

_____ 11. Fluid dram

_____ 12. Quart

_____ 13. Pint

_____ 14. Minim

_____ 15. Cup

_____ 16. Tablespoon

_____ 17. Teaspoon

_____ 18. Drops

Column II

a. T

b. g

c. mL

d. gr

e. fl oz

f. mg

g. L or l

h. fl dr

i. minim

j. gtt

k. kg

l. mcg

m. ng

n. t

o. c

p. pt

q. qt

r. m

Complete the following.

19. The most frequently used conversions within the metric system are:

    A. 1 g = _____ mg

    B. 1 L = _____ mL

    C. 1 mg = _____ mcg

Complete the unit equivalent for the following measurements.

20. 3 grams = _____ milligrams

21. 1.5 liters = _____ milliliters

22. 0.1 gram = _____ milligrams

23. 2500 milliliters = _____ liters

24. 250 milliliters = _____ liter

25. 500 milligrams = _____ gram

26. 2 quarts = _____ pints

27. 2 pints = _____ fluid ounces

28. 1½ quarts = _____ fluid ounces

29. 32 fluid ounces = _____ pints

30. 2 fluid ounces = _____ fluid drams

Metric, Apothecary, and Household Systems

31. When converting a unit of measurement from one system to another, convert to the unit on the drug container.
    Example:
    Order: V-Cillin K 0.5 g, PO, q8h.
    Available:

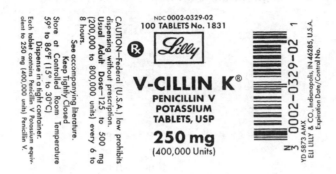

Convert _____ to _____ (unit of measurement to unit of measurement)

Convert the following units of measurement to metric, apothecary, and household equivalents. Refer to Table 14A-3 in the textbook as needed.

32. 1 g = _____ mg, or _____ gr

33. _____ g = 500 mg, or _____ gr

34. 0.1 g = _____ mg, or _____ gr

35. 1 gr = _____ mg

36. 0.4 mg = _____ gr

37. _____ L = 1000 mL, or _____ qt

38. 240 mL = _____ fl oz, or _____ glass

39. 30 mL = _____ fl oz, or _____ T, or _____ t

40. 5 mL = _____ t

41. 3 T = _____ fl oz, or _____ t

42. 5 fl oz = _____ mL, or _____ T

Section 14B—Methods for Calculation

Select the best response.

1. Before calculating drug dosages, all units of measurement must be converted to one system. Which system should the nurse use?
   a. Any one he or she prefers.
   b. One that fits with how he or she will administer the drug.
   c. One that is easy to convert to.
   d. The one on the drug label.

Interpretation of Drug Label

Give information concerning the following drug label.

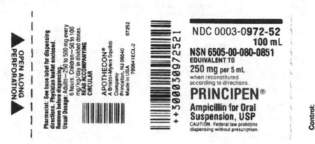

2. What is the brand name of this drug?
   a. Ampicillin
   b. Principen

3. What is the generic name of this drug?
   a. Ampicillin
   b. Principen

4. What is the dosage of this drug? _____

5. What is the form of this drug?
   a. Tablet
   b. Liquid
   c. Capsule
   d. Suspension

Methods for Drug Calculation

Use the basic formula, ratio and proportion, or dimensional analysis methods to calculate the following drug problems.

6. Order: ritonavir (Norvir) 0.2 g, PO, b.i.d.
   Available:

NDC 0074-9492-54
84 Capsules

NORVIR™
RITONAVIR CAPSULES
100 mg

Caution: Federal (U.S.A.) law prohibits dispensing without prescription.

TM-Trademark

Store in refrigerator between 36° - 46°F (2° - 8°C). Protect from light.
02-7878-2/R2
Exp.
Lot

Do not accept if seal over bottle opening is broken or missing.

Dispense in a USP tight, light-resistant container.

Each capsule contains: 100 mg ritonavir.

See enclosure for prescribing information.

©Abbott
Abbott Laboratories
North Chicago,
IL 60064, U.S.A.

   A. Is conversion needed to give this medication?
      a. No; it may be administered in grams.
      b. No; the pill may be broken if needed.
      c. Yes; it should be converted to grains.
      d. Yes; it should be converted to milligrams.

   B. How much of this medication should the nurse administer?
      a. 1 capsule
      b. 2 capsules
      c. 3 capsules
      d. 4 capsules

7. Order: Benadryl (diphenhydramine) 25 mg, PO, q6h, PRN.
   Available: Benadryl 12.5 mg/5 mL

   A. Is conversion needed to give this drug?
      a. No; it can be administered in milligrams as ordered.
      b. No; you cannot mix mg and mL.
      c. Yes; it should be converted to grains.
      d. Yes; it should be converted to grams.

   B. How many mL should the nurse give? Calculate the drug problem using the method selected.
      a. 5 mL
      b. 10 mL
      c. 15 mL
      d. 20 mL

8. Order: clarithromycin (Biaxin) 0.25 g, PO, b.i.d.
    Available:

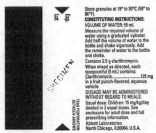 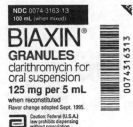

A. Is conversion needed to give this medication?
    a.   No; it may be administered in grams.
    b.   No; you cannot mix mg and mL.
    c.   Yes; it should be converted to grains.
    d.   Yes; it should be converted to milligrams.

B. How many mL should be administered?
    a.   5 mL
    b.   10 mL
    c.   15 mL
    d.   20 mL

9. Order: hydroxyzine (Vistaril) 100 mg, IM, q6h.
    Available:

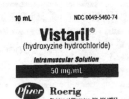

How many mL should be administered?
a.   ½ mL
b.   1 mL
c.   1½ mL
d.   2 mL

10. Order: cefazolin (Kefzol) 500 mg, IM, q8h.
    Available: (NOTE: Redi-vial container has diluent in a separate compartment of the vial. Push plug to release diluent for reconstitution.)

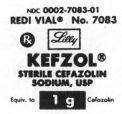

How many mL should be administered?
a.   1 mL
b.   1.5 mL
c.   2 mL
d.   2.5 mL

Additional Dimensional Analysis

11.   Order: acarbose (Precose) 50 mg, PO, t.i.d.
       Available:

      A.   How many tablets should be administered?
            a.   1 tablet
            b.   2 tablets
            c.   3 tablets
            d.   4 tablets

      B.   Which drug label(s) should be selected?
            a.   25 mg per tablet
            b.   100 mg per tablet

12.   Order: losartan potassium (Cozaar) 0.1 g, daily.
       Available:

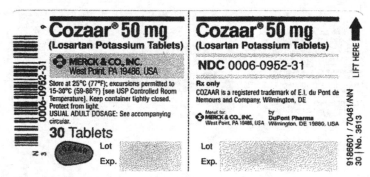

How many tablets should the patient receive per day?
a.   1 tablet
b.   2 tablets
c.   3 tablets
d.   4 tablets

Section 14C—Calculations of Oral Dosages

Drug calculation problems include oral dosages for adults.

1. Order: benztropine (Cogentin) 1 mg, PO, daily.
    Available:

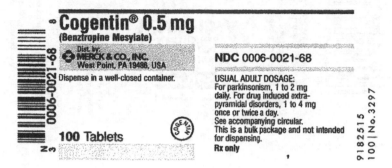

How many tablets should be administered?
a.   1 tablet
b.   1½ tablets
c.   2 tablets
d.   2½ tablets

2. Order: codeine sulfate 60 mg, PO, q6h, PRN.
    Available: Tablets are available in two forms (see drug labels).

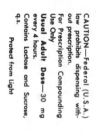 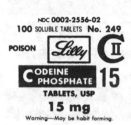 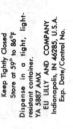 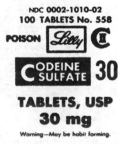

Which form should be used? Why?
a.   15-mg tablets; the patient will take more pills.
b.   30-mg tablets; the patient will take fewer pills.
c.   15-mg tablets; the patient will take fewer pills.
d.   30-mg tablets; the patient will take more pills.

3. Order: propranolol (Inderal) 15 mg, PO, q6h.
    Available: propranolol 10-mg and 20-mg tablets.

    A.   Which tablet strength should be administered?
         a.   10-mg tablets
         b.   20-mg tablets

    B.   How many tablets should be administered?
         a.   1 tablet
         b.   1½ tablets
         c.   2 tablets
         d.   2½ tablets

4.   Order: penicillin V potassium 250 mg, PO, q6h.
     Available: (NOTE: The generic name of the drug may be given instead of the brand name. Check the label for both names.)

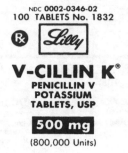

How many tablets should be administered?
a.   ½ tablet
b.   1 tablet
c.   1½ tablets
d.   2 tablets

5.   Order: cimetidine (Tagamet) 600 mg, PO, hour of sleep.
     Available:

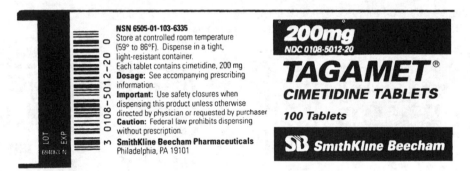

How many tablets should be administered?
a.   1 tablet
b.   2 tablets
c.   3 tablets
d.   4 tablets

6.   Order: verapamil 60 mg, PO, q.i.d.
       Available:

NDC 0005-3447-23

Verapamil HCl
Tablets

120 mg

CAUTION: Federal law prohibits
dispensing without prescription.

100 TABLETS   *Lederle* STANDARD PRODUCTS

Each tablet contains 120 mg of
verapamil hydrochloride
USUAL ADULT DOSAGE: See
accompanying circular for
complete directions for use.
This package not for household
dispensing.
Store at Controlled Room Temperature
15-30°C (59-86°F).
Dispense in a tight, light resistant con-
tainer using a child-resistant closure.
Control No.   Exp. Date

LEDERLE LABORATORIES
DIVISION
American Cyanamid Company
Pearl River, NY 10965   24256   D1

NDC 0005-3446-43

Verapamil HCl
Tablets   **80 mg**

CAUTION: Federal law prohibits
dispensing without prescription.

100 TABLETS   *Lederle*

Each tablet contains 80 mg of verapamil
hydrochloride.
USUAL ADULT DOSAGE: See accompanying circular.

Store at controlled room
temperature 15-30°C (59-86°F).
Dispense in a tight, light resistant
container using a child-resistant closure.
LEDERLE LABORATORIES DIVISION   25985 D3
American Cyanamid Company, Pearl River, NY 10965

Control No.   Exp. Date

N 3 0005-3446-43 6

    A.   Which strength of verapamil should be selected?
        a.   120-mg tablet
        b.   80-mg tablet

    B.   Tablets are scored. How many tablets should be administered?
        a.   ½ tablet
        b.   1 tablet
        c.   1½ tablets
        d.   2 tablets

7.   Order: Artane SR 10 mg, PO, daily.
       Available:

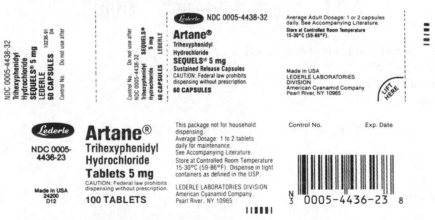

NDC 0005-4438-32
Trihexyphenidyl
Hydrochloride
SEQUELS® 5 mg
LEDERLE   10236-91
60 CAPSULES
Control No.   Do not use after

Do not use after
Control No.
NDC 0005-4438-32
Trihexyphenidyl
Hydrochloride
SEQUELS®
5 mg
LEDERLE
60 CAPSULES

Lederle NDC 0005-4438-32
Artane®
Trihexyphenidyl
Hydrochloride
SEQUELS® 5 mg
Sustained Release Capsules
CAUTION: Federal law prohibits
dispensing without prescription.
60 CAPSULES

Average Adult Dosage: 1 or 2 capsules
daily. See Accompanying Literature.
Store at Controlled Room Temperature
15-30°C (59-86°F).

Made in USA
LEDERLE LABORATORIES
DIVISION
American Cyanamid Company
Pearl River, NY 10965

Lederle **Artane®**
NDC 0005-
4436-23
Trihexyphenidyl
Hydrochloride
Tablets 5 mg
Made in USA   CAUTION: Federal law prohibits
24200   dispensing without prescription.
D12   **100 TABLETS**

This package not for household
dispensing.
Average Dosage: 1 to 2 tablets
daily for maintenance.
See Accompanying Literature.
Store at Controlled Room Temperature
15-30°C (59-86°F). Dispense in tight
containers as defined in the USP.
LEDERLE LABORATORIES DIVISION
American Cyanamid Company,
Pearl River, NY 10965

Control No.   Exp. Date

N 3 0005-4436-23 8

    A.   Which container of Artane 5 mg should be selected?
        a.   5-mg sustained-release tablets
        b.   5-mg tablets

    B.   How many tablet(s)/sequel(s) should be administered?
        a.   ½ tablet
        b.   1 tablet
        c.   1½ tablets
        d.   2 tablets

8.   Order: trazodone (Desyrel) 150 mg, PO, daily.
      Available: Desyrel in 50-mg tablets and 100-mg tablets.

    A.   How many tablets should be administered if the 50-mg tablet is used?
        a.   1 tablet
        b.   2 tablets
        c.   3 tablets
        d.   4 tablets

    B.   How many tablets should be administered if the 100-mg tablet is used?
        a.   ½ tablet
        b.   1 tablet
        c.   1½ tablets
        d.   2 tablets

9.   Order: Coumadin (warfarin) 7.5 mg, PO, daily.
      Available: (NOTE: Tablet is scored.)

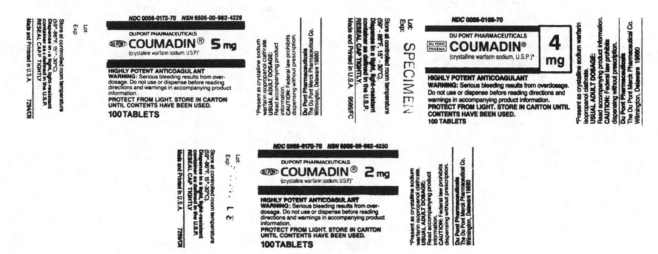

    A.   Which container of Coumadin should be selected?
        a.   Coumadin 2 mg
        b.   Coumadin 4 mg
        c.   Coumadin 5 mg

    B.   How many tablets should be administered?
        a.   ½ tablet
        b.   1 tablet
        c.   1½ tablets
        d.   2 tablets

10.   Order: lithium carbonate, 300 mg, PO, t.i.d.
      Available: lithium carbonate in 150- and 300-mg capsules, and 300-mg tablets. The patient's lithium level is
      1.8 mEq/L (normal value is 0.5-1.5 mEq/L).

      What is the best action by the nurse?
      a.   Give 150 mg (half the dose).
      b.   Give 300-mg tablet and not the capsule.
      c.   Advise the patient not to take the dose for a week.
      d.   Withhold the drug and contact the health care provider.

11. Order: carvedilol (Coreg) 25 mg, PO, b.i.d.
    Available:

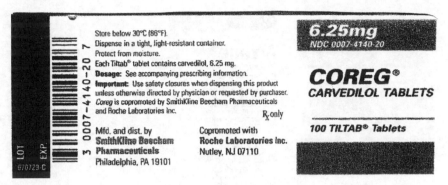

A. How many tablets should be administered per dose?
   a.   3 tablets
   b.   4 tablets
   c.   5 tablets
   d.   6 tablets

B. How many tablets should the patient receive in 24 hours?
   a.   4 tablets
   b.   6 tablets
   c.   8 tablets
   d.   10 tablets

12. Order: azithromycin (Zithromax) 400 mg, daily first day, then 200 mg, daily next 4 days.
    Available:

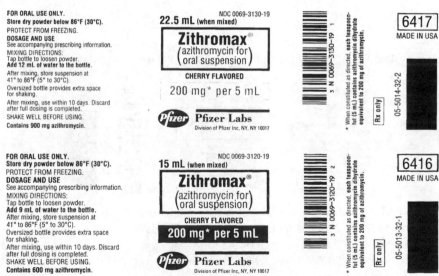

A. How many mL should be administered the first day?
   a.   10 mL/day
   b.   15 mL/day
   c.   20 mL/day
   d.   25 mL/day

B. How many mL should be administered per day for the next 4 days?
   a.   5 mL/day
   b.   8 mL/day
   c.   10 mL/day
   d.   15 mL/day

13. Order: trihexyphenidyl (Artane) Elixir 1 mg, PO, b.i.d.
    Available: Artane 2 mg/5 mL.

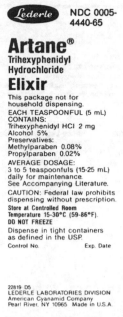

What amount should be administered?
a. 1/2 teaspoon
b. 2 teaspoons
c. 3 teaspoons
d. 4 teaspoons

14. Order: doxycycline (Vibra-Tabs), 0.2 g, PO first day, then 0.1 g, PO daily for 6 days.
    Available:

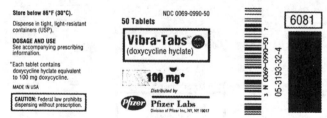

How many tablets should the patient receive the first day, then how many tablets per day for 6 days?
a. 2 for the first day and then 2 tablets for each of the following days
b. 2 for the first day and then 1 tablet for each of the following days
c. 3 for the first day and then 2 tablets for each of the following days
d. 3 for the first day and then 1 tablet for each of the following days

15. Order: digoxin 0.25 mg, PO, daily.
    Available: digoxin (Lanoxin) 0.125-mg tablets. The drug comes in 0.25-mg tablets, but that strength of tablet is not available.

    How many tablets should be administered?
    a. 1 tablet
    b. 1½ tablets
    c. 2 tablets
    d. 2½ tablets

16. A patient is scheduled to take Lanoxin 0.25 mg. The hospital is currently out of stock of Lanoxin 0.25 and only has 0.125-mg doses on hand. The patient is concerned as she receives the pills because they are a different color and a different amount from what she takes daily. When the patient questions the tablets, what is the nurse's best response?

   a. "Please don't worry; it is because we use generic drugs."
   b. "Please don't worry; I calculated this carefully and it is your regular dose."
   c. "We don't have the 0.25-mg tablets available, so you must take two pills of a different strength."
   d. "You are right, this is the wrong dosage. I will be right back with the correct one."

17. Order: Augmentin, 400 mg, PO, q6h.
   Available:

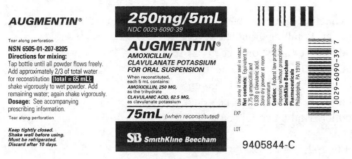

   How many mL should be administered?
   a. 4 mL
   b. 8 mL
   c. 12 mL
   d. 16 mL

18. Order: cefadroxil (Duricef) 1 g, PO, daily.
   Available:

   How many mL should be administered?
   a. 5 mL
   b. 10 mL
   c. 15 mL
   d. 20 mL

19. Order: prazosin (Minipress) 10 mg, PO, daily.
    Available: prazosin 1-mg, 2-mg, and 5-mg tablets.

    Which tablet should be selected, and how many should be administered?
    a. The 1-mg tablet; 5 pills should be given.
    b. The 5-mg tablets; 2 pills should be given.
    c. The 5-mg tablets; 5 pills should be given.
    d. The 2-mg tablets; 3 pills should be given.

20. Order: carbidopa-levodopa (Sinemet), 12.5-125 mg, PO, b.i.d.
    Available: Sinemet 25-100–mg, 25-250–mg, and 10-100–mg tablets.

    Which tablet should be selected, and how many should be administered?
    a. The 25-100–mg tablet; ½ tablet should be given.
    b. The 25-100–mg tablet; 1 tablet should be given.
    c. The 10-100–mg tablet; 2 tablets should be given.
    d. The 10-100–mg tablet; 1 tablet should be given.
    e. The 25-250–mg tablet; ½ tablet should be given.
    f. The 25-250–mg tablet; 1 tablet should be given.

21. Order: Ceclor 150 mg, PO, q8h.
    Available:

    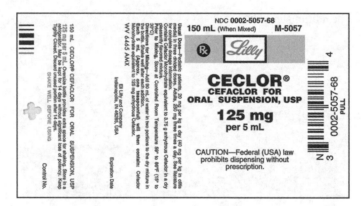

    How many mL should the patient receive per dose?
    a. 4 mL
    b. 6 mL
    c. 8 mL
    d. 10 mL

22. Order: ampicillin (Principen) 0.5 g, PO, q6h.
    Available:

    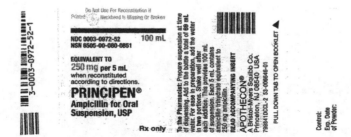

    How many mL should the patient receive per dose?
    a. 10 mL
    b. 15 mL
    c. 20 mL
    d. 25 mL

Section 14D—Calculations of Injectable Dosages

Select the best response.

1. What is/are the method(s) for administering medications by parenteral routes? *(Select all that apply.)*
    a.   Via a nasogastric tube
    b.   Subcutaneous
    c.   Intramuscular
    d.   Intradermal
    e.   Intravenous
    f.   Any liquid medication via all routes

2. What is/are the route(s) of administration for insulin and heparin? *(Select all that apply.)*
    a.   Oral
    b.   Intramuscular
    c.   Subcutaneous
    d.   Intravenous
    e.   Intradermal

3. Vials are glass containers with (self-sealing rubber tops/tapered glass necks). Vials are usually (discarded/reusable if properly stored). *(Circle correct answer.)*

4. Before drug reconstitution, the nurse should check the drug circular and/or drug label for instructions. After a drug has been reconstituted and additional dose(s) are available, what should the nurse write on the drug label? *(Select all that apply.)*
    a.   Date to discard
    b.   Initials
    c.   The health care provider's order
    d.   What it is reconstituted with

5. A tuberculin syringe (is/is not) used for insulin administration. *(Circle correct answer.)*

6. Insulin syringes are calibrated in (units/mL). *(Circle correct answer.)*

7. After use of a prefilled cartridge and Tubex injector, which piece(s) of equipment should be discarded?
    a.   Cartridge
    b.   Cartridge and Tubex injector
    c.   Neither cartridge nor Tubex injector
    d.   Tubex injector

8. The nurse is preparing an IM injection for an adult. What should be used for the needle gauge and length?
    a.   20, 21 gauge; ½, ⅝ inch in length
    b.   23, 25 gauge; ½, ⅝ inch in length
    c.   19, 20, 21 gauge; 1, 1½, 2 inches in length
    d.   25, 26 gauge; 1, 1½ inches in length

9. Which two parts of a syringe must remain sterile?
    a.   Outside of syringe and plunger
    b.   Tip of the syringe and plunger
    c.   Both the tip and outside of the syringe
    d.   Tip and outside of syringe and plunger

10. Subcutaneous injections can be administered at which degree angle(s)?
    a.   10-degree and 15-degree angles
    b.   45-degree, 60-degree, and 90-degree angles
    c.   45-degree angle only
    d.   90-degree angle only

11. The nurse calculates the drug dosage to be 0.25 mL. What type of syringe should be selected?
    a.   3-mL syringe
    b.   Insulin syringe
    c.   Tuberculin syringe
    d.   10-mL syringe

12. To mix 4 mL of sterile saline solution in a vial containing a powdered drug, which size syringe should be selected?
    a.   Tuberculin syringe
    b.   Insulin syringe
    c.   3-mL syringe
    d.   5-mL syringe

Determine how many mL to give.

13. Order: heparin 3000 units, subQ, q6h.
    Available:

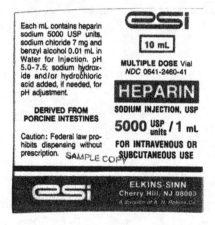 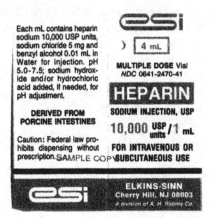

    A.   Which heparin should be selected?
          a.   The 10,000 units/mL vial
          b.   The 5000 units/mL vial

    B.   If the 5000 units/mL is chosen, how many mL should be administered?
          a.   0.2 mL
          b.   0.4 mL
          c.   0.6 mL
          d.   0.8 mL

14. Order: codeine ½ gr q4-6h, subQ, PRN.
    Available: Prefilled drug cartridge contains 60 mg/1 mL.

    How many mL should be administered?
    a.   ½ mL
    b.   1 mL
    c.   1½ mL
    d.   2 mL

15. Order: morphine sulfate 1/6 gr subQ, STAT.
    Available:

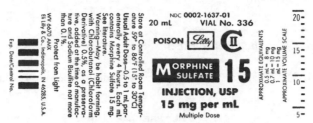

How many mL would you give?
a.   0.5 mL
b.   0.6 mL
c.   0.7 mL
d.   0.8 mL

16. Order: Humulin L insulin 36 units, subQ, qAM.
    Available:

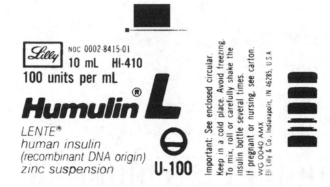

Indicate on the insulin syringe the amount of insulin to be withdrawn.

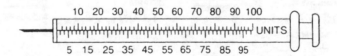

17. Order: regular insulin 8 units and NPH 44 units, subQ, qAM.
    Available: (NOTE: These insulins can be mixed together in the same insulin syringe.)

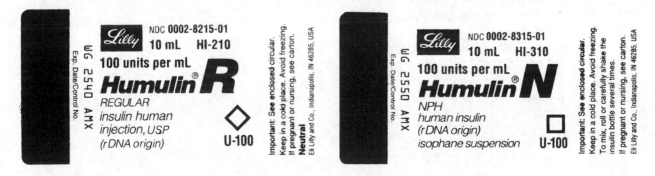

A.   Indicate on the insulin syringe the amount of each insulin to be withdrawn.

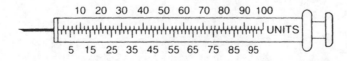

B.   Which insulin should be drawn up first?
    a.   Either one can be drawn first
    b.   The NPH insulin
    c.   The regular insulin
    d.   Neither; they should not be given together

18.   Order: digoxin 0.25 mg, IM, STAT. (NOTE: Usually digoxin is administered intravenously; however, in this problem, IM is indicated.)
Available:

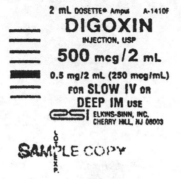

How many mL should be administered?
    a.   ½ mL
    b.   1 mL
    c.   1½ mL
    d.   2 mL

19.   Order: vitamin B_{12} (cyanocobalamin) 400 mcg, IM, daily for 5 days.
Available:

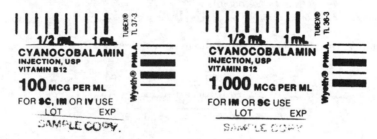

A.   Which prefilled cartridge should be selected?
    a.   Select the 1000-mcg cartridge.
    b.   Select the 100-mcg cartridge.

B.   How many mL should be administered?
    a.   0.4 mL
    b.   0.6 mL
    c.   0.8 mL
    d.   1 mL

20.   Order: clindamycin 300 mg, IM, q6h.
      Available:

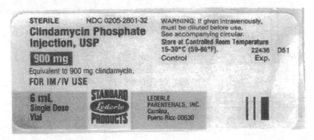

How many mL should be administered?
a.   1 mL
b.   2 mL
c.   3 mL
d.   4 mL

21.   Order: meperidine (Demerol) 60 mg, IM, and atropine 0.5 mg, IM, preoperatively.
      Available: (NOTE: These drugs are compatible and can be mixed in the same syringe.)

A.   How many mL of meperidine should be discarded?
      a.   0.2 mL
      b.   0.3 mL
      c.   0.4 mL
      d.   0.5 mL

B.   How many mL of meperidine and how many mL of atropine should be administered?
      a.   meperidine 0.4 mL and atropine 1.25 mL
      b.   meperidine 0.6 mL and atropine 0.7 mL
      c.   meperidine 0.6 mL and atropine 1.25 mL
      d.   meperidine 0.4 mL and atropine 0.7 mL

22.   Order: naloxone (Narcan) 0.8 mg, IM, for narcotic-induced respiratory depression. Repeat in 3 minutes if needed.
      Available:

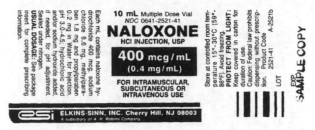

How many mL should be administered?
a.   1 mL
b.   2 mL
c.   3 mL
d.   4 mL

23.   Order: hydroxyzine (Vistaril) 35 mg, IM, preoperatively.
      Available:

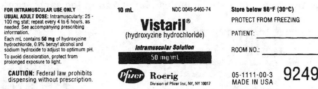

How many mL should be administered?
a.   0.25 mL
b.   0.5 mL
c.   0.7 mL
d.   0.9 mL

24.   Order: oxacillin sodium 500 mg, IM, q6h.
      Available: Drug in powdered form. (NOTE: Convert to the unit system on the bottle.)

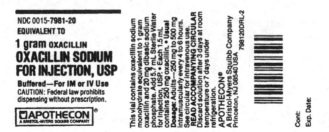

How many mL should be administered?
a.   2 mL
b.   3 mL
c.   4 mL
d.   5 mL

25. Order: oxacillin sodium 300 mg, IM, q6h.
    Available:

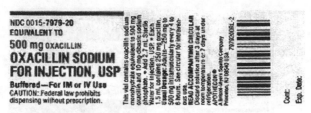

A. The nurse must add _____ mL of sterile water to yield _____ mg of drug solution. Each 1.5 mL contains 250 mg.

B. How many mL should be administered?
    a. 0.5 mL
    b. 1 mL
    c. 1.8 mL
    d. 2 mL

26. Order: nafcillin (Nafcil) 250 mg, IM, q4h.
    Available:

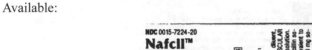
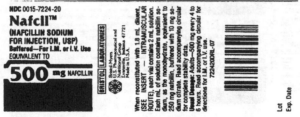

A. The nurse must add _____ mL of diluent to yield _____ mL of drug solution.

B. How many mL should be administered?
    a. 1 mL
    b. 2 mL
    c. 3 mL
    d. 4 mL

27. Order: trimethobenzamide (Tigan) 100 mg, IM, STAT.
    Available: trimethobenzamide (Tigan) ampule, 200 mg/2 mL.

    How many mL should be administered?
    a. 0.3 mL
    b. 0.5 mL
    c. 0.8 mL
    d. 1 mL

28.   Order: chlorpromazine (Thorazine) 20 mg, deep IM, t.i.d.
       Available:

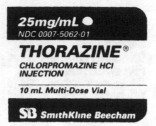

       How many mL should be administered?
       a.   0.3 mL
       b.   0.5 mL
       c.   0.8 mL
       d.   1 mL

29.   Order: ticarcillin (Ticar) 400 mg, IM, q6h.
       Available:

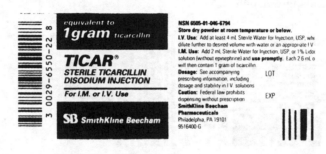

       A.   The nurse must add _____ mL of diluent to yield _____ mL of drug solution.

       B.   How many mL should be administered?
             a.   0.4 mL
             b.   1 mL
             c.   1.4 mL
             d.   2 mL

30. Order: cefonicid (Monocid) 750 mg, IM, daily.
    Available:

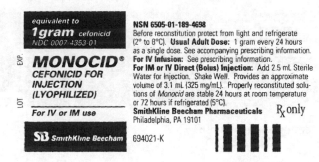

A. How many grams is 750 mg?
   a. 0.25 g
   b. 7.5 g
   c. 0.75 g
   d. 75 g

B. How many mL of diluent should be injected into the vial? (See drug label.)
   a. 1 mL
   b. 1.5 mL
   c. 2 mL
   d. 2.5 mL

C. How many mL of cefonicid should the patient receive per day?
   a. 1.3 mL
   b. 2.3 mL
   c. 3.3 mL
   d. 4.3 mL

31. Order: cefotetan disodium (Cefotan) 750 mg, IM, q12h.
    Available: (NOTE: Mix 2 mL of diluent; drug solution will equal 2.4 mL.)

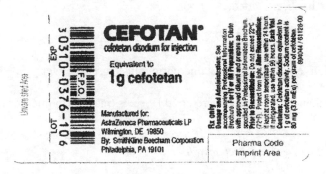

How many mL should be administered per dose?
   a. 1 mL
   b. 1.8 mL
   c. 2 mL
   d. 2.8 mL

32.   Order: Unasyn (ampicillin sodium/sulbactam sodium) 1 g, IM, q6h.
       Available: (NOTE: Mix 2.2 mL of diluent; drug solution will equal 2.6 mL.)

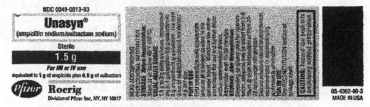

How many mL should be administered per dose?
a.   1.3 mL
b.   1.4 mL
c.   1.7 mL
d.   1 mL

Section 14E—Calculations of Intravenous Fluids

Select the best response.

1.   The health care provider orders the type and amount of intravenous (IV) solutions per 24 hours. What should the
      nurse use to calculate the IV flow rate? *(Select all that apply.)*
      a.   Drop factor
      b.   Amount of fluid to be infused
      c.   Time of administration
      d.   Weight of the patient

2.   When should drugs such as potassium chloride (KCl) and multiple-vitamin solutions be injected into the IV bag or
      bottle?
      a.   As soon as the order is written.
      b.   When one-half of the bag has been administered.
      c.   Before the infusion is started.
      d.   Just after the infusion has been started.

Complete the following.

3.   Macrodrip infusion sets deliver _____ gtt/mL; microdrip infusion sets deliver _____ gtt/mL.

4.   If the infusion rate is less than 100 mL/hr, the preferred IV set is (macrodrip/microdrip). *(Circle correct answer.)*

5.   KVO means _____. The preferred size of IV bag for KVO is
      (1000 mL/500 mL/250 mL). *(Circle correct answer.)*

Give the abbreviations for the following solutions.

6.   5% dextrose in water: _____

7.   Normal saline solution or 0.9% sodium chloride (NaCl): _____

8.   5% dextrose in ½ normal saline solution (0.45% NaCl): _____

9.   5% dextrose in lactated Ringer's: _____

Complete the following.

10. Intermittent IV administration is prescribed when a drug is administered in a (small/large) volume of IV fluid over a (long/short) period of time. *(Circle correct answers.)*

11. The Buretrol is a (calibrated cylinder with tubing/small IV bag of solution with short tubing). It is used in (continuous IV drug administration/intermittent IV drug administration). *(Circle correct answers.)*

12. The pump infusion regulator that delivers mL/hr is a (volumetric/nonvolumetric) IV regulator. *(Circle correct answer.)*

13. Patient-controlled analgesia (PCA) is a method used to administer drugs intravenously. The purpose/objective is to provide _____.

Continuous Intravenous Administration

Select step method I, II, or III from the text to calculate the continuous IV flow rate. Memorize the step method.

14. Order: 1 liter or 1000 mL of D_5W to infuse over 6 hours.
     Available: Macrodrip set: 10 gtt/mL.

     The IV flow rate should be regulated as _____ gtt/min.

15. Order: 1000 mL of $D_5\frac{1}{2}$ NS with multiple vitamins and KCl 10 mEq to infuse over 8 hours.
     Available: Macrodrip set: 15 gtt/mL

     KCl (potassium chloride) 20 mEq/10 mL ampule
     Multiple vitamin (MVI) vial

     Calculate the IV flow rate in gtt/min. _____

16. Order: 1 L of 0.9% NaCl (normal saline solution) to infuse over 12 hours.
     Available: Macrodrip set: 10 gtt/mL
                 Microdrip set: 60 gtt/mL

     A. Which IV set should be used?
         a. Macrodrip set
         b. Microdrip set

     B. Calculate the IV flow rate in gtt/min according to the IV set selected. _____

17. Order: 2.5 L of IV fluids to infuse over 24 hours. This includes 1 L of D_5W, 1 L of $D_5\frac{1}{2}$ NS, and 500 mL of 5% D/LR.
     Available: The three above solutions.

     A. One liter is equal to _____ mL.

     B. Total number of mL of IV solutions to infuse in 24 hours is _____ mL.

C.   Approximate amount of IV solution to administer per hour is _____ mL.

D.   Which type of IV set would you select? _____

E.   Calculate the IV flow rate according to the IV set you selected. _____ gtt/min

18.   A liter of IV fluid was started at 7:00 AM and was to run for 8 hours. The IV set delivers 10 gtt/mL. At 12:00 PM, only 500 mL were infused.

   A.   How much IV fluid is left?
   a.   100 mL
   b.   200 mL
   c.   300 mL
   d.   400 mL
   e.   500 mL

   B.   Recalculate the flow rate for the remaining IV fluids. Keep in mind that if the patient has a cardiovascular problem, rapid IV flow rate may not be desired. _____

Intermittent Intravenous Administration

(NOTE: Only add the volume of drug solution ≥ 5 mL to IV fluid to determine final drip rate.)

19.   Order: cimetidine (Tagamet) 200 mg, IV, q6h.
      Available:

Store at controlled room temperature (59° to 86°F). Do not refrigerate. Each 2 mL contains, in aqueous solution, cimetidine hydrochloride equivalent to cimetidine, 300 mg; phenol, 10 mg. For I.M. injection; dilute for slow I.V. use. **Dosage:** See accompanying prescribing information. **Caution:** Federal law prohibits dispensing without prescription. U.S. Patents 3,950,333 and 4,024,271 **SmithKline Beecham Pharmaceuticals** Philadelphia, PA 19101

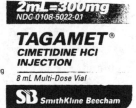

2mL=300mg
NDC-0108-5022-01

TAGAMET®
CIMETIDINE HCl
INJECTION

8 mL Multi-Dose Vial

SB SmithKline Beecham

Set and solution: Buretrol (calibrated cylinder set) with drop factor 60 gtt/mL; 500 mL of NSS.
Instruction: Dilute cimetidine 200 mg in 50 mL of NSS and infuse in 20 minutes.

   A.   How much cimetidine will be infused per mL?
   a.   2 mg
   b.   3 mg
   c.   4 mg
   d.   5 mg

   B.   IV flow calculation (determine gtt/min):
   a.   50 gtt/min
   b.   100 gtt/min
   c.   150 gtt/min
   d.   200 gtt/min

20.   Order: cefamandole (Mandol) 500 mg, IV, q6h.
      Available:

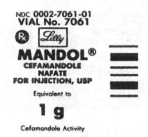

   A.   How many mL of diluent should be added? _____

   B.   Drug solution equals: _____ mL

Set and solution: Calibrated cylinder with drop factor, 60 gtt/mL; 500 mL of D_5W.
Instruction: Dilute cefamandole 500 mg reconstituted solution in 50 mL of D_5W and infuse in 30 minutes.

   C.   IV flow calculation (determine gtt/min):
        a.   100 gtt/min
        b.   110 gtt/min
        c.   120 gtt/min
        d.   130 gtt/min

21.   Order: nafcillin (Nafcil) 1000 mg, IV, q6h.
      Available:

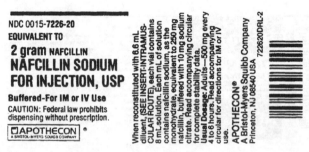

   A.   How many mL of diluent should be added? _____

   B.   Drug solution equals: _____ mL

Set and solution: Secondary set with drop factor 15 gtt/mL; 100 mL of D_5W.
Instruction: Dilute nafcillin 1000 mg in 100 mL of D_5W and infuse in 40 minutes.

   C.   IV flow calculation (determine gtt/min):
        a.   20-22 gtt/min
        b.   37-38 gtt/min
        c.   50-53 gtt/min
        d.   68-69 gtt/min

22.   Order: kanamycin (Kantrex) 250 mg, IV, q6h.
       Available:

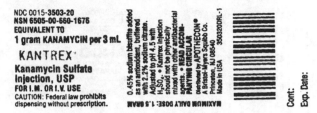

Set and solution: Secondary set with drop factor 15 gtt/mL; 100 mL of D₅W.

Set and solution: Secondary set with drop factor 15 gtt/mL; 100 mL of D$_5$W.
Instruction: Dilute kanamycin 250 mg in 100 mL of D$_5$W and infuse in 45 minutes.

A.   Drug calculation (convert to the unit on the drug label):
       a.   250 mg = 1 g
       b.   250 mg = 0.5 g
       c.   250 mg = 0.25 g
       d.   250 mg = 0.15 g

B.   IV flow calculation (determine gtt/min):
       a.   25-27 gtt/min
       b.   33-34 gtt/min
       c.   51-54 gtt/min
       d.   75-76 gtt/min

23.   Order: ticarcillin (Ticar) 750 mg, IV, q4h.
       Available:

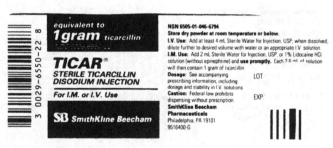

A.   How many mL of diluent would you add? _____

B.   Drug solution equals: _____ mL

Set and solution: Buretrol set with drop factor 60 gtt/mL; 500 mL of D$_5$W.
Instruction: Dilute ticarcillin 750-mg solution in 75 mL of D$_5$W and infuse in 30 minutes.

C.   Drug calculation (convert to the unit on the drug label):
       a.   1 mL of ticarcillin
       b.   2 mL of ticarcillin
       c.   3 mL of ticarcillin
       d.   4 mL of ticarcillin

D.   IV flow calculation (determine gtt/min):
       a.   100 gtt/min
       b.   135 gtt/min
       c.   150 gtt/min
       d.   175 gtt/min

Volumetric IV Regulator

24.   Order: Septra (trimethoprim 80 mg and sulfamethoxazole 400 mg), IV, q12h.
Available: Septra (trimethoprim 160 mg and sulfamethoxazole 800 mg/10 mL).

Set and solution: Volumetric pump regulator and 125 mL of D_5W.
Instruction: Dilute Septra 80/400 mg in 125 mL of D_5W and infuse in 90 minutes.

A.   Drug calculation:
    a.   5 mL
    b.   10 mL
    c.   12 mL
    d.   15 mL

B.   Volumetric pump regulator (How many mL/hr?):
    a.   50 mL/hr
    b.   72 mL/hr
    c.   87 mL/hr
    d.   94 mL/hr

25.   Order: doxycycline (Vibramycin) 75 mg, IV, q12h.
Available: Add 8 mL of diluent = 10 mL.

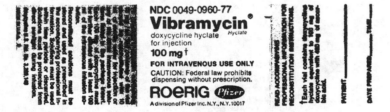

A.   How many mL would equal the Vibramycin 75 mg? _____

Set and solution: Volumetric pump regulator; 100 mL of D_5W.
Instruction: Dilute Vibramycin 75-mg solution in 100 mL of D_5W and infuse in 1 hour.

B.   Volumetric pump regulator (How many mL/hr?):
    a.   75 mL/hr
    b.   95 mL/hr
    c.   108 mL/hr
    d.   118 mL/hr

26. Order: amikacin sulfate 400 mg, IV, q12h.
    Adult weight: 64 kg
    Adult drug dosage: 7.5 mg/kg/q12h
    Available:

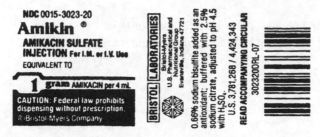

A.   How many mL would equal amikacin 400 mg? _____

Set and solution: Volumetric pump regulator; 125 mL of D₅W.
Instruction: Dilute amikacin 400 mg in 125 mL of D₅W and infuse in 1 hour.

B.   Volumetric pump regulator (How many mL/hr?):
      a.   100 mL/hr
      b.   125 mL/hr
      c.   150 mL/hr
      d.   200 mL/hr

27. Order: minocycline 75 mg, IV, q12h.
    Available: Add 5 mL of diluent.

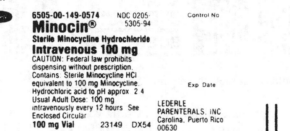

Set and solution: Volumetric pump regulator; 500 mL of D₅W.
Instruction: Dilute minocycline 75 mg in 500 mL of D₅W and infuse in 2 hours.

A.   How many mL would equal minocycline 75 mg?
      a.   1.25 mL
      b.   2.50 mL
      c.   3.75 mL
      d.   4 mL

B.   Volumetric pump regulator (How many mL/hr?):
      a.   150 mL/hr
      b.   200 mL/hr
      c.   250 mL/hr
      d.   300 mL/hr

28. Order: cefepime hydrochloride (Maxipime) 500 mg, IV, q12h.
    Available:

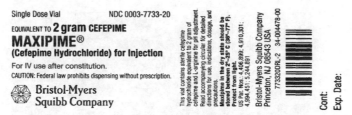

Set and solution: Calibrated cylinder set with drop factor.
Instruction: 60 gtt/mL; 100 mL of D$_5$W.

The drug label does not indicate the amount of diluent to use. This may be found in the pamphlet insert. Usually, if 2.6 mL of diluent is injected, the amount of drug solution should be 3 mL. If 3.4 or 3.5 mL of diluent is injected, the amount of drug solution should be 4 mL.

How many mL of drug solution should the patient receive?
a. 1 mL
b. 2 mL
c. 3 mL
d. 4 mL

29. Order: Unasyn (ampicillin sodium/sulbactam sodium) 1.5 g, IV, q6h.
    Available: (NOTE: Mix 3 g in 10 mL of diluent.)

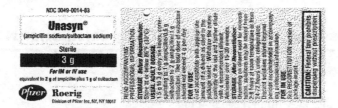

Set and solution: Buretrol or like set with drop factor of 60 gtt/mL; 500 mL of D$_5$W.
Instruction: Dilute Unasyn 1.5-g solution in 100 mL of D$_5$W and infuse in 30 minutes.

A. Drug calculation:
   a. 2.5 mL
   b. 5 mL
   c. 7.5 mL
   d. 10 mL

B. IV flow calculation (determine gtt/min):
   a. 175 gtt/min
   b. 210 gtt/min
   c. 225 gtt/min
   d. 250 gtt/min

30. Order: cefoxitin (Mefoxin) 500 mg, IV, q6h.
    Available: (NOTE: Mix 1 g in 10 mL of diluent.)

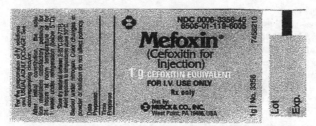

Set and solution: Volumetric pump regulator; 60 gtt/mL; 100 mL of D_5W.
Instruction: Dilute Mefoxin 500 mg in 100 mL of D_5W and infuse in 45 minutes.

A. Drug calculation:
   a. 2.5 mL
   b. 5 mL
   c. 7.5 mL
   d. 10 mL

B. IV flow calculation (determine gtt/min):
   a. 120 gtt/min
   b. 140 gtt/min
   c. 180 gtt/min
   d. 200 gtt/min

Section 14F—Pediatric Drug Calculations

Orals

1. Order: penicillin V potassium (V-Cillin K) 200,000 units, PO, q6h.
   Child weighs 46 pounds or 21 kg.
   Child's drug dosage: 25,000-90,000 units/kg/day in 3-6 divided doses.
   Available: (NOTE: The dosage per 5 mL is in mg and units.)

A. Is the prescribed dose in a safe range?
   a. No
   b. Yes

B. How many mL should the child receive for each dose?
   a. 1 mL
   b. 1.5 mL
   c. 2 mL
   d. 2.5 mL

2.   Order: cefuroxime axetil (Ceftin), 200 mg, PO, q12h.
     Child's age: 8 years; weight: 75 pounds.
     Child's drug dosage (3 months-12 years): 10-15 mg/kg/day.
     Available:

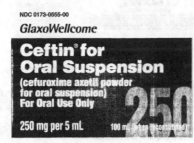

NDC 0173-0555-00
GlaxoWellcome
Ceftin® for
Oral Suspension
(cefuroxime axetil powder
for oral suspension)
For Oral Use Only
250 mg per 5 mL   100 mL (when reconstituted)
250

Contains 6.6 g of cefuroxime axetil equivalent to 5.5 g of cefuroxime.
Caution: Federal law prohibits dispensing without prescription.
See package insert for Dosage and Administration.
Directions for Mixing Oral Suspension: Prepare the suspension at time of dispensing. Shake the bottle to loosen the powder. Remove the cap. Add **35 mL** of water for reconstitution and replace the cap. Invert bottle and vigorously rock it from side to side so that water rises through the powder. Once the sound of the powder against the bottle disappears, turn the bottle upright and vigorously shake it in a diagonal direction.
Before reconstitution, store dry powder between 2° and 30°C (36° and 86°F). After reconstitution, store suspension between 2° and 25°C (36° and 77°F), at room temperature or in a refrigerator. **SHAKE WELL BEFORE EACH USE.** Replace cap securely after each opening. Discard after 10 days.
Glaxo Wellcome Inc.
Research Triangle Park, NC 27709
Made in England
4087836   Rev. 11/97

A.   Is the prescribed dose appropriate?
     a.   No
     b.   Yes

B.   If the 200-mg dose is given, how many mL should the child receive per dose?
     a.   1 mL
     b.   2 mL
     c.   3 mL
     d.   4 mL

3.   Order: amoxicillin 75 mg, PO, q6h.
     Child weighs 5 kg.
     Child's drug dosage: 50 mg/kg/day in divided doses.
     Available:

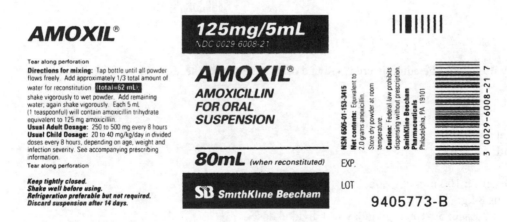

AMOXIL®

Tear along perforation
Directions for mixing: Tap bottle until all powder flows freely. Add approximately 1/3 total amount of water for reconstitution (total=62 mL); shake vigorously to wet powder. Add remaining water; again shake vigorously. Each 5 mL (1 teaspoonful) will contain amoxicillin trihydrate equivalent to 125 mg amoxicillin.
Usual Adult Dosage: 250 to 500 mg every 8 hours
Usual Child Dosage: 20 to 40 mg/kg/day in divided doses every 8 hours, depending on age, weight and infection severity. See accompanying prescribing information.
Tear along perforation

Keep tightly closed.
Shake well before using.
Refrigeration preferable but not required.
Discard suspension after 14 days.

125mg/5mL
NDC 0029-6008-21
AMOXIL®
AMOXICILLIN
FOR ORAL
SUSPENSION
80mL (when reconstituted)
EXP.
LOT
SB SmithKline Beecham

NSN 6505-01-153-3415
Net contents: Equivalent to 2.0 grams amoxicillin.
Store dry powder at room temperature.
Caution: Federal law prohibits dispensing without prescription.
SmithKline Beecham
Pharmaceuticals
Philadelphia, PA 19101

3 0029-6008-21 7

9405773-B

A.   Is the prescribed dose safe?
     a.   No
     b.   Yes

B.   According to the drug order, how many mg should the child receive per day (24 hours)?
     a.   250 mg
     b.   300 mg
     c.   350 mg
     d.   400 mg

4.   Order: acetaminophen 250 mg, PO, PRN.
     Available: 160 mg/5 mL.

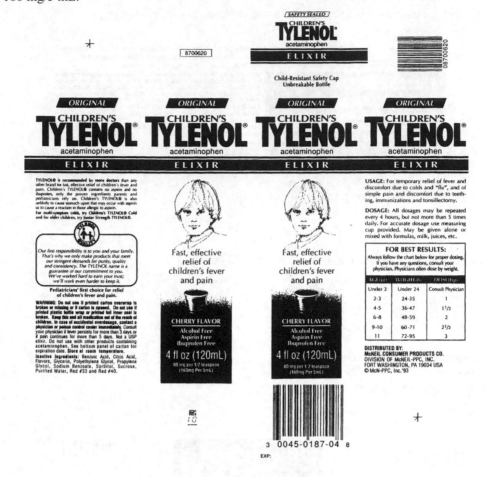

How many mL should be administered? (Round off numbers when necessary.)
a.   4 mL
b.   6 mL
c.   8 mL
d.   10 mL
e.   12 mL

5.   Order: cloxacillin 100 mg, PO, q6h.
     Child weighs 8 kg.
     Child's drug dosage: 50-100 mg/kg/day in 4 divided doses.
     Available: cloxacillin (Tegopen), 125 mg/5 mL.

A.   Is the prescribed dose appropriate?
     a.   Yes
     b.   No

B.   How many mL should the child receive per dose?
     a.   2 mL
     b.   4 mL
     c.   6 mL
     d.   8 mL
     e.   10 mL

6. Order: erythromycin suspension 160 mg, PO, q6h.
    Child weighs 25 kg.
    Child's drug dosage: 30-50 mg/kg/day in divided doses, q6h.
    Available:

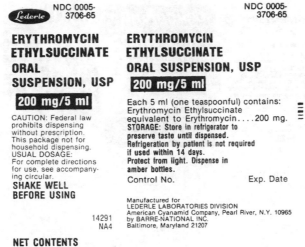

    Is the prescribed dosage within dose parameters?
    a.   Yes, the dosage is safe.
    b.   No, the dosage is too low.
    c.   No, the dosage is too high.

7. Order: cefaclor (Ceclor) 75 mg, PO, q8h.
    Child weighs 22 pounds.
    Child's drug dosage: 20-40 mg/kg/day in 3 divided doses.
    Available:

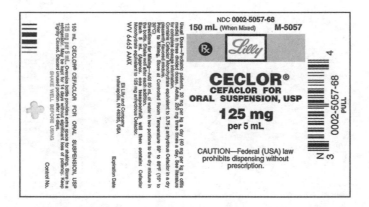

    How many mL per dose should be given?
    a.   2 mL
    b.   3 mL
    c.   4 mL
    d.   5 mL
    e.   6 mL

8.   Order: Augmentin 150 mg, PO, q8h.
      Child weighs 26 pounds.
      Child's drug dosage: 40 mg/kg/day in 3 divided doses.
      Available:

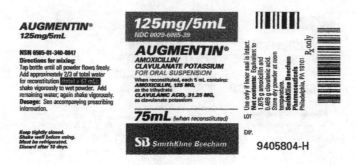

A.   How many kg does the child weigh?
      a.   10 kg
      b.   12 kg
      c.   14 kg
      d.   15 kg

B.   Is the prescribed dosage within dose parameters?
      a.   Yes, the dosage is safe.
      b.   No, the dosage is too low.
      c.   No, the dosage is too high.

C.   How many mL of Augmentin should the child receive per dose?
      a.   2 mL
      b.   3 mL
      c.   4 mL
      d.   5 mL
      e.   6 mL

9.   Order: phenytoin (Dilantin).
Child's weight is 50 pounds; height is unknown.

A.   Child's BSA is _____ m². Use the center graph of the nomogram because the height is unknown.

Child's drug dosage: 250 mg/m² in 3 divided doses.
Available: Dilantin 30 mg/5 mL.

B.   How many mL should be given per dose? Round off numbers.
a.   8 mL
b.   10 mL
c.   12 mL
d.   14 mL

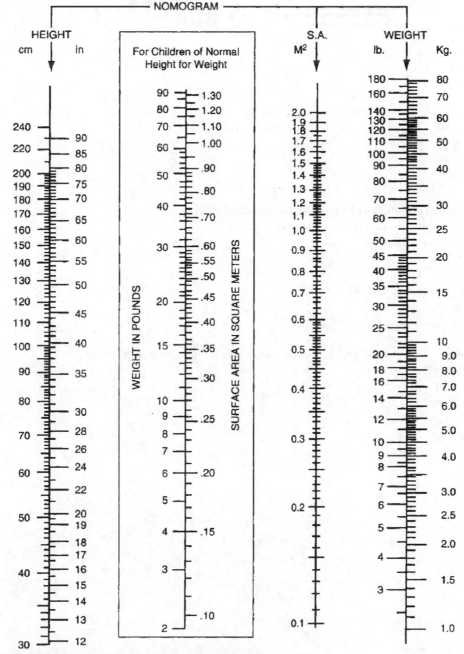

West Nomogram for Infants and Children
Directions: (1) Find height. (2) Find weight. (3) Draw a straight line connecting the height and weight.
Where the line intersects on the SA column is the body surface area (m²). (Modified from data by
Boyd E, West CD. In Behrman RE, Kliegman RM, Jensen HB: *Nelson Textbook of Pediatrics*,
ed 18, Philadelphia, 2007, Saunders.)

Injectables

10. Order: ampicillin (Polycillin-N) 100 mg, IM, q6h.
    Child's weight: 26 pounds. (Convert pounds to kilograms [kg].)
    Child's drug dosage: 25-50 mg/kg/day.
    Available:

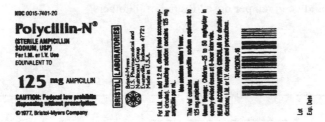

    A. Is the drug dose safe?
       a. Yes
       b. No

    B. How many mL per dose should the child receive?
       a. 0.8 mL
       b. 1.5 mL
       c. 1.8 mL
       d. 2 mL

11. Order: pentobarbital (Nembutal) 25 mg, IM, preoperatively.
    Child's weight: 40 pounds. (Convert pounds to kilograms.)
    Child's drug dosage: 3-5 mg/kg
    Available: Nembutal 50 mg/mL

    A. Is the drug dose safe and effective?
       a. Yes
       b. No

    B. If the dose is given as ordered, how many mL per dose should the child receive?
       a. 0.25 mL
       b. 0.5 mL
       c. 0.75 mL
       d. 1 mL

12. Order: kanamycin (Kantrex) 50 mg, IM, q12h.
    Child's weight: 10 kg.
    Child's drug dosage: 15 mg/kg/day in 2 divided doses.
    Available:

A. Is the drug dose within safe range?
    a. Yes
    b. No

B. How many mL per dose should the child receive?
    a. 1.1 mL
    b. 1.3 mL
    c. 1.6 mL
    d. 1.9 mL

13. Order: amikacin sulfate (Amikin) 50 mg, IM, q12h.
    Child's weight: 9 kg.
    Child's drug dosage: 5 mg/kg/q8h *OR* 7.5 mg/kg/q12h.
    Available:

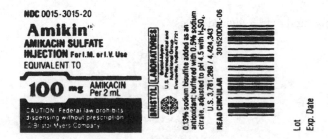

A. Is the drug dose within safe range?
    a. Yes
    b. No

B. How many mL per dose should the child receive?
    a. 0.5 mL
    b. 1 mL
    c. 1.6 mL
    d. 2 mL

14. Order: cefazolin sodium (Kefzol) 125 mg, IM, q6h.
    Child's weight: 48 pounds.
    Child's drug dosage: 25-50 mg/kg/day in 3-4 divided doses.
    Available:

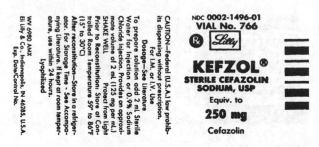

   A. The nurse must add _____ mL of diluent to yield _____ mL of drug solution.

   B. Is the drug dose appropriate?
       a. Yes
       b. No

   C. How many mL per dose should the child receive?
       a. 0.5 mL
       b. 1 mL
       c. 1.6 mL
       d. 2 mL

15. Order: tobramycin (Nebcin) 25 mg, IM, q8h.
    Child's weight: 22 kg.
    Child's drug dosage: 3-5 mg/kg/day in 3 divided doses.
    Available:

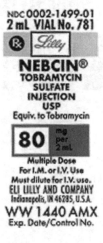

   A. Is the drug dose appropriate?
       a. Yes
       b. No

   B. How many mL per dose should the child receive?
       a. 0.3 mL
       b. 0.6 mL
       c. 0.9 mL
       d. 1.3 mL

15 Vitamin and Mineral Replacement

Study Questions

Match the letter of the fat- or water-soluble vitamins in Column II with the appropriate word or phrase in Column I.

Column I

_____ 1. Vitamin A

_____ 2. Vitamin B complex

_____ 3. Vitamin C

_____ 4. Vitamin D

_____ 5. Vitamin E

_____ 6. Vitamin K

_____ 7. Toxic in excessive amounts

_____ 8. Metabolized slowly

_____ 9. Minimal protein binding

_____ 10. Readily excreted in urine

_____ 11. Slowly excreted in urine

Column II

a. Fat-soluble vitamins
b. Water-soluble vitamins

Match the letter of the common food sources in Column II with the appropriate vitamin in Column I.

Column I

_____ 12. Vitamin A

_____ 13. Vitamin B_{12}

_____ 14. Vitamin C

_____ 15. Vitamin D

_____ 16. Vitamin E

Column II

a. Salmon, egg yolk, milk
b. Wheat germ, egg yolk, avocado
c. Fish, liver, egg yolk
d. Green and yellow vegetables
e. Tomatoes, pepper, citrus fruits
f. Whole grains and cereals
g. Milk and cream

NCLEX Review Questions

Select the best response.

17. What food group(s) is/are included in the ChooseMyPlate guidelines? *(Select all that apply.)*
    a. Dairy
    b. Fruits
    c. Grains
    d. Oils
    e. Proteins
    f. Sugars
    g. Vegetables

18. Regulation of calcium and phosphorus metabolism and calcium absorption from the intestine is a major role of which of the following vitamins?
    a. A
    b. B_{12}
    c. C
    d. D

19. The patient has just given birth, and the nurse is preparing to administer vitamin K to the newborn. The patient asks, "Why do you have to give that to my baby?" What is the nurse's best response?
    a. "It will help the baby's digestive tract work better."
    b. "Vitamin K helps a baby maintain its temperature."
    c. "Newborns are vitamin K–deficient at birth."
    d. "This will help prevent infections for the first month."

20. Protection of red blood cells from hemolysis is a role of which vitamin?
    a. A
    b. D
    c. E
    d. K

21. The patient presents for her annual well-woman exam. She states that she does not take any medications but she knows she is supposed to take "some supplement in case I get pregnant." What is the nurse's best response?
    a. "Folic acid supplements are recommended in women who may become pregnant to prevent neural tube defects."
    b. "Vitamin A 8000 units should be taken to promote bone growth."
    c. "Megadoses of iron are important for blood formation."
    d. "Vitamin C 1600 mg should be taken to prevent colds, which are more common in pregnancy."

22. The patient has been involved in a motorcycle collision and has lost 1500 mL of blood due to a pelvic fracture. Which mineral is essential for regeneration of hemoglobin?
    a. Chromium
    b. Copper
    c. Iron
    d. Selenium

23. The patient has a history of heavy alcohol abuse. He presents to the emergency department confused, combative, and complaining of double vision. The patient's family states he has become very forgetful recently. The nurse will anticipate that the provider will order which substance for this patient?
    a. Vitamin C
    b. Vitamin B_1
    c. Dextrose
    d. Vitamin B_6

24. Which vitamin or mineral is responsible for collagen synthesis?
    a. Vitamin C
    b. Vitamin D
    c. Iron
    d. Zinc

25. The patient takes an antacid for reflux and an iron supplement for anemia. What information will the nurse be sure to include in patient education regarding these medications?
    a. "The medications have a synergistic effect."
    b. "Iron and antacids must be taken on alternate days."
    c. "Antacids will decrease iron absorption."
    d. "Iron will decrease the effectiveness of the antacids."

26. A patient is advised to drink a liquid iron preparation through a straw because it may cause which effect?
    a. Bleeding gums
    b. Esophageal varices
    c. Corroded tooth enamel
    d. Teeth discoloration

27. Which patient might be most at risk for vitamin A deficiency?
    a. A 36-year-old pregnant patient
    b. An 18-year-old patient with celiac disease
    c. A 74-year-old patient with a urinary tract infection
    d. A 33-year-old patient with sickle cell anemia

28. Vitamin A is stored in the liver, kidneys, and fat. How is it excreted?
    a. Rapidly through the bile and feces
    b. Slowly through the urine and feces
    c. Rapidly through the bile only
    d. Slowly through the feces only

29. A 24-year-old patient has been prescribed large doses of vitamin A as treatment for acne. What will the nurse advise this patient? *(Select all that apply.)*
    a. Contact the health care provider concerning drug dosing.
    b. Report peeling skin, anorexia, or nausea and vomiting to the health care provider.
    c. Do not to exceed the recommended dosage without consulting the health care provider.
    d. Avoid alcohol consumption.
    e. Megadoses of vitamin A are necessary for several months to alleviate acne.

30. The patient has a history of tuberculosis and is on isoniazid (INH) therapy. The patient presents to the clinic with complaints of numbness and weakness in his hands and feet. He has no other medical history. Which vitamin supplement might be considered for his condition?
    a. Niacin
    b. Pyridoxine
    c. Riboflavin
    d. Thiamine

31. The patient has sustained burns to 40% of his body and is receiving total parenteral nutrition (TPN). This patient is at risk for which mineral deficiency?
    a. Copper
    b. Iron
    c. Selenium
    d. Zinc

32. Chromium is thought to be helpful in control of which condition?
    a. Alzheimer's disease
    b. Common cold
    c. Type 2 diabetes
    d. Raynaud's phenomenon

33. Which food is high in copper?
    a. Broccoli
    b. Grapefruit
    c. Lamb
    d. Shellfish

34. The patient presents to the emergency department with an overdose of warfarin (Coumadin). The nurse will anticipate administration of which vitamin for this patient?
    a. Vitamin B_2
    b. Vitamin C
    c. Vitamin E
    d. Vitamin K

16 Fluid and Electrolyte Replacement

Study Questions

Match the electrolyte in Column I with its normal value in Column II.

Column I

_____ 1. Magnesium

_____ 2. Calcium

_____ 3. Sodium

_____ 4. Potassium

_____ 5. Chloride

_____ 6. Phosphorus

Column II

a. 95-108 mEq/L

b. 135-145 mEq/L

c. 1.7-2.6 mEq/L

d. 1.5-2.5 mEq/L

e. 3.5-5.3 mEq/L

f. 4.5-5.5 mEq/L

Match the terms in Column II with the descriptions in Column I.

Column I

_____ 7. Similar to plasma concentration

_____ 8. Based on milliosmoles per kilogram of water

_____ 9. Fluids contain fewer particles and more water

_____ 10. Fluids have a higher solute/particle concentration

Column II

a. Osmolality

b. Osmolarity

c. Iso-osmolar

d. Hypo-osmolar

e. Hyperosmolar

Match the electrolyte in Column II with the related drug in Column I (answers may be used more than once).

Column I

_____ 11. Normal saline

_____ 12. Potassium chloride

_____ 13. Epsom salt

_____ 14. Calcium chloride

_____ 15. Slow-K

Column II

a. Potassium

b. Sodium

c. Calcium

d. Magnesium

NCLEX Review Questions

16. The nurse has taught the patient how to take his oral potassium supplement. Which statement by the patient indicates that he requires more education on taking this medication?
    a. "I can take this with a few sips of water."
    b. "It may upset my stomach"
    c. "I should drink at least six ounces of water or juice when I take it."
    d. "I must not chew up the tablet."

17. The patient has been diagnosed with hypokalemia and will be admitted to the hospital for IV potassium replacement. What is the nurse's best action when preparing to give this medication?
    a. Prepare the syringe with the ordered amount of medication to give IV push.
    b. Push the potassium into the IV bag and keep it still before administration.
    c. Push the potassium chloride into the IV bag and shake vigorously.
    d. Obtain an IV pump and pump tubing since this drip must be controlled.

18. A patient has been receiving IV potassium therapy and the nurse notices that the site has become erythematous and edematous. What is the nurse's best action?
    a. Flush the IV site with normal saline and increase the rate.
    b. Flush the IV site with heparin.
    c. Stop the IV and check for blood return.
    d. Discontinue the IV and restart in another site.

19. A patient has been receiving IV potassium supplements. The nurse notices that the patient's heart rate is now 116 beats/minute. What other symptom(s) might the nurse expect to see if the patient is becoming hyperkalemic? *(Select all that apply.)*
    a. Abdominal distention
    b. Nausea
    c. Numbness in extremities
    d. Polyurea
    e. Confusion

20. The patient presents to the hospital and is found to be hyperkalemic. What will the nurse anticipate administering?
    a. 10 mEq/L magnesium mixed in 1000 mL of normal saline
    b. 0.9% normal saline bolus of 500 mL
    c. A fluid challenge of 250 mL of high molecular-weight dextran
    d. Sodium bicarbonate

21. The patient has been started on a potassium supplement. What should be included in the teaching plan for this patient? *(Select all that apply.)*
    a. List the signs and symptoms of both hypokalemia and hyperkalemia.
    b. Regular testing of serum potassium levels is required.
    c. The patient should increase his intake of potassium-rich foods.
    d. The medication must be taken on a full stomach or with a glass of water.
    e. The patient should sit up for 30 minutes after taking the medication.

22. What is the normal range for serum osmolality?
    a. 175-195 mOsm/kg
    b. 280-300 mOsm/kg
    c. 330-350 mOsm/kg
    d. 475-495 mOsm/kg

23. What is the term used to describe the body fluid when the serum osmolality is 285 mOsm/kg?
    a. Hypo-osmolar
    b. Hyperosmolar
    c. Iso-osmolar
    d. Neo-osmolar

24. A patient with severe head trauma is receiving 3% saline. It has an osmolality of 900 mOsm/kg. This is considered to be what type of solution?
    a. Hypotonic
    b. Hypertonic
    c. Isotonic
    d. Neotonic

25. How is the majority of potassium excreted?
    a. Feces
    b. Kidneys
    c. Liver
    d. Lungs

26. The patient has pancreatitis. The nurse knows he is at risk for which electrolyte abnormality?
    a. Hypocalcemia
    b. Hypernatremia
    c. Hypomagnesemia
    d. Hyperkalemia

27. The nurse is teaching the patient about calcium absorption and includes the health teaching that vitamin D is needed for calcium absorption. Where in the body is calcium absorbed?
    a. Colon
    b. GI tract
    c. Kidneys
    d. Liver

28. Calcium is distributed intercellularly and intracellularly in what proportions?
    a. 25% : 75%
    b. 50% : 50%
    c. 75% : 25%
    d. 90% : 10%

29. A patient is prescribed 2 L of IV fluids: 1000 mL D_5W followed by 1000 mL of $D_5\frac{1}{2}$ NS. What are these fluids classified as?
    a. Colloids
    b. Crystalloids
    c. Lipids
    d. Parenteral nutrition

30. The patient is in the hospital overnight after having surgery and the nurse has received an order to start an IV of $D_5\frac{1}{2}$ NS. What type of fluid is $D_5\frac{1}{2}$ NS?
    a. Hypotonic
    b. Hypertonic
    c. Isotonic
    d. Normotonic

31. A patient is receiving high molecular-weight dextran after an explosion. What is the purpose of this fluid?
    a. Temporarily restore circulating volume
    b. Serve as a line to infuse blood into
    c. Piggyback fluid for antibiotics
    d. Whole blood substitute

32. Which body fluid has a similar composition to lactated Ringer's IV solution?
    a. Plasma
    b. Skin
    c. Tears
    d. White blood cells

33. The patient is taking Slow-K. She is also taking hydrochlorothiazide (HCTZ) 50 mg daily to control her hypertension. The patient's serum potassium level is 2.8 mEq/L. What clinical manifestations would the nurse expect to see in this patient?
    a. Bradycardia
    b. Headache
    c. Muscle weakness
    d. Nausea

34. Magnesium deficiencies are frequently associated with which other electrolyte imbalance?
    a. Hypocalcemia
    b. Hyperkalemia
    c. Hyponatremia
    d. Hyperphosphatemia

35. The patient has a serum potassium level of 3.2 mEq/L and has been prescribed K-Dur. She asks the nurse why she has to take the supplement. What is the nurse's best response?
    a. "A low potassium level can be dangerous, and 3.2 mEq/L is considered too low."
    b. "You will only be on the medication for a few days, so don't worry."
    c. "You obviously aren't taking enough in your diet, so you have to take this."
    d. "Have you been constipated lately? Constipation will cause a low potassium level."

36. The patient has the following lab results: Na^+ 150 mEq/L, K^+ 4.2 mEq/L, Cl^- 100 mEq/L, iCa 2.2 mEq/L, Mg^{2+} 1.8 mg/dL, PO_4^- 1.9. What electrolyte abnormality is present?
    a. Hypocalcemia
    b. Hyperkalemia
    c. Hypernatremia
    d. Hypomagnesemia

37. The patient has a serum potassium level of 6.1 mEq/L. What clinical manifestation(s) should the nurse expect to assess in this patient? *(Select all that apply.)*
    a. Abdominal cramps
    b. Muscle weakness
    c. Oliguria
    d. Paresthesias of face
    e. Tachycardia and later bradycardia

38. Which drug(s) is/are used to treat hyperkalemia? *(Select all that apply.)*
    a. Digoxin and furosemide
    b. Glucagon and magnesium
    c. Glucose and insulin
    d. Kayexalate and sorbitol
    e. Sodium bicarbonate and calcium gluconate

39. The patient has had diarrhea for several days and
has a serum calcium level of 3.6 mEq/L. What
clinical manifestations will the nurse expect to see
in this patient? *(Select all that apply.)*
a. Hyperactive deep tendon reflexes
b. Irritability
c. Numbness of the fingers
d. Pathologic fractures
e. Tetany

Case Study

**Read the scenario and answer the following questions
on a separate sheet of paper.**

D.M., 28 years old, has been stabbed multiple times in
the chest and abdomen. His vital signs on arrival are
blood pressure 84/62 mm Hg, heart rate 118 beats/min-
ute, respiratory rate 30 breaths/minute, pulse oximetry
94%, and temperature 35.2° C.

1. What is the priority assessment for this patient?

2. What type of fluids would the nurse anticipate to be
ordered?

3. Explain the advantage of using whole blood versus
packed red blood cells.

17 Nutritional Support

Study Questions

Crossword puzzle: Use the definitions to determine the correct terms.

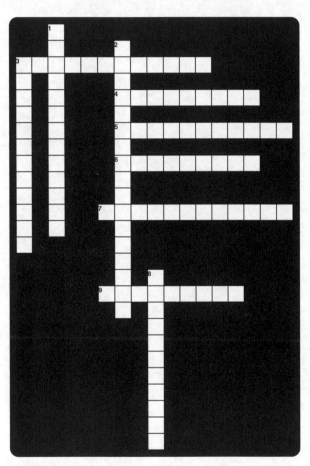

Across

3. May be caused by sudden interruption of total parenteral nutrition (TPN)
4. Provides partially digested nutrients for feedings
5. May occur during changing of IV tubing when the Valsalva maneuver is not used (2 words)
6. May occur if poor technique is used during IV insertion
7. Accidental puncture of the pleural cavity
9. Supplements prescribed for patients who have normal or near-normal gastrointestinal (GI) function

Down

1. May occur as a result of the hypertonic dextrose solution when TPN is initiated
2. Another name for total parenteral nutrition
3. Fluid shift from cellular to vascular spaces because of hypertonic solutions
8. Occurs when the catheter perforates the vein, releasing solution into the chest

10. Label the routes for enteral feedings.

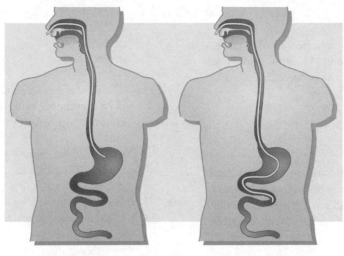

a. _____   b. _____

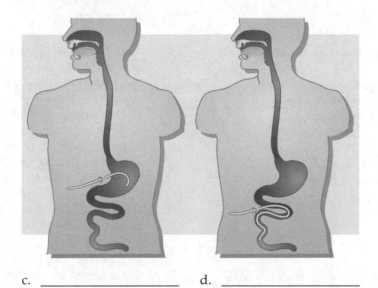

c. _____   d. _____

Match the terms in Column I with the descriptions in Column II.

Column I

____ 11. Bolus

____ 12. Intermittent

____ 13. Continuous

____ 14. Cyclic

Column II

a. Feeding given every 3-6 hours for 30-60 minutes by gravity infusion

b. Feeding given continuously into the small intestine

c. Feeding infused over 8-16 hours per day

d. 250-400 mL given at one time, used for ambulatory patients

NCLEX Review Questions

Select the best response.

15. The older adult patient has a history of hypertension, arthritis, and diabetes. Which formula does the nurse anticipate will be ordered?
    a. Glucerna
    b. Nepro
    c. NutriHep
    d. Respalor

16. The patient is a heavy smoker and has just been intubated for his chronic obstructive pulmonary disease (COPD). He will require enteral nutrition. Which formula does the nurse anticipate will be ordered?
    a. Glucerna
    b. Nepro
    c. NutriHep
    d. Respalor

17. Ensure and Isocal are examples of which type of solution?
    a. Blenderized solutions
    b. Elemental or monomeric solutions
    c. Polymeric, lactose-free solutions
    d. Polymeric, milk-based solutions

18. What type of enteral feeding is administered over 30-60 minutes by pump infusion?
    a. Bolus
    b. Continuous
    c. Gravity
    d. Intermittent

19. The patient is a full-time college student who sustained full-thickness burns to her face 2 months ago. She is now undergoing skin grafting and wound repair and requires nutritional support. The nurse understands that which is the best way to administer nutrition to this patient?
    a. Continuous
    b. Cyclic
    c. Gravity
    d. TPN

20. The patient has ulcerative colitis and is in the midst of a flare-up. He has been prescribed TPN. Which site will the nurse select to administer TPN?
    a. Basilic vein
    b. Brachiocephalic vein
    c. Radial vein
    d. Subclavian vein

21. What is the average percentage of dextrose in TPN?
    a. 3%
    b. 5%
    c. 10%
    d. 25%

22. The patient has sustained a severe head injury and is on continuous tube feedings. These feedings are commonly infused at which rate?
    a. 15-50 mL/hour
    b. 50-125 mL/hour
    c. 125-160 mL/hour
    d. 160-200 mL/hour

23. What is a common side effect associated with enteral nutrition?
    a. Constipation
    b. Diarrhea
    c. Urinary retention
    d. Yeast infection

24. The patient is receiving enteral nutrition by means of continual feeding. The nurse is checking for gastric residual and withdraws 70 mL. What is the best action by the nurse?
    a. Discontinue enteral nutrition and change to TPN.
    b. Immediately notify the health care provider.
    c. Stop the feeding for 30-60 minutes and recheck.
    d. Switch to a formula with more fiber.

25. What are the best reasons enteral feedings should be used before TPN? *(Select all that apply.)*
    a. Less costly
    b. Less risk of aspiration
    c. Lower risk of infection
    d. Maintenance of GI integrity
    e. Promotes better wound healing

26. Which complication(s) is/are associated with the use of TPN? *(Select all that apply.)*
    a. Air embolism
    b. Aspiration
    c. Hyperglycemia
    d. Pneumothorax

Case Study

Read the scenario and answer the following questions on a separate sheet of paper.

M.B., 35 years old, sustained severe trauma from a roll-over motor vehicle collision. He has been on TPN for several weeks and is being transitioned to enteral feeding through a nasogastric tube prior to a gastrostomy being placed.

1.   What steps must be performed to transition a patient from TPN to enteral nutrition?

2.   What precautions will the nurse take to prevent aspiration?

18 Adrenergic Agonists and Adrenergic Blockers

Study Questions

Match the description in Column I with the letter of the reference in Column II.

Column I

_____ 1. Alpha blocker

_____ 2. Beta blocker

_____ 3. Selectivity

_____ 4. Sympathomimetic

_____ 5. Sympatholytic

Column II

a. Blocks action of sympathetic nervous system
b. Has a greater affinity for certain receptors
c. Causes vasodilation
d. Causes decreased heart rate
e. Similar in action to stimulation of the sympathetic nervous system

Complete the following.

6. Adrenergic receptors are located on the cells of _____ muscle.

7. Urinary retention may occur with high doses of _____ agonists.

8. Nasal sprays should be used with the patient (sitting up/lying down). *(Circle correct answer.)*

9. Sympathomimetics (do/do not) pass into the breast milk. *(Circle correct answer.)*

10. Adrenergic blockers are the same as _____.

11. The antidote for IV infiltration of alpha- and beta-adrenergic drugs such as norepinephrine and dopamine is _____.

12. The adrenergic neuron blocker that may cause impotence or decreased libido is _____.

13. Mood changes such as depression and suicidal tendencies are possible when taking which type of adrenergic blocker? _____

14. Abruptly stopping a beta blocker can cause rebound _____.

15. Nonselective beta blockers such as propranolol (Inderal) are contraindicated in patients with _____ and _____.

16. What is most likely to occur if a patient is taking an adrenergic agonist with an adrenergic blocker? _____

Match the letter of the receptor in Column II with the associated adrenergic response in Column I. (Answers may be used more than once.)

Column I

_____ 17. Increases gastrointestinal relaxation

_____ 18. Increases force of heart contraction

_____ 19. Dilates pupils

_____ 20. Decreases salivary secretions

_____ 21. Inhibits release of norepinephrine

_____ 22. Dilates bronchioles

_____ 23. Increases heart rate

_____ 24. Promotes uterine relaxation

_____ 25. Dilates blood vessels

Column II

a. Alpha$_1$
b. Alpha$_2$
c. Beta$_1$
d. Beta$_2$

NCLEX Review Questions

Select the best response.

26. A patient with asthma asks the nurse how his albuterol inhaler will work to help him breathe better. What is the best response for the nurse to explain the action of the medication?
  a. "Albuterol will increase your heart rate so you will feel like you are able to breathe better."
  b. "Albuterol causes bronchodilation in the lungs, improving function."
  c. "Albuterol will cause an increase in urinary output to remove extra fluid from the lungs."
  d. "Albuterol causes bronchial smooth muscle contraction that forces air into the lungs."

27. A patient presents to the clinic with a swollen face and tongue, difficulty breathing, and audible wheezes after eating a peanut butter sandwich for lunch. What is the first action the nurse should take?
  a. Assure a patent airway.
  b. Obtain an electrocardiogram (ECG).
  c. Administer 1 mg of 1:1000 epinephrine subQ.
  d. Start an IV of normal saline.

28. A patient calls the home health agency to tell the nurse she is having a reaction to her albuterol (Proventil) inhaler. She tells the nurse she is shaking and trembling. What is the first question the nurse should ask the patient?
  a. "Are you having any other symptoms?"
  b. "How long ago did this start?"
  c. "When was the last time you took your inhaler?"
  d. "How many puffs on the inhaler did you take?"

29. Which medication(s) is/are classified as beta blockers? (*Select all that apply.*)
  a. Albuterol (Ventolin)
  b. Atenolol (Tenormin)
  c. Propranolol (Inderal)
  d. Amphetamine, dextroamphetamine (Adderall)
  e. Acebutolol (Sectral)

30. The nurse is teaching the patient about clonidine (Catapres), which the patient will begin taking for high blood pressure. What statement by the patient indicates understanding of why she should take her medication with food?
  a. "If I eat a big meal, I won't get diarrhea."
  b. "Having even something small to eat will prevent nausea and vomiting."
  c. "This medicine might make me get ulcers, so I have to eat."
  d. "Lots of fiber in my diet will prevent constipation."

31. When completing the patient health history, the nurse finds a history of narrow-angle glaucoma. When performing the medication reconciliation, which medication would concern the nurse? (*Select all that apply.*)
  a. Pseudoephedrine (Sudafed)
  b. Midodrine (ProAmatine)
  c. Albuterol (Ventolin)
  d. Carvedilol (Coreg)

32. Some over-the-counter (OTC) medications for cold symptoms contain substances that have sympathetic properties. These medications are contraindicated in patients with which disease process?
    a. Allergic rhinitis
    b. Hypertension
    c. Orthostatic hypotension
    d. Chronic bronchitis

33. Which adrenergic agent used in emergency settings does not decrease renal function?
    a. Norepinephrine (Levophed)
    b. Dopamine (Intropin)
    c. Phenylephrine
    d. Dobutamine (Dobutrex)

34. Where are beta$_1$ receptors located? (*Select all that apply.*)
    a. Gastrointestinal tract
    b. Lungs
    c. Kidneys
    d. Brain
    e. Heart

35. A patient tells the nurse during the admitting history that he utilizes alternative and complementary health care to help manage his medical conditions. Which medication would raise a concern in a patient taking St. John's wort?
    a. Reserpine
    b. Albuterol (Proventil)
    c. Propranolol (Inderal)
    d. Pseudoephedrine (Sudafed)

36. The nurse has been floated to the cardiac telemetry unit and is preparing to give a new medication to the patient. The health care provider's order is for timolol (Blocadren) 100 mg b.i.d. Which is the nurse's best action?
    a. Give the patient the medication after proper identification.
    b. Hold the medication and contact the health care provider regarding the dosage.
    c. Give the medication now and request a new order during patient rounds.
    d. Assess the patient's vital signs and give the medication.

37. What is a catecholamine?
    a. A substance that can produce a sympathomimetic response
    b. Another name for a beta blocker
    c. A type of decongestant
    d. A receptor site in the lungs

Case Study

Read the scenario and answer the following questions on a separate sheet of paper.

R.G. is a 34-year-old patient who sustained a beesting and had an allergic reaction. He has been prescribed an EpiPen.

1. What are the mechanism of action and indications for the EpiPen?

2. How should the EpiPen be stored?

3. Describe how the patient should administer the EpiPen.

19 Cholinergic Agonists and Anticholinergics

Study Questions

Match the term in Column I with the definition in Column II.

Column I

_____ 1. Acetylcholine

_____ 2. Anticholinergic

_____ 3. Cholinergic

_____ 4. Cholinesterase

_____ 5. Muscarinic receptor

_____ 6. Nicotinic receptor

_____ 7. Parasympathomimetic

_____ 8. Anticholinesterase

Column II

a. Stimulates smooth muscle and slows heart rate
b. Impacts skeletal muscles
c. Stimulates muscarinic receptors
d. Types of drugs that stimulate the parasympathetic system
e. Blocks the action of acetylcholine
f. Mimics cholinergic actions
g. Blocks the breakdown of acetylcholine
h. Causes the breakdown of acetylcholine

NCLEX Review Questions

Select the best response.

9. The patient has ingested an organophosphate poison in a suicide attempt. What medication does the nurse anticipate the health care provider will order to treat this patient?
   a. Bethanechol (Urecholine)
   b. Edrophonium chloride (Tensilon)
   c. Metoclopramide (Reglan)
   d. Pralidoxime Cl (Protopam)

10. The pediatric patient has urinary retention. Which cholinergic drug does the nurse anticipate will be prescribed to increase urination?
    a. Bethanechol (Urecholine)
    b. Edrophonium chloride (Tensilon)
    c. Metoclopramide (Reglan)
    d. Neostigmine bromide (Prostigmin)

11. The patient is scheduled for a comprehensive eye examination. Anticholinergic eyedrops are used for which purpose?
    a. Constrict the pupils
    b. Dilate the pupils
    c. Decrease the intraocular pressure
    d. Detect astigmatism

12. The 80-year-old patient has glaucoma and is prescribed an anticholinergic drug. What is the nurse's priority action?
    a. Administer the medication as ordered after verifying the patient's identity.
    b. Give only one-half of the prescribed dose.
    c. Hold the dose and contact the health care provider.
    d. Wait until after the patient has taken glaucoma medication and then give the medication.

13. Which type of medication is bethanecol (Urecholine)?
    a. Anticholinergic
    b. Cholinergic agonist
    c. Cholinesterase inhibitor
    d. Sympatholytic

14. How does bethanechol (Urecholine) work in the body?
    a. Inhibits muscarinic receptors
    b. Inhibits nicotinic receptors
    c. Stimulates muscarinic receptors
    d. Stimulates nicotinic receptors

15. The patient has been prescribed bethanechol and asks the nurse how it works. What is the nurse's best response?
    a. "This drug decreases bladder tone."
    b. "This drug inhibits bladder contraction."
    c. "This drug promotes contraction of the bladder."
    d. "This drug stimulates urine production."

16. How does the body respond to large doses of cholinergic drugs? *(Select all that apply.)*
    a. Decreased blood pressure
    b. Decreased salivation
    c. Increased bronchial secretions
    d. Mydriasis
    e. Urinary retention

17. The patient has been prescribed bethanechol and is experiencing decreased urinary output. What is the nurse's priority action?
    a. Catheterize the patient to drain the bladder and measure output.
    b. Encourage the patient to increase fluid intake to increase urinary output.
    c. Encourage the patient to relax when urinating.
    d. Notify the health care provider with current intake and output values.

18. The patient has been taking bethanechol and is experiencing flushing, sweating, nausea, and abdominal cramps. What is the nurse's best action?
    a. Document the patient's manifestations.
    b. Give the patient a laxative.
    c. Increase the patient's fluid intake.
    d. Prepare to administer atropine.

19. Which medication treats myasthenia gravis by increasing muscle strength?
    a. Bethanechol (Urecholine)
    b. Edrophonium chloride (Tensilon)
    c. Neostigmine bromide (Prostigmin)
    d. Pilocarpine (Pilocar)

20. The nurse is taking care of five patients in the emergency department. Which patient(s) would be candidate(s) to receive atropine? *(Select all that apply.)*
    a. A 25-year-old having surgery for appendicitis
    b. A 42-year-old with a heart rate of 38 beats/minute and dizziness
    c. A 50-year-old with diarrhea
    d. A 61-year-old with urinary retention
    e. A 68-year-old with gastric ulcers

21. The nurse would question an order for atropine for which patient?
    a. A 35-year-old with peptic ulcer
    b. A 50-year-old with parkinsonism
    c. A 55-year-old with cirrhosis
    d. A 60-year-old with glaucoma

22. The patient is admitted for evaluation of peptic ulcers. She is taking propantheline (Pro-Banthine) three times per day. The nurse is teaching this patient about nutrition while taking this medication. The priority nutrition teaching point is that the patient should eat foods that are high in which component?
    a. Calcium
    b. Fat
    c. Fiber
    d. Protein

23. What teaching point(s) will the nurse include for a 30-year-old patient who is taking hyoscyamine (Cystospaz) for irritable bowel syndrome? *(Select all that apply.)*
    a. Ensure adequate fluid intake.
    b. Do not drive until you are aware of how this medication will affect your vision.
    c. Sucking on hard candy may help with dry mouth.
    d. Increased sweating is a common side effect.
    e. Report a rapid heart rate to your health care provider.

24. Anticholinergic drugs are contraindicated in patients with which other disease processes? *(Select all that apply.)*
    a. Coronary artery disease
    b. Diabetes mellitus
    c. Gastrointestinal obstruction
    d. Supraventricular tachycardia

25. A specific group of anticholinergics may be pre-
    scribed in the early treatment of which neuromus-
    cular disorder?
    a. Multiple sclerosis
    b. Muscular dystrophy
    c. Myasthenia gravis
    d. Parkinsonism

26. The older adult patient is taking benztropine
    (Cogentin) for symptoms associated with parkin-
    sonism. The nurse will instruct the patient to report
    which clinical manifestation(s) to the health care
    provider? *(Select all that apply.)*
    a. Diarrhea
    b. Dizziness
    c. Hallucinations
    d. Hyperthermia
    e. Palpitations

Case Study

**Read the scenario and answer the following questions
on a separate sheet of paper.**

H.H., 65 years old, has just received a prescription for
tolterodine tartrate (Detrol) for treatment of urinary
incontinence.

1. What is the mechanism of action of this drug?

2. What are the some of the major side effects?

3. What are some contraindications?

4. Discuss key teaching points for the nurse to provide when educating the patient.

20 Central Nervous System Stimulants

Study Questions

Crossword puzzle: Use the definitions to determine the correct terms.

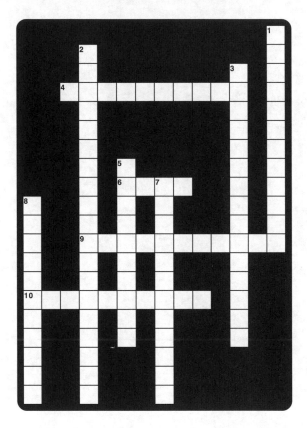

Across

4. Reliance on a substance that has reached the level that its absence will cause impairment in function
6. Attention deficit/hyperactivity disorder abbreviation
9. Used to suppress the appetite
10. Used to stimulate respirations

Down

1. Cause euphoria and alertness
2. Food and Drug Administration required its removal from over-the-counter weight-loss drugs
3. Used to correct attention deficit/hyperactivity disorder
5. Falling asleep during normal activities
7. Hypermovement; also formerly a name for attention deficit/hyperactivity disorder
8. Used to treat narcolepsy

NCLEX Review Questions

Select the best response.

11. Which medical condition(s) is/are central nervous system (CNS) stimulants approved to treat? *(Select all that apply.)*
    a. Attention deficit/hyperactivity disorder (ADHD)
    b. Anorexia
    c. Narcolepsy
    d. Obesity
    e. Posttraumatic stress disorder

12. A new nurse is admitting a patient who has received doxapam (Dopram). The nurse recognizes that this is which type of medication?
    a. Inhaled respiratory stimulant
    b. Narcotic antagonist
    c. Postanesthetic respiratory stimulant
    d. Long-acting narcotic

13. The patient has been prescribed methylphenidate for the treatment of narcolepsy. What priority teaching consideration(s) should be included for this patient? *(Select all that apply.)*
    a. Avoid operating hazardous equipment.
    b. Caffeine should be avoided.
    c. Nervousness and tremors may occur.
    d. Take the medication before meals.
    e. Report any weight gain.

14. Which drug group acts on the brainstem and medulla to stimulate respiration?
    a. Amphetamine
    b. Analeptic
    c. Anorexiant
    d. Triptan

15. The patient is being treated with methylphenidate (Ritalin) for ADHD. What common side/adverse effect(s) should the patient and family be informed might occur? *(Select all that apply.)*
    a. Euphoria
    b. Headache
    c. Hypertension
    d. Irritability
    e. Orthostatic hypotension
    f. Vomiting

16. To maintain the half-life of methylphenidate (Ritalin), how often should this medication be taken?
    a. Daily
    b. Twice per day
    c. Three times per day
    d. Every other day

17. The patient has been prescribed methylphenidate for narcolepsy. The patient also has migraines and takes amitriptyline as a preventive. What should the nurse advise the patient to do before starting the new medication?
    a. "Contact your primary health care provider to verify compatibility."
    b. "Have baseline lab work drawn to assess liver function."
    c. "Immediately stop taking the amitriptyline."
    d. "Increase fluid intake with the next meal."

18. The patient has a history of migraines, depression, and hypertension and has been started on phentermine-topiramate (Qsymia). For which condition is phentermine-topiramate used?
    a. ADHD
    b. Asthma
    c. Narcolepsy
    d. Short-term weight management

19. The pediatric patient has been started on methylphenidate for ADHD. What information should the nurse include in the health teaching?
    a. Constipation is a common side effect.
    b. Counseling should be combined with medication.
    c. This medication will only be used for a few weeks.
    d. Weight gain is to be expected.

20. Which statement(s) is/are true of methylphenidate? *(Select all that apply.)*
    a. If taken with monoamine oxidase inhibitors (MAOIs), it may increase a hypertensive crisis.
    b. The effects of anticoagulants may increase.
    c. Hyperglycemia may occur.
    d. Insulin will be more effective.
    e. There may be increased effects if taken with caffeinated beverages.

21. The 18-year-old patient is brought to the emergency department by her roommates. Her blood pressure is 220/136 mm Hg, heart rate 142 beats/minute, and respiratory rate 20 breaths/minute. She is responsive only to deep pain. Her roommates say she has been trying to lose weight and has been taking "these pills she gets over the Internet." What will the nurse consider as the most likely cause for this patient's symptoms?
    a. Cardiac arrest
    b. Food poisoning
    c. Hemorrhagic stroke
    d. Pregnancy-induced hypertension

22. CNS stimulants are absolutely contraindicated for patients with a history of which condition(s)? *(Select all that apply.)*
    a. Coronary artery disease
    b. Diabetes
    c. Hypothyroidism
    d. Hypertension
    e. Liver failure

23. The patient is born at 28 weeks gestation and is scheduled to receive caffeine citrate 20 mg IV shortly after birth. The patient's mother asks, "Why are you giving my baby stuff that is in coffee?" What is the nurse's best response?
    a. "Caffeine can help your baby breathe better."
    b. "It will help your baby gain weight faster."
    c. "The baby's temperature will be warmer with caffeine."
    d. "This isn't the same substance that is in coffee."

Case Study

Read the scenario and answer the following question on a separate sheet of paper.

There is a new school nurse at Countryside Middle School, at which there are more than 75 students who take either methylphenidate (Ritalin) or dexmethylphenidate (Focalin) for a diagnosis of ADHD. The majority of the patients come in between 11:30 AM and 12:30 PM for their medication.

1. What are the nursing implications for giving these medications at school regarding timing, monitoring, and health teaching for the students, families, and teachers?

Study Questions

Crossword puzzle: Use the definitions to determine the correct terms.

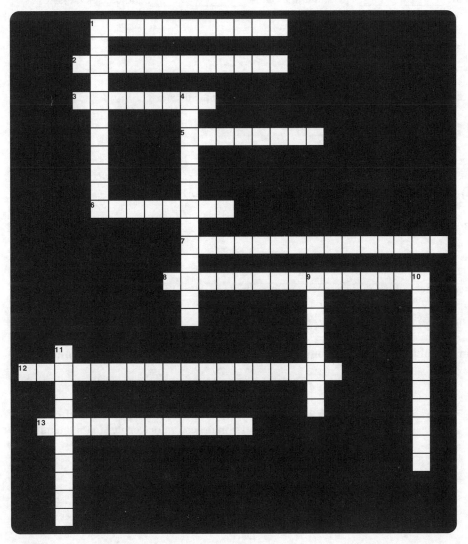

Across

1. Given at the lower end of the spinal column to block the perineal area (2 words)
2. The first anesthetic (2 words)
3. Residual drowsiness resulting in impaired reaction time
5. Inability to fall asleep
6. Herb that should not be taken with barbiturates (2 words)
7. Increase the action of the neurotransmitter GABA
8. Used to block pain at the site while consciousness is maintained (2 words)
12. Combination of drugs used in general anesthesia (2 words)
13. Should be restricted to short-term (2 weeks or less)

Down

1. Penetration of the anesthetic into the subarachnoid membrane (2 words)
4. Placement of a local anesthetic in the outer covering of the spinal cord (2 words)
9. Mildest form of central nervous system (CNS) depression
10. Placed near the sacrum (2 words)
11. Benzodiazepine marketed under the trade name Dalmane

Complete the following.

14. The broad classification of CNS depressants includes the following seven groups: _____, _____, _____, _____, _____, _____, and _____.

15. The two phases of sleep are _____ and _____.

16. The mildest form of CNS depression is _____.

17. Anesthesia (may/may not) be achieved with high doses of sedative-hypnotics. *(Circle correct answer.)*

18. Thiopental is used in general anesthesia as a(n) _____ anesthetic.

19. General anesthesia depresses the _____ system, alleviates _____, and causes a loss of _____.

20. Surgery is performed during the _____ stage of anesthesia. The other three stages are _____, _____, and _____.

21. Bupivacaine and tetracaine are drugs commonly used for _____ anesthesia.

22. A major potential adverse effect of spinal anesthesia is _____.

23. A type of spinal anesthesia used for patients in labor is a(n) _____.

24. Muscle relaxants (are/are not) part of balanced anesthesia. *(Circle correct answer.)*

25. Drugs used to induce sleep in those who have difficulty getting to sleep are _____-acting barbiturates.

26. A popular nonbenzodiazepine for the treatment of insomnia is _____.

27. The drug of choice for the management of benzodiazepine overdose is _____.

28. Local anesthetics are divided into two groups: _____ and _____.

Match the letter of the description in Column II with the common side effect of sedative-hypnotics in Column I.

Column I

_____ 29. Hangover

_____ 30. REM rebound

_____ 31. Dependence

_____ 32. Tolerance

_____ 33. Respiratory depression

_____ 34. Hypersensitivity

Column II

a. Need to increase dosage to get desired effect
b. Suppression of respiratory center in the medulla
c. Skin rashes
d. Residual drowsiness
e. Results in withdrawal symptoms
f. Vivid dreams and nightmares

NCLEX Review Questions

Select the best response.

35. What is the most commonly prescribed medication to aid patients with sleep disorders?
    a. Analeptic
    b. Anesthetic
    c. Sedative-hypnotic
    d. Triptan

36. The patient has been diagnosed with a seizure disorder. The nurse knows that which drugs may be prescribed to control seizures?
    a. Intermediate-acting barbiturates
    b. Long-acting barbiturates
    c. Short-acting barbiturates
    d. Ultra-short–acting barbiturates

37. A patient returns to the unit after having surgery with spinal anesthesia. What does the nurse know is/are the best action(s) to take to decrease the possibility of spinal headache? *(Select all that apply.)*
    a. Administer morphine 1 to 2 mg IV.
    b. Ambulate the patient as soon as she gets feeling back.
    c. Encourage the patient to stay flat in bed.
    d. Increase fluid intake.
    e. Position the patient in high-Fowler's position.

38. The 61-year-old patient will be receiving spinal anesthesia for surgery. She states, "Why do I have to sit a certain way? Why can't I just be comfortable?" What is the nurse's best response?
    a. "It is easier for the anesthesiologist if you sit this way."
    b. "Because of your age, you have to sit straight up."
    c. "The anesthesia is injected in a specific area so it distributes evenly."
    d. "You can sit however you like."

39. The patient is postoperative day 3 from major orthopedic surgery and is unable to sleep. If non-pharmacologic measures have not been effective, what medication does the nurse anticipate may be ordered?
    a. Flumazenil (Romazicon)
    b. Phenobarbital (Luminal)
    c. Triazolam (Halcion)
    d. Zolpidem (Ambien)

40. Which type(s) of anesthesia is/are administered using lidocaine? *(Select all that apply.)*
    a. General
    b. Inhaled
    c. Intravenous
    d. Local
    e. Spinal

41. The patient works 12-hour night shifts one week and 12-hour day shifts the next week. He tells the nurse he has been taking "some kind of sleeping pill from the drugstore." What does the nurse suspect is the most likely main ingredient in the over-the-counter sleep medication?
    a. Antihistamines
    b. Barbiturates
    c. Benzodiazepines
    d. Melatonin

42. The 71-year-old patient presents to the health care provider with complaints of inability to go to sleep and inability to stay asleep. What question(s) will the nurse ask to further evaluate her complaint? *(Select all that apply.)*
    a. "Do you have a bedtime routine?"
    b. "How many caffeinated beverages do you drink per day?"
    c. "Do you take naps?"
    d. "Do you sleep with the windows open?"
    e. "Are you taking diuretics?"

43. What is/are the possible complication(s) of spinal anesthesia? *(Select all that apply.)*
    a. Drowsiness
    b. Dysrhythmias
    c. Dizziness
    d. Headache
    e. Hypertension
    f. Respiratory distress

Case Study

Read the scenario and answer the following questions on a separate sheet of paper.

F.B., 42 years old, is scheduled for a laparoscopic cholecystectomy next week. She has had a bad experience with anesthesia before and is very anxious.

1. What medications might be prescribed prior to her surgery for anxiety?

2. Explain the principles of balanced anesthesia.

22 Anticonvulsants

Study Questions

Crossword puzzle: Use the definitions to determine the correct terms.

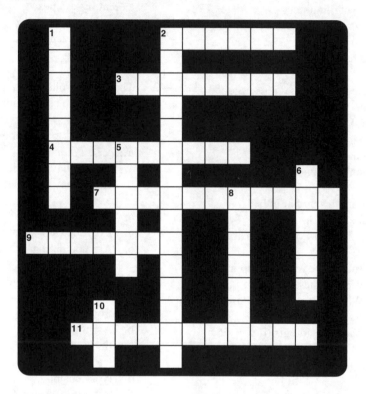

Across

2. Seizure that involves head drop, loss of posture, and sudden loss of muscle tone
3. Absence seizure (2 words)
4. Seizure that involves isolated clonic contraction or jerks lasting 3-10 seconds
7. Involuntary paroxysmal muscular contractions
9. Seizure that involves one hemisphere of the brain
11. The type of effect that results from drugs that have a negative impact on the fetus

Down

1. Tonic-clonic seizure (2 words)
2. Drugs used for epileptic seizures
5. Dysrhythmic muscle contraction seizure
6. Absence of oxygen to the brain
8. Results from abnormal electrical discharges from the cerebral neurons
10. Useful in diagnosing epilepsy

Complete the following.

12. To diagnose epilepsy, results of a(n) _____ are useful.

13. Seventy-five percent of all epilepsy is considered to be primary or _____.

14. The international classification of seizures describes the two categories of seizures as _____ and _____.

15. Anticonvulsant drugs suppress abnormal electrical impulses, thus _____ the seizure, but they (do/do not) eliminate the cause. *(Circle correct answer.)*

16. Anticonvulsants (are/are not) used for all types of seizures. *(Circle correct answer.)*

17. The first anticonvulsant used to treat seizures was _____, discovered in 1938, and today is the most commonly used drug for this condition.

18. It is strongly recommended that the patient check with the health care provider before taking _____ preparations.

19. Administration of phenytoin via the (oral/intramuscular/intravenous) route is not recommended because of its erratic absorption rate. *(Circle correct answer.)*

NCLEX Review Questions

Select the best response.

20. The patient has not responded to other oral anticonvulsant drug therapy. Which drug would the nurse expect to be prescribed for this patient?
    a. Carbamazepine (Tegretol)
    b. Diazepam (Valium)
    c. Ethosuximide (Zarontin)
    d. Valproic acid

21. The patient has a seizure disorder and has just discovered that she is pregnant. At her first prenatal visit, she tells the nurse, "I quit taking all of my medications because I don't want anything to be wrong with my baby." What is the nurse's best response?
    a. "You can't do that. You have to take your medications."
    b. "What medications have been prescribed for you?"
    c. "How long have you had seizures?"
    d. "When was your last seizure?"

22. Which anticonvulsant(s) is/are classified as pregnancy category C? *(Select all that apply.)*
    a. Acetazolamide (Diamox)
    b. Carbamazepine (Tegretol)
    c. Phenobarbital
    d. Pregabalin (Lyrica)
    e. Topiramate (Topamax)

23. The patient has just been diagnosed with epilepsy and will be starting phenytoin. The patient's spouse asks how this medication works in the body. What is the nurse's best response?
    a. "It inhibits the enzyme that destroys one of the neurotransmitters."
    b. "It helps stop the entry of sodium into the cell."
    c. "It has not been determined exactly how it prevents seizures."
    d. "It increases the amount of calcium that enters the cell."

24. The patient has just been diagnosed with a seizure disorder and has been started on valproic acid. What statement(s) by the patient indicate(s) to the nurse the patient needs more instruction regarding his medication? *(Select all that apply.)*
    a. "I just have to remember to take it once a day."
    b. "I have to take it with lots of water."
    c. "I need to take it at the same times every day."
    d. "I can't drink grapefruit juice anymore."

25. The nurse has received an order to administer an initial dose of IV phenytoin to a patient with new-onset seizures. What will the nurse check before administering this medication? *(Select all that apply.)*
    a. Hourly urine output
    b. Blood glucose levels
    c. Cardiac rhythm
    d. Blood pressure

26. The nurse is working on a neurosurgery unit. The patient calls the desk to complain that his arm is really burning and feels hot. The patient is receiving IV phenytoin for his grand mal seizures. What is the nurse's best action?
    a. Call the health care provider immediately to change the medication to oral.
    b. Continue the infusion and reassure the patient.
    c. Flush the line with 10 mL of normal saline and continue the infusion.
    d. Discontinue the IV and restart the IV infusion in a different site.

27. A patient has been started on an anticonvulsant for a seizure disorder and asks how long he will need to take the medication. What is the nurse's best response?
    a. "You will need to take an anticonvulsant of some type for your lifetime."
    b. "This medication should be taken until you haven't had a seizure for a month."
    c. "Seizures are unpredictable and so is the duration of the treatment."
    d. "You will only need to take it for a short period of time because anticonvulsants will cure the seizure disorder."

28. Phenytoin levels must be monitored carefully as there is a narrow therapeutic range. Which result is within therapeutic range?
    a. 8 mcg/mL
    b. 18 mcg/mL
    c. 28 mcg/mL
    d. 38 mcg/mL

29. A nurse working triage in the emergency department witnesses a patient having a seizure. What information will be included in the nurse's documentation? *(Select all that apply.)*
    a. Type of movements
    b. Duration of movements
    c. Ability to stop movements
    d. Progression of movements
    e. Preceding events

30. The nurse is preparing discharge teaching for a patient who has been started on phenytoin for a seizure disorder. What information about side effects of this medication should the nurse provide to the patient and his family?
    a. "There may be a green discoloration of the patient's urine."
    b. "It is best to use a hard-bristle toothbrush for dental care."
    c. "Nosebleeds and sore throats should be reported to the health care provider."
    d. "The patient should get up slowly to prevent fainting."

31. What would the nurse expect to see if the patient is experiencing a common side effect of phenytoin?
    a. Gingival hyperplasia
    b. Excessive thirst
    c. Weight gain
    d. Muscle tremors

32. A patient presents to the emergency department in status epilepticus. Which medication would the nurse anticipate to be ordered first?
    a. Diazepam (Valium)
    b. Midazolam (Versed)
    c. Propofol (Diprivan)
    d. Phenobarbital

33. Which statement(s) is/are true about seizures and anticonvulsant use in pregnancy? *(Select all that apply.)*
    a. Seizures may increase up to 25% in epileptic women.
    b. Many anticonvulsants have teratogenic properties.
    c. Anticonvulsant use increases loss of folic acid.
    d. Anticonvulsants increase the effects of vitamin K.
    e. Valproic acid causes malformation in 40% to 80% of fetuses.

34. Which anticonvulsant may also be used as prophylaxis for migraine headaches?
    a. Diazepam (Valium)
    b. Phenytoin (Dilantin)
    c. Valproic acid (Depakote)
    d. Clorazepate (Tranxene)

Case Study

Read the scenario and answer the following question on a separate sheet of paper.

A 30-year-old elementary school teacher has missed several appointments with her primary care provider. She has a history of tonic-clonic seizure activity. She states, "I just can't take the carbamazepine (Tegretol). I can't function with it." Her provider prescribes oxcarbazepine (Trileptal).

1. What will the nurse discuss with the patient regarding oxcarbazepine?

23 Drugs for Neurologic Disorders: Parkinsonism and Alzheimer's Disease

Study Questions

Match the description in Column I with the letter of the reference in Column II.

Column I

_____ 1. Acetylcholinesterase inhibitor

_____ 2. Dopamine agonist

_____ 3. Dystonic movement

_____ 4. Bradykinesia

_____ 5. Pseudoparkinsonism

Column II

a. Stimulates dopamine receptors

b. Adverse reaction to antipsychotic medications

c. Allows more acetylcholine in the neuron receptors

d. Involuntary abnormal movements

e. Slowed movements

Complete the following.

6. The two neurotransmitters within the neurons of the striatum of the brain that have opposing effects are _____ and _____.

7. Which of the neurotransmitters is deficient in parkinsonism? _____

8. The drug prescribed to treat parkinsonism by replacing the neurotransmitter is _____.

9. The substance that inhibits the enzyme dopa decarboxylase and allows more levodopa to reach the brain is _____.

10. An example of an acetylcholinesterase inhibitor is _____.

11. Acetylcholinesterase inhibitors _____ transmission at the cholinergic synapses, both peripheral and central.

12. The drug _____ prolongs action of levodopa and can decrease "on-off" fluctuations in patients with parkinsonism.

13. The medication that is a combination of dopaminergics and a COMT inhibitor that provides the greatest dosing flexibility is called _____.

14. An example of a Food and Drug Administration (FDA)–approved anticholinergic drug used for parkinsonism is _____.

NCLEX Review Questions

Select the best response.

15. The nurse is administering carbidopa-levodopa to an older adult patient with parkinsonism. Which order(s) would the nurse question before administering the medication? (*Select all that apply.*)
    a. Carbidopa 5 mg/levodopa 50 mg t.i.d./q.i.d.
    b. Carbidopa 10 mg/levodopa 100 mg t.i.d./q.i.d.
    c. Carbidopa 15 mg/levodopa 150 mg t.i.d./q.i.d.
    d. Carbidopa 20 mg/levodopa 200 mg t.i.d./q.i.d.
    e. Carbidopa 25 mg/levodopa 250 mg t.i.d./q.i.d.

16. A patient taking carbidopa-levodopa for parkinsonism is complaining of dizziness, diarrhea, anxiety, and nasal stuffiness. Which of these complaints does the nurse recognize as a possible side effect of carbidopa-levodopa?
    a. Dizziness
    b. Diarrhea
    c. Anxiety
    d. Nasal stuffiness

17. The nurse is teaching a patient with parkinsonism about carbidopa-levodopa. Which statement(s) by the patient indicate(s) the need for further teaching? (*Select all that apply.*)
    a. "This medication may make my movements smoother."
    b. "My skin may turn yellow if I miss too many doses."
    c. "I need to take vitamin B$_6$ supplements with this medication."
    d. "I should take this medicine on an empty stomach."
    e. "I need to check my blood sugar regularly while taking this medication."

18. The nurse is helping a family prepare for a grocery shopping trip for a patient who has been prescribed selegiline (Eldepryl). Which food(s) should be avoided? (*Select all that apply.*)
    a. Aged cheeses
    b. Chocolate
    c. Peanut butter
    d. Wheat bread
    e. Yogurt

19. A patient with Alzheimer's disease is taking rivastigmine (Exelon) and has also been started on medication for depression. Which order will the nurse question prior to administering the new drug?
    a. Atypical antidepressant
    b. Monoamine oxidase inhibitor (MAOI) antidepressant
    c. Selective serotonin reuptake inhibitor (SSRI) antidepressant
    d. Tricyclic antidepressant

20. A patient with parkinsonism currently takes carbidopa-levodopa, and the patient's health care provider adds the medication entacapone to the patient's drug regimen. What would the nurse expect to occur with the carbidopa-levodopa dosing?
    a. There should be no change in the medication dosage.
    b. Both carbidopa and levodopa dosages should be decreased.
    c. The levodopa dosage alone should decrease.
    d. The carbidopa dosage alone should decrease.

21. Anticholinergics are contraindicated for which patient(s)? (*Select all that apply.*)
    a. A 45-year-old with glaucoma
    b. A 60-year-old with shingles
    c. A 65-year-old with urinary frequency
    d. A 71-year-old with diabetes
    e. A 77-year-old with angina

22. A patient with a history of parkinsonism is brought into the emergency department after the family reports the patient is talking to "rabbits coming out of the walls" at home. Which medication does the nurse suspect may have caused this symptom?
    a. Bromocriptine mesylate
    b. Selegiline HCl (Eldepryl)
    c. Pramipexole dihydrochloride (Mirapex)
    d. Tolcapone (Tasmar)

23. A patient's wandering and hostility levels have increased per family reports. What should concern the nurse in this patient who is taking memantine (Namenda) 10 mg/d?
    a. The patient is taking too high a daily dose to maintain mental status.
    b. The patient has taken an overdose of the medication.
    c. The patient is not taking enough of the medication.
    d. The patient needs to take a combination of memantine and amantadine.

24. What statement by the patient indicates an understanding of how to relieve some of the side effects associated with the use of benztropine mesylate (Cogentin)?
   a. "I can suck on hard candy or chew sugarless gum to prevent dry mouth."
   b. "I need to take my medication every 6 hours so I don't get constipated."
   c. "I should decrease the doses of all of my other medications so I don't get dizzy."
   d. "I should urinate after meals so I do not retain urine."

Case Study

Read the scenario and answer the following questions on a separate sheet of paper.

J.T. is a 75-year-old woman who has been diagnosed with stage 3 Alzheimer's disease. She will be living with her daughter and granddaughter. J.T.'s health care provider has prescribed tacrine (Cognex) 10 mg q.i.d.

1. Explain the stages of cognitive decline and progression of Alzheimer's disease.

2. How does tacrine work?

3. What are some safety measures the daughter and granddaughter can utilize to help the patient stay safe in her new home?

Drugs for Neuromuscular Disorders:
Myasthenia Gravis, Multiple Sclerosis,
and Muscle Spasms

Study Questions

Crossword puzzle: Use the definitions to determine the correct terms.

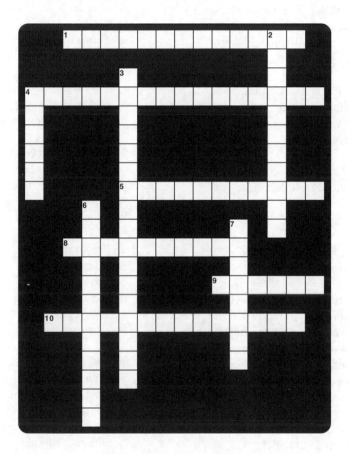

Across

1. Myasthenia gravis (MG) patients have inadequate secretion of this neurotransmitter
4. Generalized muscular weakness of the patient with MG (2 words)
5. Drug used to diagnose MG
8. Paralysis of one side of the body
9. Drooping eyelid
10. Involuntary muscle twitching

Down

2. First acetylcholinesterase inhibitor used to control MG
3. An acute exacerbation of MG symptoms (2 words)
4. Abnormal pupil constriction
6. Multiple sclerosis (MS) forms plaques on this area of the nerve (2 words)
7. A direct-acting drug that is effective in reducing spasticity in patients with MS

NCLEX Review Questions

Select the best response.

11. The patient is receiving treatment for MG with pyridostigmine (Mestinon). The nurse is assessing the patient. What clinical manifestations would be noted if the medication is working?
    a. Increased salivation
    b. Maintenance of muscle strength
    c. Miosis
    d. Tachycardia

12. The patient is receiving treatment for MG with an acetylcholinesterase inhibitor. The nurse observes that the patient is drooling, her eyes are tearing, and she is diaphoretic. What will concern the nurse about the patient exhibiting these clinical manifestations?
    a. She is having an anaphylactic reaction.
    b. She is having a cholinergic crisis.
    c. She is in the early stages of myasthenic crisis.
    d. She is having a vascular spasm.

13. What emergency medication will be administered to a patient exhibiting the signs of cholinergic crisis?
    a. Atropine
    b. Diazepam (Valium)
    c. Edrophonium (Tensilon)
    d. Pyridostigmine (Mestinon)

14. The patient presents to her health care provider with complaints of double vision, headache, and muscle weakness. She states that these symptoms come and go every few weeks, but her "spells" seem to be getting closer together. If her health care provider is considering a diagnosis of MS, what test is likely to be ordered?
    a. Angiography
    b. Computerized tomography (CT) scan
    c. Magnetic resonance imaging (MRI)
    d. Myelogram

15. The patient has been receiving pyridostigmine (Mestinon). Which medication when ordered by the health care provider should the nurse question before administering to the patient?
    a. Histamine₂ blocker
    b. Propranolol
    c. Cephalosporin
    d. Tetracycline

16. The patient has had MS for several years, during which time he has had many remissions and exacerbations. He has been prescribed azathioprine (Imuran) and interferon-β (Betaseron). The patient inquires, "How will this help me feel better?" What is the nurse's best response?
    a. "These medications will help form new neurons and axons."
    b. "They will improve muscle strength."
    c. "They will reduce spasticity and improve muscular movement."
    d. "They will stop the progression of the disease."

17. The patient has MS and is experiencing muscle spasms. How will centrally acting muscle relaxants improve his status?
    a. They affect mu receptors to decrease pain.
    b. They decrease pain and increase range of motion.
    c. They decrease inflammation of the peripheral nerves.
    d. They speed conduction to improve flexibility.

18. The patient has been involved in a motor vehicle collision and has been prescribed methocarbamol (Robaxin) for muscle spasms in her neck and back. What side effect(s) should the nurse discuss with the patient prior to discharge? *(Select all that apply.)*
    a. Brown urine
    b. Diarrhea
    c. Drowsiness
    d. Increased appetite
    e. Tachycardia
    f. Urinary retention

19. The nurse is administering medications to her patients on a medical-surgical floor. Which medication order should the nurse question before administration?
    a. Dantrolene sodium (Dantrium) for a 50-year-old with muscle spasms
    b. Diazepam (Valium) for a 60-year-old who also has glaucoma
    c. Edrophonium (Tensilon) for a 30-year-old who is undergoing diagnostic testing for MG
    d. Chlorzoxazone (Parafon Forte DSC) for a 33-year-old with muscle trauma

Case Study

Read the scenario and answer the following questions on a separate sheet of paper.

G.D., 24 years old, was involved in a high-speed roll-over motor vehicle accident and has a spinal cord injury. He has muscle spasms and some spasticity in his lower extremities bilaterally. He has intermittently been prescribed carisoprodol (Soma) and will be started on baclofen (Lioresal).

1. Why do muscle spasms occur in patients with spinal cord injuries?

2. What is the mechanism of carisoprodol (Soma)? How does baclofen (Lioresal) work?

3. What are the side effects of each medication?

25 Antiinflammatory Drugs

Study Questions

Match the term in Column I with the definition in Column II.

Column I

_____ 1. Acetylsalicylic acid

_____ 2. *Para*-chlorobenzoic acid

_____ 3. Ketorolac

_____ 4. Fenamates

_____ 5. Oxicams

_____ 6. Immunomodulators

_____ 7. Colchicine

_____ 8. Allopurinol

_____ 9. Celecoxib

Column II

a. Disrupts the inflammatory process and delays disease progression

b. Indicated for long-term arthritic conditions

c. One of the first nonsteroidal antiinflammatory drugs (NSAIDs) introduced

d. Oldest antiinflammatory agent

e. The first injectable NSAID

f. The first drug used to treat gout

g. Drug of choice for patients with chronic tophaceous gout

h. Potent NSAID used for acute and chronic arthritic conditions

i. Cyclooxygenase inhibitor

Complete the following.

10. Inflammation is a response to tissue _____ and _____.

11. The five cardinal signs of inflammation are _____, _____, _____, _____, and _____.

12. Leukocyte infiltration of the inflamed tissue occurs during the _____ phase of inflammation.

13. The half-life of each NSAID (does/does not) differ greatly. *(Circle correct answer.)*

14. When using NSAIDs for inflammation, the dosage is generally _____ than for pain relief.

15. The half-life of corticosteroids is greater than _____ hours.

NCLEX Review Questions

Select the best response.

16. What occurs during the vascular phase of inflammation?
    a. Leukocyte and protein infiltration into inflamed tissue
    b. Vasoconstriction with leukocyte infiltration into inflamed tissue
    c. Vasoconstriction and fluid influx into the interstitial space
    d. Vasodilation with increased capillary permeability

17. A patient who is taking NSAIDs for arthritis complains of persistent heartburn. What further question(s) should the nurse ask the patient about the heartburn? *(Select all that apply.)*
    a. "Do you take your medication with food?"
    b. "Have you been drinking an increased amount of water?"
    c. "Have you noticed a change in the color of your bowel movements?"
    d. "What dosage of the NSAID are you taking?"
    e. "Where is the heartburn located?"

18. When preparing discharge teaching for a patient who has been prescribed ibuprofen for arthritis, how does the nurse explain the mode of action?
    a. "Ibuprofen is a COX-2 inhibitor, so it blocks prostaglandin synthesis."
    b. "Ibuprofen inhibits prostaglandin synthesis."
    c. "Ibuprofen binds with opiate receptor sites."
    d. "Ibuprofen promotes vasodilation to increase blood flow."

19. A patient with a complicated medical history including hypertension, atrial fibrillation, and arthritis calls the health care provider's office to speak with a nurse about "all of these bruises I have all of a sudden." Which potential drug interaction should concern the nurse with these symptoms?
    a. Aspirin and warfarin
    b. Sulfasalazine and acetaminophen
    c. Tolmetin and propranolol
    d. Meloxicam and amlodipine

20. A father presents to the emergency department with his 4-year-old son. The father explains that his son had a fever, so he gave the child baby aspirin to decrease the fever and it has not worked. What should concern the nurse about a 4-year-old receiving aspirin?
    a. Aspirin has the potential to cause gastrointestinal (GI) bleeding in children.
    b. Aspirin has the potential to cause ringing in the ears in children.
    c. Aspirin has the potential to cause hyperglycemia in children.
    d. Aspirin has the potential to cause Reye's syndrome in children.

21. The patient with a history of asthma has been prescribed ibuprofen for arthritis. What can ibuprofen cause that should concern the nurse?
    a. Tachycardia
    b. Increased secretions
    c. Bronchospasm
    d. Fluid retention

22. Ibuprofen is a frequently prescribed antiinflammatory, analgesic, and antipyretic. What is a positive aspect of this drug in relation to other NSAIDs?
    a. It tends to cause less GI irritation.
    b. It may be taken between meals.
    c. It has a long half-life of 20-30 hours.
    d. It has no drug-drug interactions.

23. A 35-year-old female patient has been prescribed ibuprofen 400 mg t.i.d. for arthritis. What statement by the patient would indicate a need for further education?
    a. "This medication should cause less GI upset than other NSAIDs."
    b. "Now I won't have to drink so much water."
    c. "I know this medicine might cause some diarrhea."
    d. "I will need to stop taking this medication if I get pregnant."

24. What advantage does piroxicam (Feldene) have over other NSAIDs?
    a. No GI irritation
    b. Few drug-drug interactions
    c. Long half-life
    d. Rapid onset

25. By which action does colchicine (Colcrys) relieve the symptoms of gout?
    a. It inhibits the migration of leukocytes to the inflamed area.
    b. It blocks reabsorption of uric acid.
    c. It blocks prostaglandin release.
    d. It inhibits uric acid synthesis.

26. Uricosuric agents such as probenecid (Benemid) are used in the treatment of gout. What is the mechanism of action?
    a. Retention of urate crystals in the body
    b. Inhibition of the reabsorption of uric acid
    c. Promotion of uric acid removal in the ureters
    d. Increased release of uric acid

27. A patient has been switched to the immunomodulator etanercept (Enbrel) for severe rheumatoid arthritis. What is the mechanism of action for etanercept?
    a. It neutralizes tumor necrosis factor (TNF), thereby delaying the inflammatory disease process.
    b. It inhibits IL-1 from binding to interleukin receptor sites in cartilage and bone.
    c. It blocks COX-2 receptors, which are needed for biosynthesis of prostaglandins.
    d. It promotes uric acid reabsorption.

28. When discontinuing steroid therapy, the dosage should be tapered over a period of how many days?
    a. No taper is necessary
    b. 1-4 days
    c. 5-10 days
    d. More than 10 days

29. A patient has started on corticosteroids for an arthritic condition. What information should the nurse include in a health teaching plan? (*Select all that apply.*)
    a. Corticosteroids are used to control arthritic flare-ups in severe cases.
    b. Corticosteroids have a short half-life.
    c. Corticosteroids are usually administered once a day.
    d. Corticosteroids are tapered over the course of 5-10 days.
    e. Corticosteroids may not be taken with prostaglandin inhibitors.

30. The nurse is planning teaching regarding antigout medication. What information should be included? (*Select all that apply.*)
    a. Include large doses of vitamin C supplements.
    b. Increase fluid intake.
    c. Avoid alcoholic beverages.
    d. Avoid foods high in purine.
    e. Take medication with food.
    f. Avoid direct sunlight.

31. The patient has been prescribed infliximab (Remicade) for severe rheumatoid arthritis. Her spouse calls the clinic and states his wife has a fever of 101.9° F, chills, nausea and vomiting, and is very dizzy. What will the nurse advise the patient's spouse to do?
    a. Nothing. These are common side effects of infliximab.
    b. Have the patient take a cool bath.
    c. Wait 24 hours and if symptoms continue, call back.
    d. Bring the patient to the emergency department or clinic for further evaluation.

Case Study

Read the scenario and answer the following questions on a separate sheet of paper.

F.E., 54 years old, comes to the clinic for treatment of an inflammatory condition. He reports that he has been taking 975 mg of aspirin combined with 65 mg of caffeine q4h for the past week. He states that his joint pain is getting worse and he now has noticed some blood in his stools. F.E.'s vital signs are blood pressure 90/62 mm Hg, heart rate 118 beats/min, respiratory rate 24 breaths/min, temperature 37.8° C, and pulse oximetry 98% on room air. His skin is pale and cool.

1. What is the therapeutic dosage range for aspirin?

2. What are the side effects of aspirin? What are the signs and symptoms of aspirin overdose?

3. Discuss the possible etiology of the patient's vital signs.

26 Nonopioid and Opioid Analgesics

Study Questions

Complete the following.

1. Opioids act primarily on the _____ and nonopioid analgesics act on the _____ at the pain receptor sites.

2. In addition to suppressing pain impulses, opioids also suppress _____ and _____.

3. In addition to pain relief, many opioids have _____ and _____ effects.

4. Opioids are contraindicated for use in patients with _____ and _____.

5. The patient taking meperidine reports blurred vision. The nurse knows this is a(n) _____ and would report this finding to the _____.

6. Pentazocine, an opioid agonist-antagonist, is classified as a Schedule _____ drug.

NCLEX Review Questions

Select the best response.

7. The patient has returned to the floor from surgery after a hip arthroplasty. For the first 48 hours postoperatively, meperidine (Demerol) is ordered for pain control. During the time the patient is taking meperidine, frequent monitoring of what is required?
    a. Blood pressure
    b. Pulse
    c. Temperature
    d. Urine output

8. The nurse is assessing a patient for a possible overdose of opioids. The pupils are pinpoint. What is this called?
    a. Diplopia
    b. Meiosis
    c. Miosis
    d. Mitosis

9. Which nursing assessment would be least important when monitoring a patient who is receiving hydromorphone (Dilaudid)?
    a. Bowel sounds
    b. Fluid intake
    c. Pain scale
    d. Vital signs

10. What information should the nurse include in a teaching plan for a patient who is being discharged home after knee surgery with a prescription for hydrocodone? *(Select all that apply.)*
    a. Dietary restrictions while taking hydrocodone
    b. Instructions not to exceed recommended dosage
    c. Instructions not to use alcohol or CNS depressants while taking hydrocodone
    d. Instructions on how to prevent constipation
    e. Side effects to report

11. Which factor is most relevant to the relief of chronic pain?
    a. Administration of drugs at patient's request
    b. Opioid analgesics
    c. Use of injectable medications
    d. Use of drugs with long half-lives

12. The patient is brought to the emergency department with a reported overdose of morphine. Which drug does the nurse anticipate will be prescribed?
    a. Butorphanol (Stadol)
    b. Naloxone (Narcan)
    c. Flumazenil (Romazicon)
    d. Pentazocine (Talwin)

13. Mixed opioid agonist-antagonists were developed in hopes of decreasing what problem?
    a. Chronic pain
    b. Opioid abuse
    c. Renal failure
    d. Respiratory depression

14. The patient has been taking oxycodone (OxyContin) for 8 weeks for a back injury he sustained at work. He has stopped taking his medication. How many hours after he last takes his medication does the nurse anticipate his withdrawal symptoms will begin?
    a. 6-12 hours
    b. 24-48 hours
    c. 48-72 hours
    d. 72-96 hours

15. The patient has breast cancer and is in hospice care. She has been taking morphine (MS Contin) for pain control. What is the duration of pain relief for controlled-release morphine?
    a. 1-2 hours
    b. 4-5 hours
    c. 8-12 hours
    d. 24-48 hours

16. The 72-year-old patient is scheduled to have major surgery. In his preoperative evaluation, his daughter shares with the nurse that she is concerned he will not have his pain relieved. What does the nurse tell the patient and his daughter regarding postoperative pain control? *(Select all that apply.)*
    a. "You will only be able to receive acetaminophen because you are over age 70."
    b. "We will be able to adjust your pain medication to an appropriate dose for your age."
    c. "Please let us know when you are having pain so we can work together to stay on top of it."
    d. "Older patients do not have pain as much as middle-aged patients do."
    e. "You will be able to help him push the button for his patient-controlled analgesia (PCA) device to control his pain."

17. What will the nurse do to be more successful in treating pain in an 8-year-old patient who fell from a tree and broke his arm? *(Select all that apply.)*
    a. Assume the child hurts and administer pain medication.
    b. Discuss the child's typical responses with the caregivers.
    c. Only utilize nonpharmacologic pain control methods.
    d. Use a pain scale appropriate for children such as the Ouch Scale.
    e. Utilize developmentally appropriate communication techniques.

18. The nurse is completing the medication reconciliation for the patient who will be discharged home with a prescription for oxycodone and acetaminophen (Percocet). Which medication that the patient is currently taking raises a concern for the nurse?
    a. Ampicillin
    b. Cholestyramine
    c. Furosemide
    d. Propranolol

19. The nurse is concerned that the patient is experiencing side effects of opioid agonist-antagonists. What might the nurse assess for if this patient is experiencing side/adverse effects? *(Select all that apply.)*
    a. Cardiac standstill
    b. Constipation
    c. Dysuria
    d. Hypertension
    e. Nausea and vomiting
    f. Respiratory depression

20. The patient is taking morphine after a procedure. The patient has made his third request for pain medication in the past 4 hours. The patient's vital signs are temperature 36.4° C, heart rate 88 beats/min, respiratory rate 12 breaths/min, blood pressure 104/60 mm Hg, and oxygen saturation 98%. He rates his pain as an 8 on a scale of 1-10. Assuming that a dose of the medication is due, what is the nurse's best action?
    a. Administer the dose and contact the health care provider about his respiratory rate.
    b. Administer the dose and contact the health care provider about his pain control.
    c. Hold the dose and contact the health care provider regarding his respiratory rate.
    d. Hold the dose and contact the health care provider about his pain control.

21. The older adult patient has a fentanyl patch 50 mg for chronic pain from an injury. What does the nurse know regarding this medication for this patient?
    a. This patient should not have a fentanyl patch for chronic pain.
    b. The dose may be too low.
    c. The dose may be too high for this patient.
    d. The dose is appropriate.

22. The patient is taking Vicoprofen after reconstructive knee surgery. Which statement by the patient indicates the need for more teaching?
    a. "I must take only what is prescribed for my pain."
    b. "I may need to take a laxative if I get constipated while I am taking this medication."
    c. "Having a few beers on the weekend will help me relax and ease the pain."
    d. "I should not take anything with ibuprofen in it while I am taking this medication."

23. The patient has had major surgery and has been prescribed oral ketorolac. What is the maximum length of time this medication can be taken?
    a. 24 hours
    b. 3 days
    c. 5 days
    d. 2 weeks

24. The patient has fallen off his mountain bike and sustained multiple abrasions to both of his knees. Which would be appropriate medication(s) for pain management for this patient? *(Select all that apply.)*
    a. Acetaminophen
    b. Aspirin
    c. Hydrocodone
    d. Ibuprofen
    e. Morphine

Case Study

Read the scenario and answer the following questions on a separate sheet of paper.

G.F., 25 years old, presents to the emergency department with a severe headache on the left side of her head. She states that she has had the headache for the last day and "it just won't go away." She is nauseated and is vomiting. G.F. states that lights hurt her eyes and "everything sounds loud." Her vital signs are temperature 36.8° C, heart rate 92 beats/min, respiratory rate 18 breaths/min, blood pressure 142/76 mm Hg, and oxygen saturation 100%. She rates her pain as a "13 on a scale of 1-10." The health care provider diagnoses her with a migraine headache.

1. What is the mechanism behind the pain associated with a migraine?

2. What is the difference between a classic and a common migraine?

3. What treatment options are available for this patient?

27 Antipsychotics and Anxiolytics

Study Questions

Match the term in Column I to the corresponding statement in Column II.

Column I

_____ 1. Acute dystonia

_____ 2. Akathisia

_____ 3. Anxiolytics

_____ 4. Neuroleptic

_____ 5. Psychosis

_____ 6. Schizophrenia

_____ 7. Tardive dyskinesia

_____ 8. Pseudoparkinsonism

Column II

a. Losing contact with reality

b. Protrusion and rolling of the tongue, sucking and smacking movements of the lips, chewing motion

c. Muscle tremors, rigidity, shuffling gait

d. Restlessness, inability to sit still, foot-tapping

e. Spasms of tongue, face, neck, and back

f. Used to treat anxiety and insomnia

g. Drug that modifies psychotic behavior

h. Chronic psychotic disorder

Complete the following.

9. Antipsychotic drugs were developed to improve the _____ and _____ of patients with psychotic symptoms resulting from an imbalance in the neurotransmitter _____.

10. Typical antipsychotics are subdivided into phenothiazines and nonphenothiazines. Nonphenothiazines are divided into four classes: _____, _____, _____, and _____.

11. The most common side effect of all antipsychotics is _____.

12. Antipsychotics may lead to dermatologic side effects that include _____ and _____.

13. Phenothiazines (increase/decrease) the seizure threshold; adjustment of anticonvulsants may be required. *(Circle correct answer.)*

14. Anxiolytics (are/are not) usually given for secondary anxiety. *(Circle correct answer.)*

15. Long-term use of anxiolytics is not recommended because _____ may develop within a short time.

16. The action of anxiolytics resembles that of _____, not antipsychotics.

Match the following drugs in Column I with their drug classification in Column II.

Column I

_____ 17. clozapine (Clozaril)

_____ 18. chlorpromazine (Thorazine)

_____ 19. fluphenazine (Prolixin)

_____ 20. molindone HCl (Moban)

_____ 21. haloperidol (Haldol)

_____ 22. risperidone (Risperdal)

Column II

a. Phenothiazine

b. Nonphenothiazine

c. Atypical antipsychotic

NCLEX Review Questions

Select the best response.

23. Neuroleptic drugs are useful in the management of which type of illness?
   a. Anxiety disorders
   b. Depressive disorders
   c. Psychotic disorders
   d. Psychosomatic disorders

24. The patient has been started on an antipsychotic medication for treatment of her schizophrenia. She asks the nurse when she will start to feel better. What is the nurse's best response?
   a. "It may take up to one week to start to feel the effects."
   b. "Responses vary, but it may be about 6 weeks."
   c. "You will only feel better when you start psychotherapy, too."
   d. "You should start to feel better within 30-60 minutes."

25. The patient has been started on chlorpromazine HCl (Thorazine) for treatment of intractable pain. What information will the nurse include in patient education about this class of medication?
   a. "A therapeutic response to this medication will be immediate."
   b. "Change positions slowly from sitting to standing to prevent orthostatic hypotension."
   c. "It is all right to have alcohol when taking this medication."
   d. "This drug may be stopped abruptly as soon as your pain stops."

26. Typical or traditional antipsychotics may cause extrapyramidal symptoms (EPS) or pseudoparkinsonism. Which symptom is considered an extrapyramidal symptom?
   a. Downward eye movement
   b. Intentional tremors
   c. Loss of hearing
   d. Shuffling gait

27. What agent would the nurse expect to give to decrease EPS?
   a. Benztropine (Cogentin)
   b. Bethanechol (Urecholine)
   c. Buspirone HCl (BuSpar)
   d. Doxepin (Sinequan)

28. Phenothiazines are grouped into three categories based on their side effects. In which group is fluphenazine (Prolixin)?
   a. Aliphatic
   b. Piperazine
   c. Piperidine
   d. Thioxanthene

29. The patient has been prescribed fluphenazine (Prolixin) for treatment of schizophrenia. What information should the nurse include in the patient teaching for this medication? *(Select all that apply.)*
   a. "Blood pressure changes are not an indication of an adverse reaction."
   b. "It is all right to take all herbal medications when taking fluphenazine."
   c. "Notify your health care provider if you have dizziness, headache, or nausea."
   d. "This medication must be taken every day."
   e. "You should not drink alcohol when taking this medication."

30. The 72-year-old patient has recently been diagnosed with schizophrenia. His health care provider has prescribed fluphenazine (Prolixin) 20 mg/day. In reviewing his medications prior to discharge from the hospital, the nurse notes the dose. What should concern the nurse about the amount of the medication prescribed?
    a. Nothing. The patient is an adult and this is in the normal adult range.
    b. The patient's dose should be 10% less than the adult dose.
    c. The patient's dose should be 25% to 50% less than the adult dose.
    d. This medication is contraindicated in patients over 70 years old.

31. A patient presents to the emergency department with an overdose of chlorpromazine HCl (Thorazine). What is the priority action by the nurse?
    a. Administer activated charcoal.
    b. Administer anticholinergic medications.
    c. Establish an IV.
    d. Maintain the airway.

32. The 58-year-old patient presents to the emergency department. He is highly agitated and combative and is presenting a danger to self and others. The health care provider has ordered haloperidol (Haldol) 5 mg IM. What should the nurse know about this medication when giving it as an antipsychotic?
    a. It has a sedative effect on agitated, combative patients.
    b. It is the drug of choice for older patients with liver disease.
    c. It will not cause EPS.
    d. It can safely be used in patients with narrow-angle glaucoma.

33. What is the drug category for atypical antipsychotics?
    a. Butyrophenones
    b. Phenothiazines
    c. Serotonin/dopamine antagonists
    d. Thioxanthenes

34. The atypical antipsychotics have a weak affinity for the D_2 receptors. Consequently, what happens to the occurrence of EPS when taking these medications?
    a. An absence of EPS
    b. An increase in EPS
    c. Fewer EPS
    d. No effect on EPS

35. Atypical antipsychotics have a stronger affinity for which type of receptors that block serotonin receptors?
    a. D_1
    b. D_2
    c. D_3
    d. D_4

36. The patient has just been prescribed risperidone (Risperdal). What side effects should the nurse include in the health teaching about this medication?
    a. Hepatotoxicity
    b. Hyperglycemia
    c. Hearing loss
    d. Urinary frequency

37. The medication alprazolam belongs to which anxiolytic drug group?
    a. Antihistamines
    b. Benzodiazepines
    c. Buspirinones
    d. Phenothiazines

38. The patient has been started on IM extended-release olanzapine due to noncompliance with the oral medication regimen. What does the nurse know is/are benefit(s) of this medication? *(Select all that apply.)*
    a. Only required to be given every 2-4 weeks
    b. Few to no extrapyramidal symptoms
    c. Cures schizophrenia
    d. Completely safe in pregnancy
    e. Does not cause agranulocytosis

39. Which patient(s) should not be taking fluphenazine (Prolixin)? *(Select all that apply.)*
    a. 32-year-old with narrow-angle glaucoma
    b. 35-year-old with hepatitis C
    c. 47-year-old with subcortical brain damage
    d. 53-year-old with blood dyscrasias
    e. 62-year-old with neuromuscular pain

40. Lorazepam is an anxiolytic drug; however, it may be prescribed for other purposes. For which other condition(s) might it be prescribed? *(Select all that apply.)*
    a. Alcohol withdrawal
    b. Anxiety associated with depression
    c. Muscle spasms
    d. Preoperative medication
    e. Status epilepticus

Case Study

Read the scenario and answer the following questions on a separate sheet of paper.

H.K., 20 years old, is brought to the emergency department. Her friends say she had been trying to "cram for finals." They have been unable to awaken her in 18 hours. An empty bottle of clonazepam (Klonopin) and a bottle of vodka are found at the bedside. Vital signs are temperature 37.2° C, heart rate 64 beats/minute, respiratory rate 8 breaths/minute, blood pressure 82/40 mm Hg, O_2 saturation 78%. She is only responsive to deep pain.

1.   What kind of medication is clonazepam?

2.   What is its mechanism of action?

3.   What are the side effects associated with this category of medication?

4.   With the above history, what is concerning to the nurse, and what are the priority actions?

28 Antidepressants and Mood Stabilizers

Study Questions

Crossword puzzle: Use the definitions to determine the correct terms.

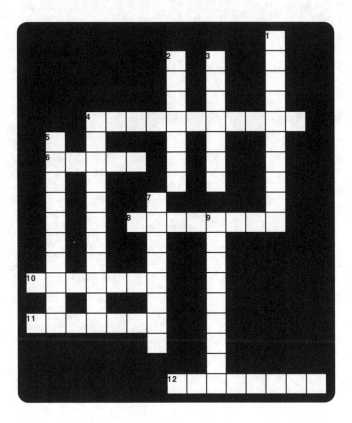

Across

4. Herbal supplement used for depression (3 words)
6. Depression that involves loss of interest in work and home
8. Depression that occurs with a sudden onset following an event
10. Depression that involves swings between two moods
11. Best time to take a tricyclic antidepressant (TCA)
12. Avoid foods with _____ when taking a monoamine oxidase inhibitor (MAOI)

Down

1. First TCA produced
2. First drug to treat bipolar affective disorder
3. Supplement that may lead to manic episodes when taken with MAOIs
4. May cause serotonin syndrome when taken with a selective serotonin reuptake inhibitor (SSRI) (3 words)
5. TCA used to treat enuresis
7. Herbal supplement that interferes with effects of fluoxetine
9. Clinical response to TCAs takes _____ weeks (3 words)

Complete the following word search. Clues are given in questions 13-19. Circle your responses.

```
T C S R V R N M J R D M J A H J H
R I Y Y V X R S A N O D J J Y E B
A N O D U O I A N N O Y N J Y V O
P I M J L R W L L D I K Q P B I I
L K F X S J G Q M O H C T W V T F
N M D S K W V O B N P I L W O C B
M A G W I G D V D L Q I T X K A U
J O T R I C Y C L I C S B U J E K
Y I Z Y M P F R F J A K P H C R V
Q S Q M U H G O U I D O F U C C X
L S T N A S S E R P E D I T N A Q
```

13. Swing-type moods
14. Abbreviation for selective serotonin reuptake inhibitors
15. Abbreviation for monoamine oxidase inhibitors
16. Type of behavior associated with the euphoric state of bipolar disorder
17. Group of drugs used to treat depression
18. Depression that has a sudden onset
19. Block the uptake of norepinephrine and serotonin in the brain

Match the drugs in Column I with their drug classification in Column II.

Column I

____ 20.   trazodone (Desyrel)

____ 21.   maprotiline (Ludiomil)

____ 22.   citalopram (Celexa)

____ 23.   amitriptyline (Elavil)

____ 24.   tranylcypromine (Parnate)

____ 25.   paroxetine (Paxil)

Column II

a.   Atypical antidepressants
b.   Selective serotonin reuptake inhibitors (SSRIs)
c.   Monoamine oxidase inhibitors (MAOIs)
d.   Tricyclic antidepressants (TCAs)

NCLEX Review Questions

Select the best response.

26. The 12-year-old patient has been evaluated for enuresis. After home remedies and other alternatives have been explored, which medication does the nurse know may be prescribed to treat this condition?
    a. Citalopram (Celexa)
    b. Fluvoxamine (Luvox)
    c. Imipramine (Tofranil)
    d. Sertraline (Zoloft)

27. The patient has been taking phenelzine (Nardil) for several months and his chronic anxiety and fear have not improved. What is the maximum daily dose for this medication?
    a. 15 mg/d
    b. 45 mg/d
    c. 60 mg/d
    d. 90 mg/d

28. The patient has been prescribed amitriptyline (Elavil) as an adjunct to therapy for depression. What information will the nurse include in the health teaching regarding this medication?
    a. "Check your heart rate daily. It may become very slow."
    b. "Stand up slowly because your blood pressure can drop suddenly."
    c. "You should start to feel less depressed within 12 hours."
    d. "Take your medication in the morning because it will make you alert."

29. Which food(s) or beverage(s) is/are contraindicated in a patient prescribed isocarboxazid (Marplan)? *(Select all that apply.)*
    a. Bananas
    b. Chocolate
    c. Grapefruit
    d. Milk
    e. Wine

30. The patient has a history of depression and is taking fluoxetine (Prozac). The patient presents to the emergency department complaining of a severe headache. She is diaphoretic and is unable to sit still. Her family tells the nurse that the patient has been taking "some herb." Which herb does the nurse suspect the patient has been taking?
    a. Ephedra
    b. Feverfew
    c. Garlic
    d. St. John's wort

31. Which is an advantage of taking SSRIs over TCAs?
    a. Fewer sexual side effects
    b. Increased appetite
    c. Less sedation
    d. Less tachycardia

32. Which nursing intervention is most important for a patient taking lithium?
    a. Advising the patient that he or she can stop taking the medication when not in a manic phase
    b. Emphasizing the importance of patient-adjusted dosage
    c. Monitoring for excessive thirst, weight gain, and increased urination
    d. Teaching the patient to limit fluid intake to prevent weight gain

33. The patient has been diagnosed with bipolar disorder and is acutely manic. The patient is currently taking lithium (Lithobid). What laboratory value is the nurse particularly concerned with?
    a. BUN
    b. Blood glucose
    c. INR
    d. Platelet count

34. The patient has been taking lithium (Lithobid) 1800 mg/day in three divided doses for 10 days. He remains agitated and hyperactive, with a lithium level of 0.8 mEq/L. He complains of feeling slow and thirsty. What does the nurse suspect is occurring?
    a. The patient is experiencing lithium toxicity.
    b. The patient's lithium level is subtherapeutic, and he is still manic.
    c. The patient's lithium level is therapeutic, and he is a nonresponder.
    d. The patient is allergic to lithium.

35. The nurse is teaching the patient about lithium (Eskalith). Which statement by the patient indicates a need for more education?
    a. "If I stop my medication, the depression will return."
    b. "I should avoid caffeine products that may aggravate the manic phase."
    c. "I should take my medication with food."
    d. "It is important that I wear or carry ID indicating that I am taking lithium."

36. The patient has been prescribed venlafaxine (Effexor) for generalized anxiety disorder. Which statement by the patient indicates the need for further health teaching?
    a. "I need to take my medication even if I am not feeling anxious."
    b. "I need to wear sunscreen when I am outdoors."
    c. "If I have any issues with my sexual performance, I can ask my health care provider."
    d. "It is OK if I keep taking my herbal medications for my depression and anxiety."

37. The patient has a history of bipolar disorder and takes lithium (Eskalith). She tells her health care provider that she would like to become pregnant in the near future. What is/are the concern(s) with taking lithium while pregnant? *(Select all that apply.)*
    a. Congenital anomaly
    b. Excessive weight gain
    c. Hyperemesis gravidarum
    d. Miscarriage
    e. Multiple gestation

Case Study

Read the scenario and answer the following questions on a separate sheet of paper.

F.K., 53 years old, has recently relocated to start a new job after the position she held for 20 years was eliminated. She started taking fluoxetine (Prozac) 40 mg at bedtime for complaints of insomnia, sadness, tearfulness, and inability to concentrate. She tells the nurse, "I can't believe I lost my job and have to start over. I feel like such a failure." She is postmenopausal and has a history of hypertension and migraines.

1. Discuss SSRIs and their mechanism of action.

2. What questions should the nurse ask in the initial interview?

3. What discharge heath education regarding fluoxetine will the nurse provide?

Study Questions

Crossword puzzle: Use the definitions to determine the correct terms.

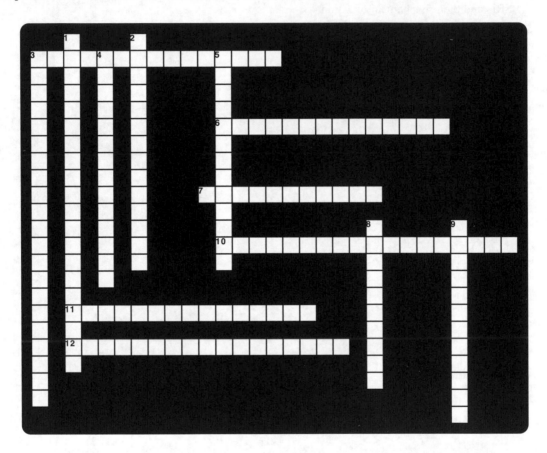

Across

3. Resistance to antibacterial drugs that have similar actions (2 words)
6. Drugs that inhibit the growth of bacteria
7. The first penicillinase-resistant penicillin
10. Caused by prior exposure to an antibacterial (2 words)
11. Antibody proteins such as IgG and IgM
12. Bacterial resistance that may occur naturally (2 words)

Down

1. Infections acquired when in a health care facility (2 words)
2. Toxicity of drugs in the kidneys
3. Should be checked before administration of antibiotics (3 words)
4. Occurrence of a secondary infection when the flora of the body are disturbed
5. Substances that inhibit bacterial growth or kill bacteria
8. Introduced during World War II
9. Drugs that kill bacteria

Match the antibiotic in Column I to its category in Column II.

Column I

_____ 13. Penicillin G

_____ 14. Amoxicillin

_____ 15. Oxacillin

_____ 16. Piperacillin-tazobactam

_____ 17. Ancef

_____ 18. Cefaclor

_____ 19. Cefdinir

_____ 20. Cefepime

Column II

a. First-generation cephalosporin
b. Second-generation cephalosporin
c. Third-generation cephalosporin
d. Fourth-generation cephalosporin
e. Basic penicillin
f. Penicillinase-resistant penicillins
g. Broad-spectrum penicillin
h. Extended-spectrum penicillins

NCLEX Review Questions

Select the best response.

21. A 28-year-old female patient presents to the clinic with complaints of severe vaginal itching and discharge. She tells the nurse that she is usually very healthy but has been taking antibiotics for an ear infection. What does the nurse recognize as a possible cause of her vaginal itching and discharge?
a. Anaphylaxis
b. Hypersensitivity
c. Nephrotoxicity
d. Superinfection

22. A patient is scheduled to receive ceftriaxone (Rocephin) for *Klebsiella pneumoniae*. What will the nurse teach the patient about this medication?
a. It is given IM or IV only.
b. There is no cross-reaction to penicillins.
c. Ceftriaxone is safe to take with anticoagulants.
d. There is no effect on lab values.

23. The nurse knows that aztreonam (Azactam) is effective against which bacteria?
a. *Escherichia coli*
b. *Haemophilus influenzae*
c. *Proteus mirabilis*
d. *Pseudomonas aeruginosa*

24. A 40-year-old patient with renal dysfunction is suffering from a *Staphylococcus aureus* infection. He is prescribed cefprozil monohydrate (Cefzil). What is the maximum dose the nurse would anticipate?
a. 250 mg/d
b. 500 mg/d
c. 750 mg/d
d. 1 g/d

25. A mother brings her 3-year-old child to the emergency department with difficulty breathing and fever. The child is admitted to the pediatric intensive care unit (PICU) with a severe lower respiratory tract infection and started on aztreonam (Azactam). The child weighs 37 pounds. What is the usual dose of aztreonam?
a. 170 mg q6h
b. 340 mg q6h
c. 510 mg q6h
d. 680 mg q6h

26.   Which class of medication would increase risk of nephrotoxicity in a patient taking ceftriaxone?
a. Angiotensin-converting enzyme (ACE) inhibitors
b. Antiarrhythmics
c. Loop diuretics
d. Nonsteroidal antiinflammatory drugs (NSAIDs)

27. The patient has been started on ceftriaxone (Rocephin). Her family is concerned regarding her recent weight loss. What can the nurse tell the family regarding side effects of ceftriaxone?
a. Loss of appetite is a common side effect.
b. Gastrointestinal bleeding may occur frequently.
c. Ceftriaxone causes nutrient absorption problems.
d. She will eat more when the infection is cured.

28. What statement by a parent indicates more discharge teaching is necessary for care of 5-year-old child who has been prescribed dicloxacillin (Dynapen) for otitis media?
    a. "Abdominal pain can be a side effect."
    b. "She needs to drink plenty of orange juice with this medication."
    c. "My child must take all of the medication until it is gone."
    d. "If my child develops a rash, I should bring her back to the doctor."

29. What category of drugs is known to increase the serum levels of cephalosporins?
    a. Antacids
    b. Laxatives
    c. Opioids
    d. Uricosurics

30. How does penicillin V potassium work?
    a. Alteration in membrane permeability
    b. Inhibition of cell wall synthesis
    c. Inhibition of protein synthesis
    d. Interference with cellular metabolism

31. A 35-year-old patient presents to the clinic with a complaint of sore throat. Vital signs are temperature 39.2° C, blood pressure 132/60 mm Hg, heart rate 98 beats/min, respiratory rate 18 breaths/min. She is allergic to dextromethorphan and takes oral contraceptives, vitamin C, and fexofenadine. She is diagnosed with strep throat and prescribed amoxicillin/clavulanate potassium (Augmentin). What instruction should the nurse include in the discharge teaching regarding this medication?
    a. "Increase calcium intake."
    b. "Wear sunscreen at all times."
    c. "Use an alternate method of birth control."
    d. "Stop the fexofenadine."

32. Which specific nursing intervention(s) should be performed for a patient taking ceftazidime (Fortaz)? *(Select all that apply.)*
    a. Obtain a culture and sensitivity.
    b. Administer IV dose over 20 minutes every day.
    c. Assess for allergic reaction.
    d. Monitor urine output.
    e. Restrict oral fluid intake.

33. Quinupristin/dalfopristin (Synercid) is marketed for IV use against life-threatening infection caused by which bacteria?
    a. Vancomycin-resistant *Enterococcus faecium*
    b. *Escherichia coli*
    c. *Proteus mirabilis*
    d. *Klebsiella pneumoniae*

34. Which patient should not be taking amoxicillin?
    a. 10-year-old patient with a staphylococcal infection of the skin
    b. 21-year-old pregnant patient
    c. 38-year-old patient with asthma
    d. 62-year-old diabetic patient

35. A patient has been prescribed cephradine (Velosef) for otitis media. What order will the nurse question?
    a. 250 mg q6h
    b. 500 mg q6h
    c. 750 mg q8h
    d. 1000 mg q12h

36. Which patient must be monitored carefully if receiving carbenicillin indanyl (Geocillin)?
    a. 34-year-old with diabetes
    b. 50-year-old with parkinsonism
    c. 58-year-old with heart failure
    d. 70-year-old with Alzheimer's disease

Case Study

Read the scenario and answer the following questions on a separate sheet of paper.

S.T. is an 18-year-old patient admitted for treatment of Pseudomonas pneumonia who has been started on piperacillin-tazobactam (Zosyn).

1. What is the mechanism of action of piperacillin-tazobactam?

2. What are the signs and symptoms of allergic reaction and superinfection?

3. What patient teaching related to the administration of this medication will the nurse provide?

30 Macrolides, Tetracyclines, Aminoglycosides, and Fluoroquinolones

Study Questions

Match the drug in Column I with the category in Column II.

Column I

_____ 1. Amikacin

_____ 2. Clindamycin

_____ 3. Tigecycline

_____ 4. Erythromycin

_____ 5. Telithromycin

_____ 6. Azithromycin

_____ 7. Doxycycline

_____ 8. Ciprofloxacin

_____ 9. Clarithromycin

_____ 10. Moxifloxacin

_____ 11. Daptomycin

Column II

a. Macrolides

b. Lincosamides

c. Ketolides

d. Lipopeptides

e. Tetracyclines

f. Glycylcyclines

g. Aminoglycosides

h. Fluoroquinolones

NCLEX Review Questions

Select the best response.

12. Which fluoroquinolone order will the nurse question?
    a. Levofloxacin 750 mg IV q day
    b. Ofloxacin 300 mg PO q12h
    c. Moxifloxacin 400 mg PO q day
    d. Norfloxacin 400 mg PO b.i.d.

13. What is the usual oral dose of a short-acting tetracycline?
    a. 250 mg q6h
    b. 500 mg q6h
    c. 750 mg q6h
    d. 1000 mg q6h

14. Which laboratory test is influenced by tetracycline?
    a. White blood count
    b. Serum calcium level
    c. Blood urea nitrogen
    d. Serum potassium levels

15. The patient has been prescribed doxycycline. What statement(s) by the patient indicate(s) that the nurse needs to provide more discharge teaching? *(Select all that apply.)*
    a. "It is best if I take this with meals."
    b. "I should drink extra milk."
    c. "I have to take this medicine on an empty stomach."
    d. "I should wait a half-hour after meals to take the medication."
    e. "I cannot eat eggs when I take this medication."

16. What will the nurse include in the teaching for a patient taking tetracycline for a respiratory tract infection? *(Select all that apply.)*
    a. Outdated tetracycline breaks down into toxic by-products and must be discarded.
    b. Observe for superinfection like vaginitis or gastritis.
    c. Avoid tetracycline during first and third trimesters of pregnancy.
    d. Anticipate urinary urgency.
    e. Wear sunscreen and limit outdoor exposure during peak daylight hours.

17. The nurse assesses a patient who is taking gentamicin (Garamycin). What assessment finding(s) should be cause for serious concern? *(Select all that apply.)*
    a. Nausea
    b. Ototoxicity
    c. Headache
    d. Photosensitivity
    e. Thrombocytopenia

18. Which drug(s), if prescribed for a patient taking doxycycline (Vibramycin), will the nurse question? *(Select all that apply.)*
    a. Prenatal vitamins
    b. Antacids
    c. Warfarin
    d. Morphine
    e. Omeprazole

19. Which specific nursing intervention(s) should be implemented for a patient taking doxycycline for chlamydia? *(Select all that apply.)*
    a. Restricting fluids
    b. Storing the drug away from light
    c. Ordering renal and liver profiles
    d. Obtaining a specimen for culture and sensitivity
    e. Advising the patient to use additional contraceptives when taking this drug

20. The patient is taking gentamicin (Garamycin) for a postsurgical infection, and the nurse needs to draw a peak level. The patient takes the medication at 0900 and at 2100. When is the correct time to draw a drug peak level?
    a. 0930
    b. 1000
    c. 2045
    d. 2130

21. The trough level that the nurse drew for a patient taking gentamicin (Garamycin) is 3.5 mcg/mL. What is the best action by the nurse?
    a. Administer the medication at the correct time.
    b. Hold the medication and contact the health care provider.
    c. Repeat the trough level after the next dose of medication.
    d. Give the patient Benadryl to decrease the risk of a reaction.

22. The patient tells the nurse that she has developed vaginal discharge since she began taking gentamicin (Garamycin). What does the nurse suspect may be occurring?
    a. The patient has been exposed to other infectious agents.
    b. The patient is experiencing an allergic reaction.
    c. A superinfection has developed.
    d. A drug-drug interaction is taking place.

23. The nurse is doing a morning assessment on a 65-year-old patient who is receiving vancomycin. The patient states that her ears have been ringing all night. What does the nurse know about vancomycin and ringing in the ears?
    a. Only low-pitched sounds are affected by vancomycin.
    b. Tinnitus is a sign of vancomycin allergy.
    c. Ototoxicity is caused by damage to cranial nerve VIII.
    d. Only female patients have ringing in their ears.

24. The nurse is noting the intake and output for a 70-year-old patient receiving vancomycin and sees that the patient's urine output has decreased to 500 mL/day. What is the best action by the nurse?
    a. Increase the patient's oral fluid intake.
    b. Increase the patient's IV rate.
    c. Contact the health care provider.
    d. Document this in the patient's chart.

25. What will the nurse routinely monitor in a 65-year-old patient taking amikacin (Amikin)? *(Select all that apply.)*
    a. Color of sclera
    b. Color and clarity of urine
    c. AST/ALT
    d. Blood glucose
    e. Visual acuity

26. The patient has been prescribed azithromycin (Zithromax) for an upper respiratory infection. What statement by the patient indicates understanding of side effects of the medication?
   a. "I need to stay out of the sun or wear sunscreen."
   b. "I have to take it on an empty stomach to prevent nausea."
   c. "If my eyes get red and itchy, I shouldn't wear my contacts."
   d. "I cannot take anything for pain if I get a headache."

Case Study

Read the scenario and answer the following questions on a separate sheet of paper.

A.B., a 24-year-old woman with medical history of asthma, migraines, and seizure disorder comes to the health care provider complaining of a productive cough, fever, and flulike symptoms. Her sputum culture is positive for *Pseudomonas aeruginosa*. Levofloxacin 500 mg/d for 10 days has been prescribed.

1. To which drug class does levofloxacin belong, and what is the mechanism of action?

2. What side effects should the nurse educate the patient about?

3. What adverse reactions are associated with this medication?

4. Are there any precautions regarding levofloxacin for this patient?

31 Sulfonamides

Study Questions

Complete the following word search. Clues are given in questions 1-8. Circle your responses.

```
W J Q I O K D N F A B U L H N R Q
W D P E N I C I L L I N O K R H K
B L R Y E D R M C P S D D O V P A
L K C O V N V E E A U L G Y Q N M
M C R C C E R M V F C L J M E C T
P A A N Y Y I U A I F I U S Q X Y
V X B J D S S C D C L F L S K K E
E Q A R G I N C R E A S E O N W S
B Q A R E N O T L Q V U Z D F D L
Y N C I T A T S O I R E T C A B E
R T R I M E T H O P R I M C J C F
```

1. Sulfonamides inhibit bacterial synthesis of _____.

2. Clinical use of sulfonamides has decreased because of the availability and effectiveness of _____.

3. The antibacterial drug that has a synergistic effect with sulfonamides is _____.

4. Sulfonamides (are/are not) effective against viruses and fungi. *(Circle correct answer.)*

5. Anaphylaxis (is/is not) common with the use of sulfonamides. *(Circle correct answer.)*

6. Sulfonamide drugs are metabolized in the _____ and excreted by the _____.

7. Sulfonamides are (bacteriostatic/bactericidal). *(Circle correct answer.)*

8. The use of warfarin with sulfonamides (increases/decreases) the anticoagulant effect. *(Circle correct answer.)*

Match the drug in Column I with its duration of action in Column II. Answers may be used more than once.

Column I

____ 9. Sulfamethoxazole

____ 10. Sulfasalazine

____ 11. Sulfadiazine

Column II

a. Short-acting
b. Intermediate-acting

NCLEX Review Questions

Select the best response.

12. The patient has sustained partial-thickness and full-thickness burns over 20% of his body in a house fire. Which medication would be useful for treatment?
    a. Sulfadiazine (Microsulfon)
    b. Sulfasalazine (Azulfidine)
    c. Sulfacetamide sodium (Cetamide)
    d. Silver sulfadiazine (Silvadene)

13. Sulfacetamide solution may be prescribed to treat conjunctivitis caused by which organism?
    a. *Escherichia coli*
    b. *Serratia marcescens*
    c. *Pseudomonas aeruginosa*
    d. *Neisseria meningitidis*

14. The patient has her first postnatal visit with her obstetrician. She is complaining of frequency and burning on urination. She has been diagnosed with a urinary tract infection (UTI) and is started on TMP-SMZ. What important question(s) should the nurse ask when teaching the patient? *(Select all that apply.)*
    a. "What kind of juice do you like to drink?"
    b. "Are you breastfeeding?"
    c. "Are you allergic to any medications?"
    d. "Do you have a history of kidney stones?"
    e. "What medications do you take regularly?"

15. What intervention(s) should the nurse implement in a 50-year-old patient with bronchitis who is receiving TMP-SMZ and lisinopril (Zestril)? *(Select all that apply.)*
    a. Encourage fluids.
    b. Monitor urinary output.
    c. Observe for undesired side effects.
    d. Assess lung sounds.
    e. Administer laxatives.

16. What is the usual adult dose of TMP-SMZ?
    a. 160 mg TMP/800 mg SMZ q6h
    b. 160 mg TMP/800 mg SMZ q12h
    c. 40 mg TMP/60 mg SMZ q6h
    d. 40 mg TMP/60 mg SMZ q12h

17. Why aren't sulfonamides classified as antibiotics?
    a. They do not inhibit cell wall growth.
    b. They are only bacteriostatic, not bactericidal.
    c. They were not obtained from biological sources.
    d. They are only effective against viruses and fungi.

18. The patient has been started on TMP-SMZ for otitis. What side effect will the nurse advise the patient about?
    a. Confusion
    b. Constipation
    c. Fever
    d. Insomnia

19. The 28-year-old patient is taking sulfasalazine (Azulfadine) for Crohn's disease. What is the maintenance dose?
    a. 500 mg q6h
    b. 1000 mg q6h
    c. 1250 mg per day
    d. 1500 mg per day

Case Study

Read the scenario and answer the following questions on a separate sheet of paper.

D.T., 72 years old, presents to the emergency department from a long-term acute care facility (LTAC) with complaints of fever, shaking chills, flank pain, and burning on urination. Vital signs are temperature 39° C, heart rate 94 beats/min, respiratory rate 16 breaths/min, and blood pressure 102/70 mm Hg. D.T. weighs 70 kg. His medical history is positive for adult-onset diabetes and cerebrovascular accident with residual left-sided weakness. His current medications include glyburide, warfarin, and a daily multivitamin. He is allergic to all cephalosporins.

He is been diagnosed with an *E. coli* urinary tract infection and he is admitted to the medical-surgical unit. Orders are received for IV trimethoprim-sulfamethoxazole (Bactrim).

1. What is the mechanism of action and standard dosage range for Bactrim?

2. What will the nurse discuss with the patient and his family regarding the plan of care as it relates to Bactrim?

3. What adverse reactions will the nurse monitor for?

32 Antituberculars, Antifungals, Peptides, and Metronidazole

Study Questions

Crossword puzzle: Use the definitions to determine the correct terms.

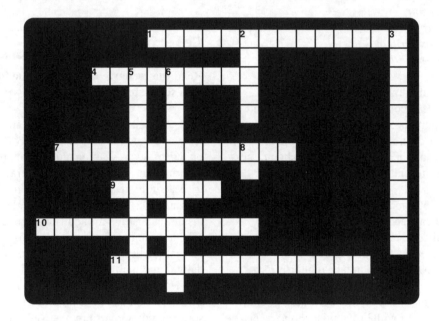

Across

1. Type of drugs that is more effective and less toxic than other drugs (3 words)
4. Drug of choice to prevent disseminated *Mycobacterium avium* complex
7. Drug of choice for severe systemic fungal infections (2 words)
9. One body area where fungi are normal flora
10. Bacitracin is effective against most bacteria (2 words)
11. Liver toxicity

Down

2. Target area for systemic fungal infections
3. First drug prescribed for tuberculosis
5. Common oral antifungal
6. Action of polymyxins
8. Preferred route for administration of polymyxins

Match the drug in Column I with its type in Column II. Answers may be used more than once.

Column I

___ 12. Ethambutol

___ 13. Pyrazinamide

___ 14. Capreomycin

___ 15. Isoniazid

___ 16. Streptomycin

___ 17. Aminosalicylate

___ 18. Ethionamide

___ 19. Amikacin

___ 20. Rifapentine

Column II

a. First-line drug

b. Second-line drug

NCLEX Review Questions

Select the best response.

21. Which outcome is a serious adverse effect of isoniazid?
     a. Crystalluria
     b. Hepatotoxicity
     c. Ototoxicity
     d. Palpitations

22. Which person should not receive prophylactic treatment for tuberculosis with isoniazid?
     a. 29-year-old concurrently taking theophylline
     b. 46-year-old with alcoholism
     c. 57-year-old taking warfarin
     d. 65-year-old with parkinsonism

23. The patient has just started taking rifapentine. The nurse knows that this medication will be taken how often?
     a. Twice per day
     b. Daily
     c. Twice per week
     d. Every other day

24. The patient is taking capreomycin in combination with another antitubercular. Which food(s) will the nurse encourage the patient to include in his diet to prevent peripheral neuropathy? *(Select all that apply.)*
     a. Apples
     b. Bran
     c. Pistachios
     d. Baked potatoes
     e. Tuna

25. The patient is immunocompromised and has recently been diagnosed with histoplasmosis. The patient has been started on ketoconazole. Which herbal preparation taken by the patient is of concern?
     a. Echinacea
     b. *Ginkgo biloba*
     c. Peppermint
     d. St. John's wort

26. During the admission interview, which information will the nurse seek to obtain from a 69-year-old patient taking isoniazid? *(Select all that apply.)*
     a. Blood glucose level
     b. Drug allergies
     c. History of TB exposure
     d. History of IV drug abuse
     e. Date of last purified protein derivative (PPD) and chest x-ray

27. The 28-year-old patient has been diagnosed with active TB. The patient weighs 80 kg. What is the initial dose of INH?
     a. 2 mg/kg/day for 2 months then 7 mg/kg/day for 6 months
     b. 5 mg/kg/day for 2 months then 15 mg/kg/day for 6 months
     c. 7.5 mg/kg/day for 2 months then 20 mg/kg/day for 6 months
     d. 10 mg/kg/day for 2 months then 25 mg/kg/day for 6 months

28. Why is it important to monitor liver function tests in a patient who is taking INH?
    a. INH is excreted by the liver.
    b. INH causes liver cancer.
    c. INH can be hepatotoxic.
    d. INH cannot be metabolized by patients who have liver disease.

29. The patient has just been prescribed INH for active tuberculosis. Which medication taken by the patient would be of concern to the nurse?
    a. Cetirizine
    b. Lisinopril
    c. Maalox
    d. Metformin

30. What priority health teaching should the nurse include for the patient who has just started a course of INH? *(Select all that apply.)*
    a. The patient may need to take vitamin B$_6$ supplements.
    b. Alcohol should be avoided.
    c. Fluid intake should be restricted.
    d. Body fluids including urine and tears may turn a brownish-orange color.
    e. Daily weights should be monitored.

31. How should rifampin be taken to decrease the incidence of resistance?
    a. Daily
    b. In conjunction with another antitubercular drug
    c. Once a week
    d. Only if patient is symptomatic

32. An immunocompromised patient has aspergillosis and has been prescribed amphotericin B. How is this medication administered?
    a. IM
    b. IV
    c. Orally
    d. Rectally

33. The 40-year-old patient has coccidioidomycosis and is in the intensive care unit. He has been prescribed amphotericin B and the nurse is preparing his first dose. He weighs 75 kg. What would be the standard dose of this medication?
    a. 10 mg in 500 mL of D$_5$W to infuse over 2-6 hours
    b. 50 mg in 500 mL of D$_5$W to infuse over 2-6 hours
    c. 100 mg in 500 mL of D$_5$W to infuse over 2-6 hours
    d. 250 mg in 500 mL of D$_5$W to infuse over 2-6 hours

34. The patient is being treated with amphotericin B for histoplasmosis. What statement by the patient would be concerning to the nurse?
    a. "I know I can only get this medicine by having an IV."
    b. "This medication may make me feel flushed."
    c. "I should not eat for 12 hours before receiving the medication."
    d. "I should let my health care provider know if I am not urinating as much."

35. The patient has been prescribed amphotericin B. What priority information should be part of the teaching plan for this patient? *(Select all that apply.)*
    a. Avoid operating hazardous machinery.
    b. Do not consume any alcohol.
    c. Follow up with health care provider as scheduled.
    d. Obtain laboratory testing as ordered.
    e. Report any weakness, fever, or chills.

36. Metronidazole is primarily used for treatment of disorders caused by organisms in which area of the body?
    a. Gastrointestinal tract
    b. Peripheral nervous system
    c. Respiratory tract
    d. Urinary tract

37. In combination with other agents, metronidazole is commonly used to treat *Helicobacter pylori* associated with which disease process?
    a. Adenomas
    b. Gastroesophageal reflux disease (GERD)
    c. Peptic ulcers
    d. Urinary retention

38. Which symptom(s) will the nurse advise the patient taking metronidazole to report to the health care provider? *(Select all that apply.)*
    a. Abdominal cramps
    b. Diarrhea
    c. Headache
    d. Photophobia
    e. Urinary urgency

39. Available:

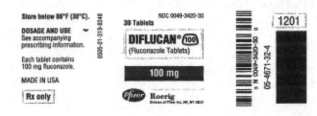

The patient's prescription is for a maintenance dose of fluconazole (Diflucan), 150 mg/day. How many tablets should the patient take per dose?
a. 1 tablet
b. 1.5 tablets
c. 2 tablets
d. 2.5 tablets

40. Which laboratory value(s) must be frequently monitored in the patient taking fluconazole? *(Select all that apply.)*
a. AST
b. ALT
c. BUN
d. Glucose
e. Potassium
f. PT

Case Study

Read the scenario and answer the following questions on a separate sheet of paper.

C.J., 22 years old, has presented to the clinic complaining of "white spots in my mouth." She has been taking multiple antibiotics during the past month for a severe lower respiratory tract infection. Nystatin (Mycostatin) is ordered, 500,000 units oral swish and swallow t.i.d.

1. What questions should the nurse ask in the assessment?

2. What is the likely source of the patient's symptoms?

3. What specific instructions will the nurse include in health teaching regarding nystatin?

33 Antivirals, Antimalarials, and Anthelmintics

Study Questions

Match the term in Column I with the appropriate definition in Column II.

Column I

_____ 1. Tissue phase

_____ 2. Erythrocyte phase

_____ 3. Prophylaxis

_____ 4. Helminthiasis

_____ 5. Opportunistic infection

Column II

a. Prevention
b. Worm infestation
c. Invasion of the body
d. Infections in an immunocompromised patient
e. Invasion of the blood cells

NCLEX Review Questions

Select the best response.

6. The patient has received an organ transplant and is being treated with ganciclovir (Cytovene). Which finding does the nurse know is a serious adverse reaction to this medication?
    a. Electrocardiogram changes
    b. Granulocytosis
    c. Ototoxicity
    d. Thrombocytopenia

7. Which is the most common site for helminthiasis?
    a. Blood
    b. Intestines
    c. Liver
    d. Urinary tract

8. The patient is receiving treatment for herpes simplex 1. Acyclovir sodium 400 mg t.i.d. is prescribed. How many milligrams will the patient have taken at the end of a 24-hour period?
    a. 800 mg
    b. 1200 mg
    c. 1600 mg
    d. 2000 mg

9. The 48-year-old patient is scheduled to receive a dose of acyclovir. Which medication on the medication administration record will concern the nurse?
    a. Amantadine
    b. Flucytosine
    c. Gentamicin
    d. Primaquine

10. The patient works as a paramedic and has a "cold sore" caused by HSV-1. What health teaching does the nurse provide to the patient regarding his treatment?
    a. "Wear sunscreen when you are outside due to photosensitivity."
    b. "You will not be able to work as a paramedic again since you have HSV-1."
    c. "You will need to take the famciclovir 125 mg twice per day for 5 days."
    d. "Your medication must be taken on an empty stomach."

11. The 61-year-old patient is taking ganciclovir (Cytovene) for an active cytomegalovirus (CMV) infection. What baseline laboratory test(s) does the nurse anticipate will be ordered? *(Select all that apply.)*
    a. Bilirubin
    b. Blood glucose
    c. BUN and creatinine
    d. Electrolytes
    e. INR

12. What is the causative agent for malaria?
    a. Bacterium
    b. Fungus
    c. Protozoan
    d. Virus

13. The patient has recently returned from an archeology dig in Belize. She presents to the emergency department with complaints of fever, chills, and body aches. She has been diagnosed with malaria. What medication does the nurse anticipate she may be prescribed?
    a. Acyclovir (Zovirax)
    b. Chloroquine HCl (Aralen)
    c. Delavirdine (Rescriptor)
    d. Tobramycin

14. Which laboratory value(s) is/are affected by chloroquine (Aralen) usage? *(Select all that apply.)*
    a. Creatinine
    b. Glucose
    c. Hemoglobin
    d. Hematocrit
    e. Red blood cell count
    f. Aspartate aminotransferase (AST)

15. The patient is planning a mission trip to Haiti, and her health care provider has prescribed chloroquine as prophylaxis for malaria. What statement by the patient indicates the need for more health education by the nurse?
    a. "I may have some abdominal cramping and nausea."
    b. "I only need to take my medication before my trip."
    c. "If my ears start ringing, I should contact my health care provider."
    d. "I should avoid taking any antacid while I am taking this medicine."

16. The patient has been diagnosed with malaria and has been treated with chloroquine (Aralen). He returns to his health care provider after he has finished his medication and states, "I still feel awful. This isn't getting any better." Vital signs are temperature 40.3° C, heart rate 120 beats/min, respiratory rate 22 breaths/min, blood pressure 138/82 mm Hg, and oxygen saturation 99%. What does the nurse anticipate the next treatment will be?
    a. Continue 5 more days of chloroquine (Aralen).
    b. Change medication to artemether/lumefantrine (Coartem).
    c. Start thiabendazole.
    d. Start zidovudine (Retrovir).

17. What priority(ies) should be included in the patient teaching for anthelmintics? *(Select all that apply.)*
    a. Bathing in hot water instead of showering
    b. Changing clothing, linen, and towels daily
    c. Taking the medicine on an empty stomach to aid in absorption
    d. The importance of hand hygiene
    e. Cook all foods containing pork thoroughly

18. The 18-year-old patient has been diagnosed with cysticercosis, which is caused by pork tapeworm. He is being treated with praziquantel (Biltricide). Which possible side effect(s) should the nurse teach the patient about? *(Select all that apply.)*
    a. Blurred vision
    b. Difficulty hearing
    c. Dizziness
    d. Headache
    e. Weakness

19. The patient, who is 80 years old, has been diagnosed with shingles. What illness in the patient's medical history will support this diagnosis?
    a. AIDS
    b. Chicken pox
    c. Measles
    d. Mumps
    e. Strep throat

Case Study

Read the scenario and answer the following questions on a separate sheet of paper.

J.C., 25 years old, has been diagnosed with the flu.

1. What is "the flu"?

2. How is it diagnosed and treated?

34 Drugs for Urinary Tract Disorders

Study Questions

Crossword puzzle: Use the definitions to determine the correct terms.

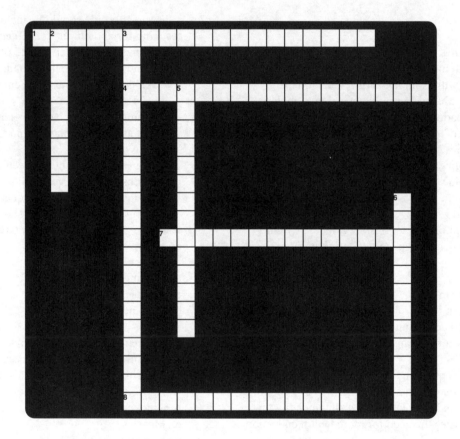

Across
1. A severe upper urinary tract infection (UTI) (2 words)
4. Agents that increase muscle tone of urinary muscles (2 words)
7. Drugs that inhibit the growth of bacteria
8. A severe lower UTI (2 words)

Down
2. Juice that decreases urine pH
3. Bacteria that cannot be treated with nitrofurantoin (2 words)
5. Stains teeth
6. Drug that kills bacteria

NCLEX Review Questions

Select the best response.

9. What may occur when methenamine (Hiprex) is given with sulfonamide?
   a. Bleeding
   b. Chest pain
   c. Crystalluria
   d. Intestinal distention

10. The patient has a urinary tract infection and has been advised to increase her fluid intake and decrease her urine pH. What information would the nurse include in discharge teaching to help the patient meet this goal?
    a. "Drinking whole milk will help."
    b. "Cranberry juice will help acidify the urine."
    c. "Be sure to drink 12-14 8-oz glasses of water per day."
    d. "Drink prune juice four times per day to make urine alkaline."

11. A 72-year-old patient has been prescribed flavoxate (Urispas) for urinary spasms. Which diagnosis in the patient's medical history would be of concern to the nurse?
    a. Dementia
    b. Glaucoma
    c. Hypoglycemia
    d. Migraines

12. The nurse is planning health teaching for a patient receiving nalidixic acid (NegGram) for chronic urinary tract infection. What information should be included? *(Select all that apply.)*
    a. Urine may turn orange.
    b. Photosensitivity may occur.
    c. Increase your fluid intake.
    d. This drug may cause drowsiness.
    e. Take the medication on an empty stomach.

13. The patient will be receiving ertapenem (Invanz) to prevent recurring UTIs. Which side effect(s) will the nurse include in patient teaching? *(Select all that apply.)*
    a. Visual disturbances
    b. Back pain
    c. Diarrhea
    d. Headache
    e. Nausea

14. Which is/are urinary antiseptic drug-drug interaction(s)? *(Select all that apply.)*
    a. Trimethoprim can be combined with sulfamethoxazole.
    b. Antacids increase absorption of ciprofloxacin (Cipro).
    c. Sodium bicarbonate inhibits the action of methenamine (Hiprex).
    d. Nalidixic acid (NegGram) inhibits the effects of warfarin (Coumadin).
    e. Nitrofurantoin (Macrodantin) should not be taken with probenecid.

15. The patient is being discharged from the emergency department after being diagnosed with a UTI. She has been prescribed nitrofurantoin (Macrodantin), 100 mg q.i.d. with meals and at bedtime. The nurse will advise the patient to contact her health care provider immediately if she experiences which side effect?
    a. Brown urine
    b. Frequency in urination
    c. Diarrhea
    d. Swelling around eyes and lips

16. For which condition(s) would the nurse expect to see urinary analgesics prescribed? *(Select all that apply.)*
    a. Burning sensation
    b. Frequency
    c. Hesitation
    d. Retention
    e. Urgency

17. Which drug is commonly prescribed as a urinary analgesic?
    a. Bethanechol (Urecholine)
    b. Flavoxate (Urispas)
    c. Phenazopyridine hydrochloride (Pyridium)
    d. Trimethoprim (Trimpex)

18. The patient has been prescribed an antibiotic and a common urinary analgesic for a UTI. She calls the clinic and is very concerned that her urine has turned bright orange. After reviewing the patient's chart and her medications, what will the nurse tell the patient?
    a. "If you do not take the antibiotic with food in your stomach, your urine will turn orange."
    b. "Inadequate liquid intake will cause your urine to turn bright orange."
    c. "This is an indication of an allergic reaction. You need to come back to the clinic."
    d. "Bright reddish-orange urine is to be expected when taking phenazopyridine."

19. What drug is commonly used to treat urinary tract spasms?
    a. Bethanechol (Urecholine)
    b. Oxybutynin (Ditropan)
    c. Phenazopyridine (Pyridium)
    d. Trimethoprim (Trimpex)

20. The patient, 68 years old, has a history of environmental allergies, narrow-angle glaucoma, depression, and overactive bladder. Which medication(s) will concern the nurse? *(Select all that apply.)*
    a. Bethanechol (Urecholine)
    b. Dimethyl sulfoxide (DMSO)
    c. Nitrofurantoin (Macrodantin)
    d. Oxybutynin (Ditropan)
    e. Tolterodine tartrate (Detrol)

21. The patient has a UTI and has been prescribed a fluoroquinolone. Which pair of symptoms would cause concern for the nurse?
    a. Chest pain and difficulty breathing
    b. Headache and dizziness
    c. Nausea and diarrhea
    d. Photosensitivity and sunburn

22. Which patient is more likely to benefit from bethanechol chloride (Urecholine)?
    a. A 44-year-old patient with prostatitis
    b. A 53-year-old with paraplegia
    c. A 65-year-old patient with pyelonephritis
    d. A 70-year-old patient with overactive bladder

Case Study

Read the scenario and answer the following questions on a separate sheet of paper.

G.H., 14 years old, sustained an injury to his urinary tract while playing football and has been prescribed oxybutynin chloride (Ditropan) 5 mg b.i.d. for spasms.

1. What is the mechanism of action of oxybutynin?

2. Which patients should not take this medication, and why?

3. What are side effects that can be expected?

4. Are there any dose adjustments that need to be made due to the patient's age?

35 HIV- and AIDS-Related Drugs

Study Questions

Crossword puzzle: Use the definitions to determine the correct terms.

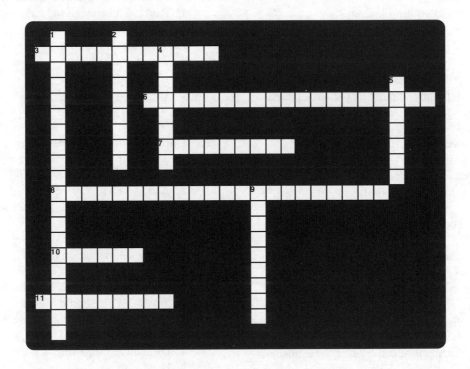

Across

3. Immunity that involves many leukocyte actions, reactions (2 words)
6. Inhibit viral enzyme reverse transcriptase (2 words)
7. The first-choice drug within the NNRTI class
8. Bind to reverse transcriptase and directly inhibit its production (2 words)
10. Genetically determined immunity
11. One of the tests used to determine when to initiate medication therapy in a patient with HIV (2 words)

Down

1. Phase 2 of the HIV replication cycle (2 words)
2. The only nucleotide analogue
4. Immunity that every person's body makes or receives
5. Phase 6 of HIV replication cycle
9. Ability to carry out the therapeutic plan

NCLEX Review Questions

Select the best response.

12. What finding is a leading AIDS indicator?
    a. *Pneumocystis jirovecii* pneumonia
    b. CD4 counts of fewer than 200 cells/mm³
    c. Kaposi's sarcoma
    d. *Mycobacterium avium* complex

13. What is/are the potential benefit(s) of early initiation of antiretroviral therapy in the asymptomatic HIV-infected patient? *(Select all that apply.)*
    a. Control of viral replication
    b. Cure the disease
    c. Decreased risk of drug toxicity
    d. Earlier development of drug resistance
    e. Prevention of progressive immunodeficiency

14. What is/are potential risk(s) of early initiation of antiretroviral therapy in patients with asymptomatic HIV infection? *(Select all that apply.)*
    a. Lower risk of drug-drug interaction
    b. Earlier development of drug resistance
    c. Reduction in quality of life from adverse effects
    d. Severe anaphylactic reaction
    e. Unknown long-term toxicity

15. What is the goal of combination antiretroviral therapy?
    a. Decrease the viral load and decrease the CD4 count
    b. Decrease the CD4 count and increase the viral load
    c. Increase the CD4 count and decrease the viral load
    d. Replace the memory cells within the immune system

16. The decision to treat asymptomatic individuals with detectable HIV RNA in plasma should include which information?
    a. Amount of time since diagnosis
    b. Patient's age and support
    c. Patient's willingness to accept therapy
    d. Probability of adherence to therapy

17. What is the goal of combination therapy [highly active antiretroviral therapy (HAART)]?
    a. To offer a cure to AIDS-diagnosed patients
    b. To offer a cure to pediatric patients
    c. To provide prophylaxis/treatment of major secondary infections
    d. To target enzymes throughout the HIV lifecycle

18. When did zidovudine receive FDA approval?
    a. 1981
    b. 1987
    c. 1994
    d. 1996

19. The patient is scheduled to begin taking zidovudine (Retrovir) 300 mg. How frequently is zidovudine generally scheduled to be taken?
    a. Daily
    b. q12h
    c. q4-6h
    d. q1-3h

20. The patient, 8 weeks old, has been diagnosed with HIV and will be receiving zidovudine. He weighs 4.5 kg. What would the nurse anticipate would be the dose for this patient?
    a. 9 mg/kg/dose b.i.d.
    b. 12 mg/kg/dose b.i.d.
    c. 120 mg/kg/dose b.i.d.
    d. 300 mg/kg/dose b.i.d.

21. During the time that a patient is taking zidovudine (Retrovir), frequent monitoring of which laboratory value(s) is required? *(Select all that apply.)*
    a. ALT/AST
    b. Complete blood count (CBC) with differential
    c. Creatinine
    d. Serum sodium
    e. Urine sedimentation rate

22. The nurse is assessing a patient taking zidovudine (Retrovir). What should the nurse expect to see if the patient is experiencing side effects? *(Select all that apply.)*
    a. Difficulty swallowing
    b. Headache
    c. Numbness and pain in lower extremities
    d. Rash
    e. Seizures

23. In what year did efavirenz (Sustiva) receive FDA approval?
    a. 1987
    b. 1992
    c. 1998
    d. 2000

24. Efavirenz is generally initially scheduled to be taken at which intervals?
    a. 600 mg q6h
    b. 600 mg q8h
    c. 600 mg q12h
    d. 600 mg q24h

25. During the time that a patient is taking efavirenz (Sustiva), periodic monitoring of which laboratory values is required?
    a. BUN/creatinine
    b. CBC and platelets
    c. Electrolytes
    d. Liver panel

26. What will the nurse assess in a patient taking efavirenz (Sustiva) if he appears to be experiencing side effects? *(Select all that apply.)*
    a. Diarrhea
    b. Difficulty swallowing
    c. Dizziness
    d. Rash
    e. Seizures

27. A patient is being discharged on efavirenz (Sustiva). What priority teaching point(s) will the nurse provide to this patient? *(Select all that apply.)*
    a. "Avoid alcohol while taking this drug."
    b. "Be sure to drink 2500 mL of fluid a day."
    c. "Don't take St. John's wort with this drug, as it will decrease its effectiveness."
    d. "This drug can cause convulsions and possibly liver failure."
    e. "Vomiting is a serious adverse reaction to efavirenz."

28. During which year did tenofovir (Viread) receive FDA approval?
    a. 1998
    b. 1999
    c. 2000
    d. 2001

29. What laboratory value(s) is/are high-priority for the nurse to monitor in a patient taking tenofovir (Viread)? *(Select all that apply.)*
    a. Blood glucose
    b. Cholesterol
    c. Liver enzymes
    d. Triglycerides
    e. Potassium

30. The patient is being discharged on tenofovir (Viread). What priority teaching information should this patient receive? *(Select all that apply.)*
    a. "You cannot take St. John's wort while taking this drug."
    b. "You can take this medication with or without food."
    c. "You will need to learn to measure your blood glucose level."
    d. "Side effects may include nausea, vomiting, and diarrhea."
    e. "Do not drive while taking this medication."

31. What is the dose of prophylactic zidovudine for the pregnant patient?
    a. 100 mg five times a day
    b. 200 mg four times a day
    c. 300 mg three times a day
    d. 400 mg two times a day

32. What side effect(s) would the nurse expect to see in a patient taking atazanavir (Reyataz)? *(Select all that apply.)*
    a. Diarrhea
    b. Nausea
    c. Rash
    d. Urinary retention
    e. Vomiting

33. Which nursing intervention(s) may help increase adherence to the therapeutic regimen? *(Select all that apply.)*
    a. Pill organizers
    b. Pill counting
    c. Scheduled pill holidays
    d. Timers/beepers
    e. Wall charts

Case Study

Read the scenario and answer the following questions on a separate sheet of paper.

D.D., 28 years old, works as a registered nurse in the trauma unit. He sustains a needle stick from a patient with HIV.

1. What should the nurse do first?

2. What is involved in postexposure prophylaxis (PEP), and how long does treatment last?

3. What are potential side effects associated with PEP?

36 Vaccines

Study Questions

Crossword puzzle: Use the definitions to determine the correct terms.

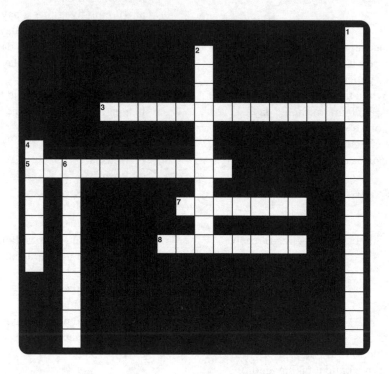

Across

3. Acquisition of detectable levels of antibodies in the bloodstream
5. A potentially life-threatening reaction
7. Transient immunity
8. Bacterium or virus that invades the body

Down

1. Weakened microorganisms (2 words)
2. Vaccines that involve the insertion of some of the genetic material of a pathogen into another cell or organism
4. A small amount of antigen that is administered to stimulate an immune response
6. Also called *immunoglobulins*

NCLEX Review Questions

Select the best response.

9. Which is the term used for vaccines made from the inactivated disease-causing substances produced by some microorganisms?
    a. Attenuated vaccines
    b. Conjugate vaccines
    c. Recombinant subunit vaccines
    d. Toxoids

10. In which situation(s) is acquired passive immunity important? *(Select all that apply.)*
    a. In newborns
    b. When time does not permit active vaccination alone
    c. When the exposed individual is at high risk for complications of the disease
    d. When a woman is pregnant
    e. When a person suffers from an immune system deficiency that renders that person unable to produce an effective immune response

11. What is the process by which antibodies are received by an individual, used for protection against a particular pathogen, and acquired from another source?
    a. Active immunity
    b. Childhood immunity
    c. Passive immunity
    d. Toxoids

12. What occurs when there is an acquisition of detectable levels of antibodies in the bloodstream?
    a. Passive immunity
    b. Acquired natural immunity
    c. Immunization
    d. Seroconversion

13. A mother of a newborn is scheduling her baby's two-month checkup. The nurse advises her that at that time some vaccinations will be given. The mother states, "I'm not really sure I want to have her vaccinated. What do most vaccines really do?" What is the nurse's best response?
    a. "Vaccines are perceived by the body as antibodies."
    b. "Vaccines cause an allergic reaction."
    c. "Vaccines produce a mild form of the disease."
    d. "Vaccines stimulate an immune response."

14. The 45-year-old patient had measles as a child. What is the type of immunity that usually persists for the remainder of the individual's life after being infected with a disease?
    a. Active natural
    b. Humoral
    c. Passive acquired
    d. Passive natural

15. When is a child's first vaccine usually administered?
    a. Birth
    b. 2 months of age
    c. 4 months of age
    d. 6 months of age

16. What is rubella commonly known as?
    a. German measles
    b. Hard measles
    c. Herpes zoster
    d. Smallpox

17. Susceptible individuals age 13 years or older receive two doses of varicella vaccine spaced how long apart?
    a. At least 4 weeks
    b. 3 months
    c. 6 months
    d. 1 year

18. In the event of an adverse reaction to a vaccine, to whom should a health care provider report the details?
    a. Centers for Disease Control and Prevention (CDC)
    b. His or her immediate supervisor
    c. Vaccine Adverse Events Reporting System
    d. Vaccine manufacturer

19. The 68-year-old patient presents to his health care provider for a routine checkup and states, "One of my friends said he was told to get a bunch of shots. I thought we were too old for shots." Which vaccines are administered to adults age 65 years and older?
    a. Tetanus-diphtheria (Td), pneumococcal (PPV), influenza, zoster
    b. Human papillomavirus (HPV), Td, influenza, PPV
    c. Rotavirus, Td, influenza
    d. Tdap, PPV, influenza, zoster

20. Which type of immunity is conferred by the Td vaccine?
    a. Active
    b. Inactive
    c. Natural
    d. Passive

21. Which immunizations are examples of live, attenuated vaccines?
    a. Influenza and hepatitis B
    b. Measles-mumps-rubella (MMR) and *Haemophilus influenzae* type B (Hib)
    c. MMR and varicella
    d. Varicella and Td

22. The patient presents to his health care provider and states, "I think I have the flu." What are the clinical manifestations of influenza?
    a. Abdominal pain, cough, and nasal congestion
    b. Fever, diarrhea, and dizziness
    c. Fever, myalgias, and cough
    d. Vomiting, diarrhea, and headache

23. A physically and medically neglected 15-month-old child has recently been placed in foster care. The foster parents present with this child today for immunization update. They have no idea what, if any, vaccines the child has previously received. What immunizations would the nurse most likely administer?
    a. No vaccines because it is assumed the child is up to date
    b. DTaP #4, Hib #4, and MMR #1
    c. DTaP, Hib, hepatitis A, hepatitis B, MMR, IPV, pneumococcal (PCV), and varicella
    d. DTaP, Hib, hepatitis B, MMR, IPV, PCV, and varicella

24. When the MMR vaccine is not given the same day as the varicella vaccine, what should be the minimum interval between administrations?
    a. 7 days
    b. 14 days
    c. 21 days
    d. 28 days

25. The 4-month-old patient was seen in the emergency department of the local hospital 3 days ago and was diagnosed with a cold and an ear infection. She is taking amoxicillin, an antibiotic, as prescribed for the ear infection and has generally improved. Her immunization record shows that she received hepatitis B vaccine on day 2 of life. At age 2 months, she received hepatitis B, DTaP, Hib, pneumococcal (PCV), rotavirus, and IPV vaccines. If the nurse elected to immunize the patient today, what vaccines should be administered?
    a. Pneumococcal and influenza
    b. Hepatitis B, DTaP, Hib, rotavirus, and IPV
    c. DTaP, Hib, and influenza
    d. DTaP, Hib, pneumococcal (PCV), rotavirus, and IPV

26. A 4-month-old patient's parent reports that after her first dose of DTaP, the patient experienced some redness and tenderness at the injection site in her left thigh. With this in mind, what should the nurse administer?
    a. DTaP again, because these are common side effects, not contraindications
    b. DT in the right thigh
    c. DTaP subcutaneously instead of intramuscularly to prevent muscle soreness
    d. Half the usual dose of DTaP to reduce the likelihood of a reaction

27. After the nurse administers immunizations to a 4-month-old patient, the nurse speaks to the patient's parent about future immunizations. When should the nurse recommend the patient return?
    a. In 2 weeks
    b. At 6 months of age
    c. At 9 months of age
    d. At 12 months of age

28. Before they leave the clinic today, what information should the nurse provide to the parent of a 4-month-old patient who just received her immunizations? *(Select all that apply.)*
    a. Appointment card for the next immunization clinic visit
    b. Immunization record
    c. List of side effects to observe for
    d. Report of adverse reaction form
    e. Vaccine Information Statements (VIS) for all vaccines administered

29. What is a good source of health and immunization information for nurses assisting patients before international travel?
    a. Centers for Disease Control and Prevention
    b. No source is necessary because there are no special immunization needs for travelers
    c. The patient's travel agent
    d. U.S. embassy in the destination country

30. In the case of an anaphylactic reaction to a vaccine, which drug should the nurse have readily available?
    a. Acetaminophen
    b. Diphenhydramine
    c. Epinephrine
    d. Ranitidine

Case Study

Read the scenario and answer the following questions on a separate sheet of paper.

M.E., 62 years old, was working in the garden and stepped on a garden tool. She sustained a deep puncture wound to her right foot. She presents to the clinic with a localized redness and swelling to her foot. She tells the nurse that she takes "only aspirin for my arthritis because I don't really like coming to the doctor much." She has no allergies. She receives an annual influenza vaccine at a local flu shot clinic but has received no other vaccinations in over 20 years. Vital signs are blood pressure 118/80 mm Hg, heart rate 70 beats/min, respiratory rate 16 breaths/min, and temperature 37.8° C oral. M.E. weighs 53 kg.

1. What is the concern for a patient who has sustained a puncture wound?

2. What are signs and symptoms of this disease process?

3. Which vaccines should be administered to the patient at this time?

37 Anticancer Drugs

Study Questions

Match the chemotherapy drugs/terms in Column I with the most appropriate description in Column II. Each answer will be used only once.

Column I

_____ 1. Alkylating agents

_____ 2. Aromatase inhibitors

_____ 3. Cyclophosphamide (Cytoxan)

_____ 4. Doxorubicin (Adriamycin)

_____ 5. Palliative chemotherapy

_____ 6. Fluorouracil (5-FU; Adrucil)

_____ 7. Hormonal agents

_____ 8. Methotrexate (Trexall)

_____ 9. Ways to reduce exposure to chemotherapy

_____ 10. Vincristine (Oncovin)

Column II

a. Associated with hemorrhagic cystitis

b. Leucovorin rescue

c. Stomatitis is early sign of toxicity

d. Associated with cardiotoxicity

e. Associated with neurotoxicity

f. Powder-free gloves, mask, impermeable gown

g. Not true chemotherapy agents

h. Cause cross-linking of DNA strands, abnormal base pairing, or DNA strand breaks

i. Used to relieve symptoms associated with advanced disease

j. Block conversion of androgens to estrogen

NCLEX Review Questions

Select the best response.

11. The nurse is caring for a patient receiving combination chemotherapy. The patient asks why she has to take more than one agent. What is the nurse's best response?
    a. "It has better response rates than single-agent chemotherapy."
    b. "It has fewer side effects than when given alone."
    c. "It is always more effective than surgery or radiation."
    d. "Survival rates are always better."

12. The nurse is teaching a community group about factors that influence the development of cancer in humans. Which information will the nurse include in this teaching?
    a. Aflatoxin is associated with cancer of the lung.
    b. Benzene is associated with cancer of the tongue.
    c. Epstein-Barr virus is associated with cancer of the stomach.
    d. Human papillomavirus is associated with cancer of the cervix.

13. A patient is receiving chemotherapy and asks the nurse about side effects. What should the nurse know concerning the side effects of chemotherapy?
    a. Side effects are minimal because chemotherapy drugs are highly selective.
    b. Side effects usually only occur during the first cycle of treatment.
    c. Side effects are caused by toxicities to normal cells.
    d. Side effects of chemotherapy are usually permanent.

14. The 65-year-old patient has metastatic cancer. He is scheduled to receive to palliative chemotherapy. He states that he does not understand why he should receive palliative chemotherapy if it won't kill the cancer cells. What is the best response?
    a. "It is done to help improve your quality of life."
    b. "It is given to limit further growth of the cancer."
    c. "It is given to slow the growth of the cancer."
    d. "It will shrink the tumors throughout your body."

15. The patient will be receiving chemotherapy that will lower her white blood cell count. Monitoring for which finding will be a nursing priority?
    a. Change in temperature
    b. Evidence of petechiae
    c. Increase in diarrhea
    d. Taste changes

16. The patient has a low platelet count secondary to chemotherapy. Which nursing actions would be the most appropriate?
    a. Apply pressure to injection site and assess for occult bleeding.
    b. Help the patient conserve energy by scheduling care.
    c. Monitor breath sounds and vital signs.
    d. Provide small frequent meals and monitor loss of fluids from diarrhea.

17. The patient has diarrhea secondary to chemotherapy. What important information should be included in patient teaching about chemotherapy-related diarrhea?
    a. Eat only very hot or very cold foods.
    b. Increase intake of fresh fruits and vegetables.
    c. Increase intake of high-fiber foods.
    d. Limit caffeine intake.

18. The 70-year-old patient is to receive cyclophospha-mide (Cytoxan) for treatment of his lymphoma. His medical history is also positive for atrial fibrilla-tion, arthritis, and cataracts. He takes digoxin 0.125 mg daily and naproxen 500 mg at bedtime. What should the nurse be aware of when giving these medications?
    a. Cyclophosphamide increases digoxin levels.
    b. Cyclophosphamide decreases digoxin levels.
    c. Digoxin increases cyclophosphamide levels.
    d. These drugs cannot be given together.

19. The patient is in the outpatient oncology clinic for treatment of her colon cancer. She is receiving fluo-rouracil (5-FU, Adrucil) as part of her treatment and has recently been started on metronidazole (Flagyl) for treatment of trichomoniasis. What should concern the nurse about this order?
    a. 5-FU may decrease the effectiveness of metronidazole.
    b. 5-FU cannot be given with metronidazole.
    c. Metronidazole may increase the side effects of 5-FU.
    d. Metronidazole may increase 5-FU toxicity.

20. The patient, 61 years old, is to receive doxorubicin (Adriamycin) as part of his chemotherapy protocol. Which assessment is the most important before ad-ministering the medication?
    a. Cardiac status
    b. Liver function
    c. Lung sounds
    d. Neurologic status

21. The patient, 69 years old, is receiving cyclophos-phamide (Cytoxan), doxorubicin (Adriamycin), and methotrexate (Trexall) (CAM) for the treatment of prostate cancer. During morning rounds, the patient complains of feeling short of breath. Physical as-sessment reveals crackles in both lungs. What is the most likely cause of this clinical manifestation?
    a. Anxiety
    b. Cyclophosphamide
    c. Doxorubicin
    d. Methotrexate

22. A patient is to receive fluorouracil (5-FU; Adrucil) as part of a treatment protocol for colon cancer. When teaching the patient about this drug, what should the nurse say concerning when the nadir usually occurs in the blood counts?
    a. 1-4 days after administration
    b. 5-9 days after administration
    c. 10-14 days after administration
    d. 15-19 days after administration

23. A patient has reached the nadir of his blood counts secondary to chemotherapy. Which nursing diagnosis is the most appropriate?
    a. Risk for cardiac failure
    b. Risk for dehydration
    c. Risk for infection
    d. Risk for malnutrition

24. Which nursing outcome would be most appropriate as part of the planning for a patient scheduled to receive cyclophosphamide (Cytoxan)?
    a. Patient will be free from symptoms of stomatitis.
    b. Patient will maintain cardiac output.
    c. Patient will show no signs of hemorrhagic cystitis.
    d. Patient will show no signs of syndrome of inappropriate antidiuretic hormone secretion (SIADH).

25. The patient is to receive cyclophosphamide (Cytoxan) as part of her cancer treatment. Which nursing intervention should the nurse expect to complete?
    a. Assess for signs of hematuria, urinary frequency, or dysuria.
    b. Decrease fluids to reduce the risk of calculus formation.
    c. Hydrate the patient with IV fluids only after administration of cyclophosphamide.
    d. Medicate with an antiemetic only after the patient complains of nausea.

26. The nurse is teaching a 29-year-old patient about cyclophosphamide (Cytoxan), which will be given as part of her treatment protocol for cancer. Which priority information should be included in the teaching?
    a. Hair loss has never been reported with the use of cyclophosphamide.
    b. Menstrual irregularities and sterility are not expected with this drug.
    c. No special isolation procedures are needed when receiving this chemotherapy.
    d. Pregnancy should be prevented during treatment with cyclophosphamide.

27. The nurse is administering IV fluorouracil (5-FU; Adrucil) to a patient in the outpatient oncology clinic. Which nursing intervention would be most appropriate?
    a. 5-FU is a vesicant, so assess for tissue necrosis at the IV site.
    b. Apply heat to the IV site if extravasation occurs.
    c. Assess for hyperpigmentation along the vein in which the drug is given.
    d. Encourage mouth rinses once every 8 hours during chemotherapy.

28. A patient receiving cyclophosphamide (Cytoxan), epirubicin (Ellence), and fluorouracil (5-FU; Adrucil) (CEF) has experienced severe nausea, vomiting, and diarrhea over the past week. He has lost 5.5 pounds. Which nursing diagnosis would be most appropriate?
    a. Knowledge deficit related to chemotherapeutic regimen
    b. Pain secondary to diarrhea
    c. Risk for altered nutrition
    d. Risk for infection secondary to low WBC counts

29. The nurse is teaching a patient about doxorubicin (Adriamycin), which she will receive as part of her treatment for breast cancer. Which statement made by the patient indicates that she needs additional teaching?
    a. "Adriamycin is a severe vesicant."
    b. "My blood counts will be checked."
    c. "My cardiac status will be closely monitored."
    d. "This drug may make my urine turn blue."

30. The nurse is administering doxorubicin (Adriamycin) to a patient in the outpatient oncology clinic. What is priority information to include in the patient teaching?
    a. Blood counts will most likely remain normal.
    b. Complete alopecia rarely occurs with this drug.
    c. Report any shortness of breath, palpitations, or edema to your health care provider.
    d. Tissue necrosis usually occurs 2-3 days after administration.

31. The nurse is administering doxorubicin (Adriamycin) to a patient diagnosed with cancer. What should the nurse keep in mind with regard to tissue necrosis associated with this drug?
    a. Tissue necrosis may occur 3-4 weeks after administration.
    b. Tissue necrosis occurs immediately after administration.
    c. Tissue necrosis occurs 2-4 days after administration.
    d. Tissue necrosis rarely occurs with this drug.

32. One week ago in the outpatient oncology clinic, a patient received his first cycle of chemotherapy consisting of cyclophosphamide (Cytoxan), doxorubicin (Adriamycin), and fluorouracil (5-FU; Adrucil) (CAF). He returns to the clinic today for follow-up. Which nursing intervention would be most appropriate at this time?
    a. Culture the IV site and send a specimen to the laboratory for analysis.
    b. Monitor blood counts and laboratory values.
    c. Offer analgesics for pain and evaluate effectiveness.
    d. Teach the patient about good skin care.

33. The nurse is preparing IV vinblastine (Velban), bleomycin (Blenoxane), and cisplatin (Platinol) (VBP) for administration to a patient on the nursing unit. Which precaution should the nurse take when hanging IV chemotherapy?
    a. Wear a clean cotton gown.
    b. Wear shoe covers.
    c. Wear a hair net.
    d. Wear powder-free gloves.

34. A patient is being discharged after receiving IV chemotherapy. Which statement made by the patient indicates a need for additional teaching?
    a. "Chemotherapy is excreted in my bodily fluids."
    b. "I will not need to know how to check my temperature."
    c. "My spouse should wear gloves when emptying my urinal."
    d. "The chemotherapy will remain in my body for 2-3 days."

35. The nurse is preparing to administer chemotherapy, which can cause severe nausea and vomiting, to a patient in the outpatient clinic. Which nursing action would be most appropriate?
    a. Give an antiemetic before administering the chemotherapy.
    b. Withhold any antiemetic drugs until the patient complains of nausea.
    c. Give an antiemetic only after the patient has vomited.
    d. Offer the patient a glass of ginger ale to prevent nausea.

36. A patient is admitted to the hospital 1 week after receiving teniposide (VP-26) in the outpatient oncology clinic. On physical assessment, the nurse notes the presence of petechiae, ecchymoses, and bleeding on the toothbrush when the patient brushes his teeth. Which nursing diagnosis would be most appropriate?
    a. Risk for fatigue
    b. Risk for infection
    c. Risk for bleeding
    d. Risk for falls

37. A patient with breast cancer is scheduled to receive anastrozole (Arimidex), an aromatase inhibitor. Which information should be included in the patient teaching?
    a. Aromatase inhibitors block the peripheral conversion of androgens to estrogens.
    b. Aromatase inhibitors are used to treat tumors that are not hormonally sensitive.
    c. Aromatase inhibitors are used only in premenopausal women with breast cancer.
    d. Aromatase inhibitors are used only in postmenopausal women with breast cancer.

38. A patient is scheduled to receive vincristine (Oncovin) as part of treatment for cancer. The medication record for the patient indicates that he is receiving phenytoin (Dilantin) to control a seizure disorder. What should the nurse monitor for in this patient?
    a. Headaches
    b. Increased blood pressure
    c. Renal failure
    d. Seizures

39. A patient is scheduled to receive vincristine as part of her treatment for non-Hodgkin's lymphoma. She reports that she likes to "rely on nature" for complementary therapy. Which herbal/supplement(s) should be avoided by this patient? *(Select all that apply.)*
    a. Bromelain
    b. Daily multivitamin
    c. Periwinkle
    d. Sheng-Mai-San
    e. Valerian

40. A patient in the outpatient oncology clinic has developed mucositis secondary to cancer therapy. Which statement made by the patient would indicate that she needs additional teaching about mucositis?
    a. "I will rinse my mouth out frequently with normal saline."
    b. "I will try using ice pops or ice chips to help relieve mouth pain."
    c. "I will use a mouthwash that has an alcohol base."
    d. "I will use a soft toothbrush."

41. A patient presents with neutropenia secondary to cancer therapy. Which nursing diagnosis would be the most appropriate?
    a. Risk for cardiac failure
    b. Risk for dehydration
    c. Risk for infection
    d. Risk for malnutrition

Case Study

Read the scenario and answer the following questions on a separate sheet of paper.

C.Z., 25 years old, is being treated for multiple myeloma with cyclophosphamide (Cytoxan).

1. To which class of drugs does cyclophosphamide belong, and how does it work?

2. What are major side effects?

3. What are key factors in the nursing assessment for this patient?

4. What are priority teaching points for this patient with regards to her medication regimen?

38 Targeted Therapies to Treat Cancer

Study Questions

Complete the following word search. Clues are given in questions 1–7. Circle your responses.

```
U S R O T C A F N O I T P I R C S N A R T B
H O Z Q M W P G H G Y G P K L G Q V V J F K
Y S G W X V E A S T R R V N I B P C Y C Q J
S N E U F S G E T O A O Y O B R X D L V M K
P I V S W P M K R H R R W K O J X N M J F Z
B L T Y T Y E X D S W J G T C F Y Y U W A N
R C B U Z Y J J Z E A A E E H Z V A D E V Z
I Y X N L A A K L K G A Y W T F F Y Q D D X
C C E W V V E J Q J S O F S R E A G P J T F
Z N O I T A L Y R O H P S O H P D C U H F Z
U R F J Z S E N M N A N B T Q Q E K T V U J
T B S P A T D E G R A D A T I O N X Z O P R
P C E L L U L A R R E C E P T O R S Y X R U
H M N O I T C U D S N A R T L A N G I S K Y
```

1. The _____ receptors on the cell membrane can activate tyrosine kinases, which then turn on signal transduction pathways promoting cell division.

2. _____ is a method of communication that allows events, conditions, and substances outside of the cell to influence it.

3. Tyrosine kinases are a family of enzymes that activate other substances by adding a phosphate molecule, a process known as _____.

4. _____ for cell division are substances that enter the nucleus and signal the cell that mitosis is needed.

5. _____ are part of a family of proteins that, when active, stimulate the cell to move through the cell cycle.

6. A(n) _____ is a large complex of proteins in cell fluid (cytoplasm) and the cell nucleus that regulates protein expression and the _____ of damaged or old proteins within the cell.

7. _____ therapy for cancer takes advantage of biological features, such as _____, _____, _____, or other molecular proteins of cancer cells that either are not present or are present in much smaller quantities in normal cells.

NCLEX Review Questions

Select the best response.

8. During the first dose of trastuzumab (Herceptin), the patient complains of shortness of breath and pruritus. What is the best action by the nurse?
   a. Decrease the infusion rate by 50% and notify the health care provider.
   b. Disconnect the IV and attach a 0.22-micron filter.
   c. Review the pretreatment multigated acquisition (MUGA) scan.
   d. Stop the infusion and manage the reaction.

9. What is the rationale for administering bevacizumab (Avastin) in a patient with metastatic colon cancer?
   a. To enhance the patient's immune response
   b. To increase apoptosis
   c. To inhibit formation of blood supply
   d. To modulate an inflammatory response

10. Gefitinib (Iressa) most frequently causes which side/adverse effect?
   a. Hypocalcemia
   b. Diarrhea
   c. Myelosuppression
   d. Seizures

11. An oncology patient is to begin treatment for non–small-cell lung cancer (NSCLC) with administration of gefitinib (Iressa). The nurse notes on his medical record that the patient is also taking warfarin daily for atrial fibrillation. What should concern the nurse about the patient taking gefitinib and warfarin?
   a. Gefitinib increases the effects of warfarin.
   b. Gefitinib may require a dose increase when taken with warfarin.
   c. Gefitinib is never given to a patient taking anticoagulants.
   d. Gefitinib may reach toxic levels when given concurrently with warfarin.

12. A patient in the outpatient oncology clinic is receiving sunitinib (Sutent) as part of his treatment for gastrointestinal stromal tumors (GIST). The health care provider prescribes ketoconazole to treat a fungal infection. What should concern the nurse about taking these medications concurrently?
   a. Ketoconazole may decrease the effectiveness of sunitinib.
   b. Ketoconazole may potentiate sunitinib toxicity.
   c. Sunitinib may decrease the effectiveness of ketoconazole.
   d. Sunitinib may lead to toxic levels of ketoconazole.

13. A patient is beginning therapy with the epidermal growth factor/receptor inhibitor (EGFRI) erlotinib (Tarceva) for NSCLC. Which is the most important status for the nurse to assess before beginning therapy with this targeted agent?
   a. Cardiac status
   b. Liver function
   c. Lung sounds
   d. Mental status

14. A patient is admitted to the hospital 1 week after receiving imatinib (Gleevec). On physical assessment, the nurse notes the presence of petechiae, ecchymoses, and bleeding gums. Which nursing diagnosis would be most appropriate?
   a. Risk for bleeding
   b. Risk for falls
   c. Risk for fatigue
   d. Risk for infection

15. Which nursing outcome(s) would be most appropriate as part of the planning for a patient about to begin therapy with the oral multikinase inhibitor (MKI) sorafenib (Nexavar)? *(Select all that apply.)*
   a. Patient will be free from symptoms of stomatitis.
   b. Patient will be free from dizziness.
   c. Patient will maintain adequate fluid balance.
   d. Patient will maintain skin integrity.
   e. Patient will maintain weight.

16. Which nursing outcome(s) would be most appropriate as part of the planning for a patient scheduled to begin treatment with imatinib (Gleevec)? *(Select all that apply.)*
   a. Patient will maintain adequate nutrition and hydration status.
   b. Patient will maintain blood counts in the desired range.
   c. Patient will maintain cardiac output.
   d. Patient will maintain renal function.
   e. Patient will maintain weight.

Case Study

Read the scenario and answer the following questions on a separate sheet of paper.

S.M., 32 years old, has been diagnosed with breast cancer and presents to the outpatient oncology clinic for treatment. She is being treated with bevacizumab (Avastin) for metastatic disease.

1.   How is bevacizumab (Avastin) administered?

2.   What is the mechanism of action?

3.   What are potential side effects?

39 Biologic Response Modifiers

Study Questions

Crossword puzzle: Use the definitions to determine the correct terms.

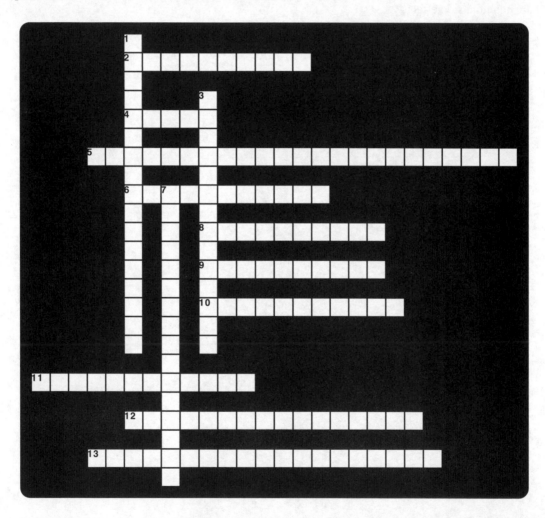

Across

2. Stimulates megakaryocyte and thrombocyte production
4. Lowest value of formed blood cells
5. (% neutrophils + % bands) × (white blood cell [WBC] count)/100,000 (3 words)
6. A family of proteins produced by WBCs when exposed to pathogens
8. Process of adding a polyethylene glycol (PEG) molecule to another molecule
9. A naturally occurring protein that was discovered in the 1950s; it has three major types
10. Destructive to tumor cells
11. Increases the number of macrophages in the body
12. Suppression of bone marrow activity
13. Process that uses mice to mass-produce monoclonal antibodies (2 words)

Down

1. Type of factor that stimulates or regulates the growth, maturation, and differentiation of bone marrow stem cells (2 words)
3. Stimulates red blood cell production in response to hypoxia
7. Condition where there are not enough platelets

Match the description in Column II with the appropriate term in Column I.

Column I

____ 14. Colony-stimulating factors (CSFs)

____ 15. Erythropoietin

____ 16. Granulocyte colony–stimulating factor (G-CSF)

____ 17. Granulocyte-macrophage colony–stimulating factor (GM-CSF)

____ 18. Oprelvekin (Neumega)

Column II

a. Glycoprotein that regulates the production of neutrophils within the bone marrow
b. Proteins that stimulate growth and maturation of bone marrow stem cells
c. Glycoprotein produced by the kidneys in response to hypoxia
d. Supports survival, clonal expression, and differentiation of hematopoietic progenitor cells
e. Indicated for prevention of severe thrombocytopenia

NCLEX Review Questions

Select the best response.

19. What is/are the primary function(s) of biologic response modifiers (BRMs)? *(Select all that apply.)*
    a. To destroy tumor activities
    b. To enhance host immunologic function
    c. To improve liver functioning
    d. To promote differentiation of stem cells
    e. To replicate red blood cells

20. The patient is receiving G-CSF therapy for treatment of severe chronic neutropenia. What is a priority assessment in this patient?
    a. Bone pain
    b. Flulike syndrome
    c. Rash
    d. Urinary retention

21. A patient is receiving GM-CSF therapy. Which system will the nurse focus attention on, both during and after these infusions?
    a. Cardiac system
    b. Central nervous system
    c. Musculoskeletal system
    d. Respiratory system

22. What special preparation and administration guideline(s) will the nurse follow with erythropoietin-stimulating agents? *(Select all that apply.)*
    a. Discard unused portions from the single-dose vial.
    b. Evaluate hemoglobin prior to administration and on a weekly basis.
    c. Multidose vials must be disposed of after 21 days of initial access.
    d. Prevent exposure to light when using Aranesp.
    e. Warm vial to room temperature between doses.

23. A patient is being treated with interferon alpha (Roferon-A) for chronic myelogenous leukemia. What is the dose-limiting side effect?
    a. Chills
    b. Fatigue
    c. Fever
    d. Malaise

24. A 64-year-old patient has hairy cell leukemia that is being treated with interferon alpha (Roferon-A). The patient reports all of the following gastrointestinal side effects. Which side effect is considered the dose-limiting toxicity for the gastrointestinal system?
    a. Anorexia
    b. Diarrhea
    c. Taste alteration
    d. Xerostomia

25. A 70-year-old patient has hairy cell leukemia that is being treated with interferon alpha (Roferon-A). The patient reports neurologic side effects. What will the nurse tell the patient about the side effects?
    a. "These side effects are reversible after the drug is stopped."
    b. "These side effects rarely occur."
    c. "These side effects will diminish as treatment goes on."
    d. "The worst effect is mild confusion."

26. The patient is starting a course of a BRM while undergoing treatment for malignant melanoma. When is the best time to administer a BRM?
    a. At bedtime
    b. 1 hour before meals
    c. 2 hours after meals
    d. With meals

27. What dermatologic effect(s) should the nurse assess for in a patient taking interferon alpha? *(Select all that apply.)*
    a. Alopecia
    b. Bruising
    c. Irritation at injection site
    d. Pruritus
    e. Rash

28. What is priority health teaching information for a 64-year-old patient who has hairy cell leukemia that is being treated with interferon alpha (Roferon-A) and her significant others? *(Select all that apply.)*
    a. Any unusual weight loss should be reported.
    b. Information on the effect of BRM-related fatigue on activities of daily living, including sexual activity
    c. She may return for another demonstration of drug administration techniques.
    d. Side effects from a BRM disappear within 24-48 hours after discontinuation of therapy.
    e. Somnolence, confusion, or problems with concentration should be reported to the health care provider.

29. For which condition(s) may GM-CSF be administered to patients? *(Select all that apply.)*
    a. Absolute neutrophil count > 1500/mm^3
    b. Autologous bone marrow transplant (BMT) recipient
    c. Allogenic BMT recipient
    d. 12 hours after high-dose chemotherapy administration
    e. Kaposi's sarcoma

Case Study

Read the scenario and answer the following questions on a separate sheet of paper.

K.U., 38 years old, has been diagnosed with acute myelogenous leukemia (AML) and will be undergoing treatment. She is scheduled to receive G-CSF and wants to know what this medication will do to cure her cancer. She will be receiving 75 mcg/kg/day IV.

1. What type of medication is G-CSF, and how does it work?

2. What are side effects experienced with this medication?

3. What priority teaching instructions will the nurse provide to the patient and her significant others?

40 Drugs for Upper Respiratory Disorders

Study Questions

Match the term in Column I to the description in Column II.

Column I

_____ 1. Antihistamines

_____ 2. Antitussives

_____ 3. Decongestants

_____ 4. Expectorants

Column II

a. Act on the cough-control center in the medulla

b. Loosen bronchial secretions so they can be removed by coughing

c. H_1 blockers or H_1 antagonists

d. Stimulate the alpha-adrenergic receptors, producing vascular constriction in the nasal capillaries

NCLEX Review Questions

Select the best response.

5. Antihistamines are another group of drugs used for the relief of cold symptoms. What properties of these medications result in decreased secretions?
   a. Analgesic
   b. Anticholinergic
   c. Antitussive
   d. Cholinergic

6. Compared to first-generation antihistamines, second-generation antihistamines have a lower incidence of which side effect?
   a. Drowsiness
   b. Headache
   c. Tinnitus
   d. Vomiting

7. The U.S. Food and Drug Administration has ordered removal of all cold remedies containing which drug?
   a. Dextromethorphan
   b. Guaifenesin
   c. Histamine
   d. Phenylpropanolamine

8. The patient has environmental allergies and asks the student health nurse about the appropriate dose of diphenhydramine. What is the recommended dosage of diphenhydramine (Benadryl)?
   a. 25-50 mg q6-8h
   b. 25-50 mg daily
   c. 50-100 mg q4-6h
   d. 100 mg daily

9. What is one of the effects of diphenhydramine (Benadryl)?
   a. Anticoagulant
   b. Anticonvulsant
   c. Antihypertensive
   d. Antitussive

10. Diphenhydramine blocks histamine receptors. Which histamine receptors does it block?
   a. H_1
   b. H_2
   c. B_1
   d. B_2

11. A patient taking diphenhydramine (Benadryl) breastfeeds her infant daughter. What advice will the nurse give her?
    a. Breastfeeding provides allergy relief to the infant.
    b. Large amounts of the drug pass into breast milk; breastfeeding is not recommended.
    c. Small amounts of the drug pass into breast milk; breastfeeding is not recommended.
    d. The drug does not affect breastfeeding.

12. The health teaching plan for a patient taking diphenhydramine (Benadryl) should include the side effects of the drug. What might the nurse assess in a patient experiencing a side effect? *(Select all that apply.)*
    a. Disturbed coordination
    b. Drowsiness
    c. Hypertension
    d. Nausea
    e. Urinary retention

13. What is the advantage of systemic decongestants over nasal sprays and drops?
    a. Fewer side effects
    b. Less costly
    c. Preferred by older patients
    d. Provide longer relief

14. Which expectorant is frequently an ingredient in cold remedies?
    a. Dextromethorphan
    b. Ephedrine
    c. Guaifenesin
    d. Promethazine

15. The patient presents to the clinic with complaints of nasal congestion, sneezing, and fever for 4 days. She has been diagnosed with a cold. What priority teaching instructions should the nurse include for this patient? *(Select all that apply.)*
    a. Instruct the patient to cover nose and mouth when sneezing.
    b. Advise the patient to discuss use of any herbal remedies with her health care provider.
    c. Encourage the patient to drink adequate fluids.
    d. Nasal sprays can be utilized q2h.
    e. Promote good hand hygiene.

16. What group(s) of drugs is/are used to treat cold symptoms? *(Select all that apply.)*
    a. Antihistamines
    b. Antitussives
    c. Decongestants
    d. Expectorants
    e. Xanthines

17. Decongestants are contraindicated or to be used with extreme caution for patients with which condition(s)? *(Select all that apply.)*
    a. Cardiac disease
    b. Diabetes mellitus
    c. Hypertension
    d. Hyperthyroidism
    e. Obesity

18. Which priority information should be included in teaching a patient who is taking medications for a common cold and also has a history of atrial fibrillation and depression? *(Select all that apply.)*
    a. Administer 4 puffs of nasal spray for a full 10 days.
    b. Antibiotics are also needed to fight a common cold virus.
    c. Do not drive during initial use of a cold remedy containing an antihistamine.
    d. Read labels of over-the-counter drugs for any interactions with current medications.
    e. Take cold remedies with a decongestant for a better night's sleep.

Case Study

Read the scenario and answer the following questions on a separate sheet of paper.

G.H., 53 years old, is preparing to fly across the country for a conference. He presents to his health care provider with nasal stuffiness. He states, "I hate to fly when my nose is this way. It just makes the trip all that much longer." A decongestant, oxymetazoline (Afrin), is ordered.

1. What is the purpose of oxymetazoline, and how does it work?

2. What is the standard dosage for this medication?

3. What is rebound congestion? What other side effects might be expected, and how can they be prevented? Are there any other options for a decongestant?

41 Drugs for Lower Respiratory Disorders

Study Questions

Match the drug in Column I with its category in Column II. Drugs may belong to more than one category.

Column I

_____ 1. Acetylcysteine

_____ 2. Zafirlukast

_____ 3. Albuterol

_____ 4. Dexamethasone

_____ 5. Epinephrine

_____ 6. Arformoterol tartrate

Column II

a. Alpha adrenergic
b. Beta adrenergic
c. Glucocorticoid
d. Mucolytic
e. Leukotriene receptor antagonist

Complete the following.

7. The substance responsible for maintaining bronchodilation is _____.

8. In acute bronchospasm caused by anaphylaxis, the drug administered subcutaneously to promote bronchodilation and elevate the blood pressure is _____.

9. The first line of defense in an acute asthmatic attack are the drugs categorized as _____.

10. Isoproterenol (Isuprel), one of the first drugs to treat bronchospasm, is a (selective/nonselective) beta$_2$ agonist. *(Circle correct answer.)*

11. Sympathomimetics cause dilation of the bronchioles by increasing _____.

12. Theophylline (increases/decreases) the risk of digitalis toxicity. *(Circle correct answer.)*

13. When theophylline and beta$_2$-adrenergic agonists are given together, a(n) _____ effect can occur.

14. The half-life of theophylline is (shorter/longer) for smokers than for nonsmokers. *(Circle correct answer.)*

15. Aminophylline, theophylline, and caffeine are _____ derivatives used to treat _____.

16. The drugs commonly prescribed to treat unresponsive asthma are _____.

17. Cromolyn (Intal) is used as _____ treatment for bronchial asthma. It acts by inhibiting the release of _____.

18.   A serious side effect of cromolyn is _____.

19.   The newer drugs for asthma are more selective for _____ receptors.

20.   The leukotriene receptor antagonist considered safe for use in children 6 years and older is
_____.

21.   The preferred time of day for the administration of leukotriene receptor antagonists is _____.

22.   The usual dose of montelukast (Singulair) for an adult is _____ and for a child is
_____.

23.   A group of drugs used to liquefy and loosen thick mucus secretions is _____.

24.   With infection resulting from retained mucus secretions, a(n) _____ may be prescribed.

NCLEX Review Questions

Select the best response.

25.   The patient is being treated for chronic obstructive
pulmonary disease (COPD). His medication is delivered via a metered-dose inhaler. Related health
teaching would include which priority information?
a. Hold the inhaler upside down.
b. Refrigerate the inhaler.
c. Shake the inhaler well just before use.
d. Test the inhaler each time to see if the spray
works.

26.   When compared to oral medication for asthma,
what information regarding a drug administered by
metered-dose inhaler should the nurse be aware of?
(Select all that apply.)
a. The inhaled dose will be lower than an oral
medication.
b. There are fewer side effects with an inhaled
medication.
c. Inhaled medication is longer-lasting.
d. Inhaled medication has a more rapid onset.
e. Some oral and inhaled medications can be taken
together.

27.   The patient has been prescribed both ipratropium
(Atrovent) and cromolyn (Nasalcrom). How many
minutes should she wait between taking the two
medications?
a. 1
b. 5
c. 10
d. Does not matter

28.   The patient is taking an inhaled beta agonist and a
steroid for his asthma. He states, "I don't have time
to wait between taking medications. I'm very busy.
Why do I have to do this?" What is the nurse's best
response to the patient?
a. "The inhaled medication will allow the bronchioles to dilate so the steroid works better."
b. "This is done so you remember which one
comes first."
c. "The inhaled medication will make your heart
circulate the steroid faster."
d. "The steroid may make your nose stuffy, so you
take the inhaled medication first."

29.   What is/are the side effect(s) of long-term use of
glucocorticoids? *(Select all that apply.)*
a. Impaired immune response
b. Insomnia
c. Hyperglycemia
d. Vomiting
e. Weight loss

30.   What anticholinergic drug has few systemic effects
and is administered by aerosol?
a. Albuterol (Proventil)
b. Ipratropium (Atrovent)
c. Isoproterenol (Isuprel)
d. Tiotropium (Spiriva)

31. Drug selection and dosage in older adults with conditions of the lower respiratory tract need to be considered. The use of large, continuous doses of a beta$_2$-adrenergic agonist may cause which side effect(s) in the older adult? *(Select all that apply.)*
    a. Bronchoconstriction
    b. Constipation
    c. Tachycardia
    d. Tremors
    e. Urinary retention

32. The 40-year-old patient has been taking theophylline for long-term treatment of his asthma. He has also been taking ephedra to stay alert while finishing a project at work. The patient presents to the clinic with complaints of feeling ill. Vital signs are temperature 36.4° C oral, heart rate 124 beats/min, respiratory rate 18 breaths/min, blood pressure 170/90 mm Hg, and oxygen saturation 99% on room air. Fingerstick blood glucose is 210. His theophylline level is 26 mcg/mL. What does the nurse suspect may be the cause of the patient's symptoms?
    a. Acute allergic reaction
    b. Asthma attack
    c. Stevens-Johnson syndrome
    d. Theophylline toxicity

33. The patient has exercise-induced bronchospasm and is being treated with a short-acting beta$_2$ agonist. Which priority information will the nurse include in a review of inhaler administration for this patient? *(Select all that apply.)*
    a. "Cleanse all washable parts of inhaler equipment daily."
    b. "Hold your breath for a few seconds, remove mouthpiece, and exhale slowly."
    c. "Keep your lips secure around the mouthpiece and inhale while pushing the top of the canister once."
    d. "Monitor your heart rate while taking this medication."
    e. "Wait 5 minutes and repeat the procedure if a second inhalation is needed."

34. The 68-year-old patient has been diagnosed with COPD. When providing health teaching for this patient, the nurse discusses the side effects that may occur with the use of bronchodilators. What possible clinical manifestation(s) should the patient be aware of? *(Select all that apply.)*
    a. Bradycardia
    b. Dry eyes
    c. Insomnia
    d. Nervousness
    e. Palpitations

35. Which medication(s) when prescribed with theophylline will concern the nurse? *(Select all that apply.)*
    a. Beta blockers
    b. Digitalis
    c. Lithium
    d. Stool softeners
    e. Phenytoin

36. Which of the following is/are side effect(s) of theophylline? *(Select all that apply.)*
    a. Cardiac dysrhythmias
    b. Diarrhea
    c. Gastrointestinal bleeding
    d. Headache
    e. Seizures

37. The patient has asthma and takes cromolyn (Nasalcrom). What statement by the patient indicates the need for more education?
    a. "I must take this medication every day."
    b. "It will stop an asthma attack that has started."
    c. "I can rinse my mouth out with water to get rid of the taste."
    d. "It is important for me to take this exactly as directed."

38. A patient presents to the health care provider's office for a follow-up visit. The patient is taking theophylline, and the nurse is reviewing the lab results. What level of theophylline would fall in the therapeutic range?
    a. 2 mcg/mL
    b. 8 mcg/mL
    c. 14 mcg/mL
    d. 23 mcg/mL

Case Study

Read the scenario and answer the following questions on a separate sheet of paper.

H.K., 35 years old, has recently been diagnosed with asthma and has been prescribed albuterol (Proventil), montelukast sodium (Singulair), and Advair Diskus 100/50.

1. What classes of drugs do each of these medications belong to? How does each medication work?

2. What are priority teaching points for this patient with a new diagnosis of asthma?

42 Cardiac Glycosides, Antianginals, and Antidysrhythmics

Study Questions

Crossword puzzle: Use the definition to determine the pharmacologic/physiologic term.

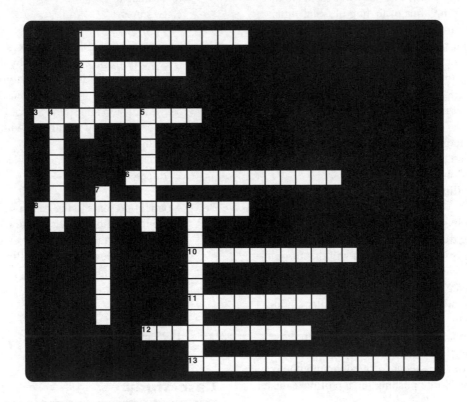

Across

1. Increased carbon dioxide in the blood
2. Amount of blood in the ventricle at the end of diastole
3. Drug category used to treat angina pectoris
6. Return of the myocardium to resting
8. Myocardial contraction
10. Low serum potassium level
11. Peripheral vascular resistance
12. Pulse rate below 60 beats/min
13. Drug group used to treat disturbed heart rhythm

Down

1. Lack of oxygen to body tissues
4. Drug group used to control angina pain by relaxing coronary vessels
5. Lack of blood supply to the (heart) muscle
7. A cardiac _____ causes cardiac muscles to contract more efficiently
9. Pulse rate above 100 beats/min

Complete the following.

14. Heart failure occurs when the myocardium (strengthens/weakens) and (shrinks/enlarges), which causes the heart to lose its ability to pump blood through the heart and circulatory system. *(Circle correct answers.)*

15. With heart failure there is a(n) (increase/decrease) in preload and afterload. *(Circle correct answer.)*

16. Another name for heart failure is _____ failure.

17. Cardiac glycosides are also called _____.

18. The action of antianginal drugs is to increase blood flow and to (increase/decrease) oxygen supply or to (increase/decrease) oxygen demand by the myocardium. *(Circle correct answers.)*

19. Name three of the four effects of digitalis preparations on the heart muscle (myocardium):
   _____, _____, and _____.

20. Beta blockers and calcium channel blockers (decrease/increase) the workload of the heart. *(Circle correct answer.)*

21. Nitroglycerin (NTG) is not swallowed because _____,
   thereby decreasing its effectiveness.

22. NTG sublingually acts within _____ minutes. Administration may be repeated _____ times.

23. The most common side effect of NTG is _____.

24. The drug group that may be used as an antianginal, antidysrhythmic, and antihypertensive is
   _____.

25. A calcium channel blocker that is effective in the long-term treatment of angina and has the side effect of bradycardia is _____.

26. Beta blockers and calcium channel blockers should not be discontinued without health care provider approval. Withdrawal symptoms may include _____ and _____.

27. Classic angina occurs when the patient is _____.

28. Unstable angina (preinfarction) has the following pattern of occurrence: _____
   _____.

29. Variant angina (Prinzmetal's angina) occurs when the patient _____.

30. Prinzmetal's angina is due to _____ of the vessels.

31. The major systemic effect of nitrates is _____.

32. Cardiac dysrhythmias can result from (hypoxia/hyperoxia) and (hypocapnia/hypercapnia). *(Circle correct answers.)*

33. Examples of types of antidysrhythmics include _____, _____, and
   _____.

34. Patients taking antidysrhythmics should avoid _____ and _____.

The nurse should obtain a history of herbs the patient is taking. This is especially true for patients taking digoxin. Match the herbs in Column I with their effects on digoxin in Column II. Answers may be used more than once.

Column I

_____ 35. St. John's wort

_____ 36. Ephedra

_____ 37. Metamucil

_____ 38. Aloe

_____ 39. Goldenseal

_____ 40. Ginseng

Column II

a. Increased risk of digitalis toxicity
b. Decreased digoxin absorption
c. Decreased effects of digoxin
d. Falsely elevated digoxin levels

NCLEX Review Questions

Select the best response.

41. What are digitalis preparations effective for treating?
    a. Asthma
    b. Heart failure (HF)
    c. Thrombophlebitis
    d. Vascular insufficiency

42. Phosphodiesterase inhibitors are used to treat HF by inhibiting phosphodiesterase enzyme. What do these agents promote?
    a. Increased serum sodium and potassium levels
    b. Negative inotropic action
    c. Positive inotropic action
    d. Vasoconstriction

43. What is an example of a phosphodiesterase inhibitor?
    a. Amlodipine
    b. Digoxin
    c. Milrinone
    d. Isosorbide dinitrate

44. The 64-year-old patient has a history of atrial flutter. His health care provider has prescribed quinidine. The patient asks the nurse how this medication will help his heart. What is the nurse's best response?
    a. "It will help your heart pump stronger."
    b. "It will prevent you from having chest pain."
    c. "It will decrease myocardial oxygen consumption."
    d. "It will slow how fast the impulses travel through your heart."

45. What type of drug is propranolol (Inderal)?
    a. Calcium channel blocker
    b. Cardioselective beta blocker
    c. Fast sodium blocker
    d. Nonselective beta blocker

46. The 61-year-old patient is in cardiac arrest. His ventricular fibrillation is refractory to other treatment. What medication is the drug of choice when other agents are ineffective?
    a. Amiodarone (Cordarone)
    b. Atropine
    c. Acebutolol HCl (Sectral)
    d. Propafenone HCl (Rythmol)

47. What is/are the action(s) of antidysrhythmics? *(Select all that apply.)*
    a. Block adrenergic stimulation to the heart
    b. Decrease conduction velocity
    c. Decrease preload
    d. Increase heart rate
    e. Increase force of myocardial contraction

48. What is lidocaine primarily used to treat?
    a. Atrial fibrillation
    b. Bradycardia with premature ventricular contractions (PVCs)
    c. Complete heart block
    d. Ventricular dysrhythmias

49. The patient has been diagnosed with angina and has been prescribed verapamil (Calan). What priority teaching point(s) should the nurse include regarding this medication? *(Select all that apply.)*
    a. "Eat lots of fiber to avoid constipation."
    b. "High blood pressure can be caused by verapamil."
    c. "This medication is taken three times per day."
    d. "Wear sunscreen due to photosensitivity."
    e. "You should not take this medication if you are diabetic."

50. Which is the most potent calcium channel blocker?
    a. Diltiazem (Cardizem)
    b. Nicardipine (Cardene)
    c. Nifedipine (Procardia)
    d. Verapamil (Calan)

51. The patient has been prescribed amlodipine (Norvasc) to help control his hypertension. What laboratory values must be monitored carefully?
    a. Arterial blood gasses
    b. Blood glucose
    c. Complete blood count
    d. Liver enzymes

52. Abnormal atrial natriuretic peptide (ANP) and brain natriuretic peptide (BNP) levels indicate which disease process?
    a. Aneurysm
    b. Cerebrovascular accident
    c. Heart failure
    d. Myocardial infarction

53. An 80-year-old patient is taking digoxin daily along with several other medications. Her BNP is 420 pg/mL. What concerns the nurse about this level?
    a. It is below the normal/reference range for her age.
    b. Nothing. It is within the normal range.
    c. It is slightly elevated.
    d. It is markedly elevated.

54. The patient presents to the emergency department and states he feels dizzy. He takes digitalis but he is unable to tell you why he is taking the medication. The nurse knows that this medication is usually prescribed for what abnormal rhythm?
    a. Atrial fibrillation
    b. Paroxysmal atrial tachycardia
    c. Second-degree heart block
    d. Ventricular tachycardia

55. What is the usual maintenance dose of digoxin?
    a. 0.125-0.5 mg/day
    b. 0.5-1.5 mg/day
    c. 2-5 mg/day
    d. 10-15 mg/day

56. The patient presents to her health care provider's office for a follow-up visit. She has been taking digoxin for approximately 2 weeks. What does the nurse know is a therapeutic digitalis level?
    a. 0.15-0.5 ng/mL
    b. 0.5-2 ng/mL
    c. 2-3.5 ng/mL
    d. 3.5-4 ng/mL

57. The 76-year-old patient has a history of heart failure and is taking digoxin 0.125 mg/day. He calls his health care provider's office with complaints of nausea, dizziness, headache, and a heart rate of 42 beats/min. He states, "I have an appointment in 2 weeks. Is it ok to wait until then?" What is the nurse's best response?
    a. "It is fine to wait until your next appointment."
    b. "You may just have the flu. Stay in bed until you are not dizzy."
    c. "Just take your digoxin every other day."
    d. "You need to be seen either here or the emergency department today."

58. What is the antidote for digitalis toxicity?
    a. Cardizem
    b. Digoxin immune Fab
    c. Gamma globulin
    d. Protamine

59. The nurse is reviewing the patient's medication administration record (MAR). Which medication(s) on the MAR will concern the nurse, given that the patient is taking digitalis? *(Select all that apply.)*
    a. Cortisone
    b. Furosemide
    c. Hydrochlorothiazide
    d. Nitroglycerin
    e. Potassium supplement

60. How often should the pulse be checked for a patient taking digoxin?
    a. Daily before taking dose
    b. Once per week
    c. Only when dosage is changed
    d. Only if the patient has symptoms

61. What parameters should concern the nurse the most in a patient taking digitalis?
    a. Heart rate of 52 beats/min and irregular
    b. Heart rate of 60 beats/min and regular
    c. Heart rate of 88 beats/min and regular
    d. Heart rate of 100 beats/min and irregular

62. The patient has been prescribed digoxin for treatment of heart failure. The nurse is providing health teaching for this patient. With regards to diet, what food(s) should the patient avoid? *(Select all that apply.)*
    a. Apples
    b. Celery
    c. Hot dogs
    d. Lettuce
    e. Potatoes

63. Which drug(s) may be used to treat heart failure? *(Select all that apply.)*
    a. Angiotensin-converting enzyme (ACE) inhibitors
    b. Beta blockers
    c. Calcium channel blockers
    d. Diuretics
    e. Vasodilators

64. What is the most commonly seen side effect a patient may experience when taking nitroglycerin (NTG)?
    a. Dizziness
    b. Headache
    c. Nausea
    d. Weakness

65. What priority health teaching should be given to a patient taking nitroglycerin? *(Select all that apply.)*
    a. Sips of water may be taken to aid in absorption.
    b. Nitroglycerin should be stored in a cool, dark place.
    c. The tablet is to be chewed and swallowed.
    d. Notify your health care provider if chest pain is not relieved after three tablets.
    e. Patients should not take vitamin C supplements while taking nitroglycerin.

66. What is the duration of action of a nitroglycerin patch?
    a. 6-8 hours
    b. 10-12 hours
    c. 20-24 hours
    d. 36-48 hours

67. The patient has been prescribed atenolol (Tenormin) 50 mg/d. What type of drug is this?
    a. Adrenergic stimulant
    b. Beta blocker
    c. Calcium channel blocker
    d. Cardiac glycoside

68. The patient has been prescribed acebutolol (Sectral) for treatment of a ventricular dysrhythmia. What is the proper dose for this medication?
    a. 200 mg q6h
    b. 200 mg q8h
    c. 200 mg q12h
    d. 200 mg q24h

69. What type of drug is acebutolol (Sectral)?
    a. Antianginal
    b. Calcium channel blocker
    c. Cardioselective beta blocker
    d. Fast sodium channel blocker

70. What priority teaching should the nurse provide to a patient who has just started taking acebutolol (Sectral)?
    a. "Do not abruptly stop this medication, or you risk an adverse reaction."
    b. "Drowsiness is a common side effect."
    c. "No laboratory work will be required while taking this medication."
    d. "Fluid intake should be increased to prevent dehydration."

71. What possible side effect(s) should be discussed with a patient who is beginning acebutolol (Sectral)? *(Select all that apply.)*
    a. Diarrhea
    b. Edema
    c. Hypertension
    d. Impotence
    e. Vomiting

72. Which herbal preparation(s) must be avoided when taking digitalis preparations? *(Select all that apply.)*
    a. Aloe
    b. Feverfew
    c. *Ginkgo biloba*
    d. Ginseng
    e. Ma-huang

73. What condition(s) can directly lead to cardiac dysrhythmias? *(Select all that apply.)*
    a. Electrolyte imbalance
    b. Excess catecholamines
    c. Hepatitis
    d. Hypocapnia
    e. Hypoxia

Case Study

Read the scenario and answer the following questions on a separate sheet of paper.

P.E., 43 years old, has a history of hypertension, diet-controlled diabetes, and vasospastic angina. He presents to the emergency department with severe left-sided chest pain, nausea, shortness of breath, and diaphoresis. Vital signs are temperature 36.5° C, heart rate 102 beats/min, respiratory rate 20 breaths/min, blood pressure 164/100 mm Hg, and oxygen saturation on room air of 99%. After administering one sublingual nitroglycerin tablet, his vital signs are heart rate 120 beats/min, respiratory rate 22 breaths/min, and blood pressure 88/60 mm Hg. He feels lightheaded and nauseated, but his pain has not been relieved. A nitroglycerin drip is started, and he is admitted to critical care.

1. What are the three different types of angina?

2. Describe nonpharmacologic and pharmacologic treatments for vasospastic angina.

3. What medications other than nitroglycerin can be used to treat angina?

4. Why did this patient's blood pressure drop?

43 Diuretics

Study Questions

Crossword puzzle: Use the definitions to determine the correct terms.

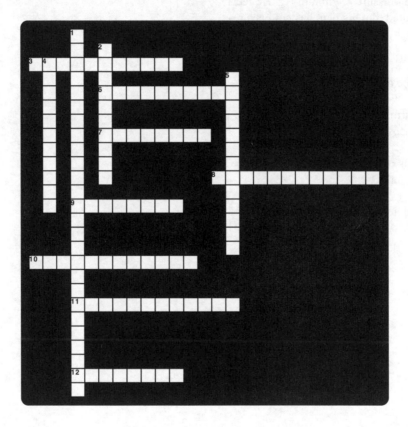

Across

3. Sodium loss in the urine
6. Concentration of body fluids
7. Most frequently prescribed osmotic diuretic
8. Main side effect of potassium-sparing diuretics
9. Increased urine flow
10. One disease for which a health care provider will prescribe diuretics
11. Term for above-normal levels of potassium
12. Term for decreased production of urine

Down

1. Decreases intraocular pressure in patients with glaucoma (3 words)
2. Potassium-wasting diuretic
4. Hormone that affects the body's sodium levels
5. Term for above-normal levels of blood glucose

List the possible abnormal serum chemistry test results associated with thiazide diuretics.

Laboratory Test	Abnormal Results
13. Potassium	
14. Magnesium	
15. Calcium	
16. Chloride	
17. Bicarbonate	
18. Uric acid	
19. Blood sugar	
20. Blood lipids	

NCLEX Review Questions

Select the best response.

21. Which group(s) of diuretics is/are frequently prescribed to treat hypertension and congestive heart failure? *(Select all that apply.)*
    a. Carbonic anhydrase inhibitors
    b. Loop diuretics
    c. Osmotic diuretics
    d. Potassium-sparing diuretics
    e. Thiazide diuretics

22. When compared with thiazides, how do loop (high-ceiling) diuretics differ?
    a. They are more effective as antihypertensives.
    b. They promote potassium absorption.
    c. They cause calcium reabsorption.
    d. They are more potent as diuretics.

23. The patient has been prescribed hydrochlorothiazide (HCTZ) for her hypertension. When she comes to the office for a follow-up appointment, the nurse observes her drinking an energy drink. Which herb, commonly found in some energy drinks, can increase blood pressure when taken with thiazide diuretics?
    a. Ginger
    b. Ginkgo
    c. Licorice
    d. St. John's wort

24. What is the pharmacologic action of spironolactone (Aldactone)?
    a. Increase potassium and sodium excretion
    b. Promote potassium retention and sodium excretion
    c. Promote potassium, sodium, and calcium retention
    d. Promote potassium excretion and sodium retention

25. What is the classification of furosemide (Lasix)?
    a. Loop diuretic
    b. Osmotic diuretic
    c. Potassium-sparing diuretic
    d. Thiazide diuretic

26. The 65-year-old patient had an acute myocardial infarction 6 months ago and has been prescribed spironolactone (Aldactone) 100 mg/d to treat an irregular heart rate. What statement by the patient indicates that he understands the medication teaching the nurse has provided?
    a. "I need sodium so my heart beats regularly."
    b. "This medication is dangerous if you have had a heart attack."
    c. "It helps keep potassium so my heart is not irregular."
    d. "I need to take it with lots of bananas to keep my potassium up."

27. The nurse has received an order to administer 40 mg furosemide (Lasix) IV to the patient. What does the nurse know about how this medication should be administered?
    a. It must be mixed in 50 mL of normal saline.
    b. It can only be given in a central line.
    c. The patient must be on a cardiac monitor.
    d. It should be given over 1-2 minutes.

28. Which lab value(s) should a nurse monitor for a patient receiving chlorothiazide (Diuril)? *(Select all that apply.)*
    a. Potassium
    b. Sodium
    c. Bicarbonate
    d. Calcium
    e. AST/ALT

29. A patient who has had an acute myocardial infarction has been started on spironolactone (Aldactone) 50 mg/d. When evaluating routine laboratory work, the nurse discovers the patient has a potassium level of 5.8 mEq/L. What is the priority intervention to be implemented?
    a. The spironolactone dose should be decreased and the patient instructed to decrease intake of foods rich in potassium.
    b. The spironolactone dose should be continued and the patient encouraged to eat fruits and vegetables.
    c. The spironolactone dose should be increased and the patient instructed to decrease foods rich in potassium.
    d. Instruct the patient to continue with the current dose of spironolactone and report any signs or symptoms of hypokalemia.

30. Which individual is the best candidate to take acetazolamide (Diamox)?
    a. A 50-year-old with open-angle glaucoma
    b. A 58-year-old with acute heart failure
    c. A 60-year-old with narrow-angle glaucoma
    d. A 75-year-old with acute glaucoma

31. What type of acid-base imbalance could occur if a patient is taking high doses of acetazolamide (Diamox) or uses the drug constantly?
    a. Metabolic acidosis
    b. Metabolic alkalosis
    c. Respiratory acidosis
    d. Respiratory alkalosis

32. The 70-year-old patient has heart failure and has been prescribed hydrochlorothiazide (Esidrix). What statement by the patient indicates understanding of the dosing regimen?
    a. "I need to take it on an empty stomach for it to work."
    b. "I really only need to take my medicine when I am having a hard time breathing."
    c. "It may take several weeks before it starts to work."
    d. "I should take it in the morning so I don't have to go to the bathroom at night."

33. The patient has a complicated medical history including heart failure, cardiac arrhythmias, arthritis, and depression. He is taking furosemide for his heart failure. Which of his other medications would be of major concern to the nurse?
    a. Amiodarone (Cordarone)
    b. Acetaminophen (Tylenol)
    c. Amitriptyline (Elavil)
    d. Zolpidem (Ambien)

34. The 62-year-old patient has been taking ethacrynic acid (Edecrin) for severe edema. The family calls to report that the patient is very weak and unable to ambulate and is complaining of severe leg cramps. Knowing the mechanism of action of ethacrynic acid, the nurse is concerned the patient may be experiencing which electrolyte imbalance?
    a. Hyponatremia
    b. Hypermagnesemia
    c. Hypokalemia
    d. Hyperchloremia

35. What is the optimal time to administer diuretics?
    a. At bedtime
    b. After arising for the day
    c. On an empty stomach
    d. With meals

36. The nurse assesses the patient who is taking hydrochlorothiazide (HCTZ) for hypertension. What might the nurse expect to see if the patient is experiencing undesired side effects? *(Select all that apply.)*
    a. Diarrhea
    b. Dizziness
    c. Headache
    d. Hypocalcemia
    e. Vomiting

37. Which drug-lab value interaction is caused by thiazide diuretics?
    a. Decreased blood glucose level
    b. Elevated lithium level
    c. Elevated BUN
    d. Decreased calcium level

38. The patient is taking furosemide 80 mg/day. She has a history of hypertension and heart failure. She presents to the emergency department after sustaining a fall at a local sports bar. She has a laceration to her posterior scalp. Vital signs are temperature 38.0° C, heart rate 98 beats/min, respiratory rate 16 breaths/min, and blood pressure 94/62 mm Hg. Her electrolytes are within normal limits. Her blood alcohol is .06, and her toxicology screen is negative. What does the nurse know about possible drug interactions?
    a. Furosemide can cause severe hypoglycemia and headache.
    b. Furosemide can cause hyperkalemia and dizziness.
    c. Furosemide can cause orthostatic hypotension when consumed with alcohol.
    d. Furosemide can lead to elevated uric acid levels causing the patient to faint.

39. In which patient are loop diuretics contraindicated?
    a. The patient with anuria
    b. The patient with asthma
    c. The patient with allergy to ceftriaxone
    d. The patient with gastric ulcers

40. The patient has been prescribed furosemide 80 mg/d as a diuretic. Which food(s) should the nurse encourage the patient to include in his diet? *(Select all that apply.)*
    a. Raisins
    b. Rice
    c. Baked potatoes
    d. Tomatoes
    e. White bread

41. The patient has been diagnosed with hypertension and diabetes and has been started on hydrochlorothiazide. What statement by the patient indicates understanding of the medication teaching the nurse has provided?
    a. "It will start working within minutes."
    b. "I don't need to monitor my blood sugar."
    c. "I should take my medicine on an empty stomach so it works better."
    d. "I need to keep track of my weight and blood pressure at home."

Case Study

Read the scenario and answer the following questions on a separate sheet of paper.

J.S., 21 years old, was involved in a motorcycle collision and has a severe traumatic brain injury. While preparing to take the patient for surgery, the neurosurgeon orders mannitol (Osmitrol) to be administered. Vital signs are temperature 37.6° C, heart rate 62 beats/min, respiratory rate controlled on a ventilator at 18 breaths/min, and blood pressure 194/132 mm Hg. The patient has an intracranial pressure (ICP) of 36 mm Hg. (The normal range for intracranial pressure is 5-15 mm Hg.) He weighs 80 kg.

1. What class of diuretic is mannitol, and how does it work?

2. What is the standard dosage range for mannitol? How is mannitol administered?

3. What would the correct dose be for this patient?

44 Antihypertensives

Study Questions

Complete the following.

1. When hypertension cannot be controlled by nonpharmacologic means, antihypertensive drugs may be prescribed. Three of the sympatholytic groups are _____, _____, and _____.

2. Two categories of antihypertensives in addition to the sympatholytics are _____ and _____.

3. The Joint National Committee on Prevention, Detection, Evaluation, and Treatment of High Blood Pressure (JNC-7) uses three classifications for defining elevated systolic blood pressure (SBP): _____, _____, and _____.

4. Thiazide diuretics may be combined with other antihypertensive agents such as _____ and _____.

5. Many antihypertensive drugs can cause fluid retention. To decrease body fluid, the drug group often administered with antihypertensive drugs is _____.

6. A patient with a blood pressure of 182/105 mm Hg has what stage of hypertension according to JNC-7? _____

7. Beta-adrenergic blockers reduce cardiac output by diminishing the sympathetic nervous system response. With continued use of beta blockers, vascular resistance is (increased/diminished) and blood pressure is (lowered/increased). *(Circle correct answers.)*

8. Atenolol and metoprolol are examples of (cardioselective/noncardioselective) antihypertensive drugs. *(Circle correct answer.)*

9. The alpha blockers are useful in treating hypertensive patients with lipid abnormalities. The effects they have on lipoproteins include _____ and _____.

Match the generic drug name in Column I with the category of antihypertensive in Column II.

Column I

_____ 10. Captopril

_____ 11. Verapamil

_____ 12. Prazosin

_____ 13. Methyldopa

_____ 14. Hydralazine

_____ 15. Candesartan

Column II

a. Beta blocker
b. Selective alpha blocker
c. Angiotensin-converting enzyme (ACE) inhibitor
d. Calcium channel blocker
e. Centrally acting alpha$_2$ agonist
f. Direct-acting vasodilator
g. Angiotensin II receptor antagonist (A-II blocker)

NCLEX Review Questions

Select the best response.

16. The patient presents to the health care provider for his annual check-up. His vital signs are blood pressure 136/82 mm Hg, heart rate 72 beats/min, respiratory rate 16 breaths/min, and temperature 36.2° C. According to the JNC-7, to which hypertension category does this patient belong?
    a. Normal
    b. Prehypertension
    c. Stage 1
    d. Stage 2

17. A cardioselective beta-adrenergic blocker is also known by which other term?
    a. Alpha-beta blocker
    b. Alpha blocker
    c. Beta-angiotensin agent
    d. Beta blocker

18. Which patient would be most suited for treatment with a nonselective alpha-adrenergic blocker?
    a. A 45-year-old with mild to moderate renal failure
    b. A 46-year-old with a severe hypertension caused by adrenal medulla tumor
    c. A 50-year-old with hyperlipidemia
    d. A 55-year-old with type 2 diabetes

19. Where in the body do direct-acting vasodilators act to decrease blood pressure?
    a. Cardiac valves
    b. Dopaminergic receptors in kidneys
    c. Renal tubules
    d. Smooth muscles of the blood vessels

20. With use of direct-acting vasodilators, sodium and water are retained, and peripheral edema occurs. Which category of drugs should be given to avoid fluid retention?
    a. Anticoagulants
    b. Antidysrhythmics
    c. Cardiac glycosides
    d. Diuretics

21. Which is/are action(s) of angiotensin II receptor blockers (ARBs)? *(Select all that apply.)*
    a. Block angiotensin II
    b. Cause vasodilation
    c. Decrease peripheral resistance
    d. Increase sodium retention
    e. Slow heart rate

22. An ARB can be combined with the thiazide diuretic hydrochlorothiazide. What is the purpose of combining these two drugs?
    a. To decrease rapid blood pressure drop
    b. To enhance the antihypertensive effect by promoting sodium and water loss
    c. To increase sodium and water retention for controlling blood pressure
    d. To promote potassium retention

23. ARBs may be prescribed for hypertensive patients instead of an ACE inhibitor. What is the most limiting factor in the use of ACE inhibitors?
    a. Coughing
    b. Dizziness
    c. Shortness of breath
    d. Sneezing

24. Which orders should the nurse question if the patient was prescribed an ACE inhibitor?
    a. A 45-year-old Hispanic man
    b. A 48-year-old Asian woman
    c. A 50-year-old white woman
    d. A 55-year-old African-American man

25. The patient, a 48-year-old African-American female, presents to her health care provider. Her blood pressure is 164/88 mm Hg, and a decision is made to start antihypertensive medication. What group of medications would be more effective than ACE inhibitors for this patient?
    a. Angiotensin II blockers
    b. Beta blockers
    c. Calcium blockers
    d. Direct renin inhibitor

26. Herb-drug interactions may occur if the patient is taking certain herbal supplements. An herb history should be obtained. What may occur in an individual who also uses ma-huang (ephedra) with an antihypertensive drug?
    a. A decrease or counteraction of the effects of the antihypertensive drug
    b. An increase in the hypertensive state
    c. An increase in the hypotensive effects of the antihypertensive drug
    d. No effect on the action of the antihypertensive drug

27. Captopril (Capoten) is from which group of antihypertensives?
    a. ACE inhibitor
    b. Beta blocker
    c. Calcium blocker
    d. Direct-acting vasodilator

28. What is the action of captopril (Capoten)?
    a. Dilation of the arteries
    b. Increase in sodium and water excretion
    c. Inhibition of the formation of angiotensin II
    d. Inhibition of the alpha receptors

29. What is the protein-binding power of valsartan (Diovan)?
    a. Highly protein-bound
    b. Moderately to highly protein-bound
    c. Moderately protein-bound
    d. Low protein-bound

30. The patient has essential hypertension. He is taking captopril (Capoten) 25 mg t.i.d. If the patient takes captopril with a highly protein-bound drug, what might occur?
    a. Captopril and the highly protein-bound drug will compete for protein sites.
    b. The concentration of captopril will be increased.
    c. There will be moderate drug displacement of captopril, which is moderately to highly protein-bound.
    d. There will be no drug displacement, because captopril is not highly protein-bound.

31. If a patient takes captopril (Capoten) with nitrates, diuretics, or adrenergic blockers, what might the nurse assess in this patient?
    a. Hypoglycemic reaction
    b. Hypotensive reaction
    c. Hyperkalemic reaction
    d. Hypertensive reaction

32. Which group(s) of individuals should absolutely not be prescribed valsartan (Diovan)? *(Select all that apply.)*
    a. African Americans
    b. Caucasians
    c. Children over age 6
    d. Older adults over age 70
    e. Pregnant women in third trimester

33. If a patient takes captopril (Capoten) with a potassium-sparing diuretic, what might occur?
    a. Hypokalemia
    b. Hyperkalemia
    c. Hypocalcemia
    d. Hypercalcemia

34. A patient states that he wishes to stop taking captopril (Capoten) for his hypertension. What is the nurse's best response?
    a. "Blood pressure can be controlled by diet and exercise, so you don't have to take medication."
    b. "It is important to keep taking your medication as directed until you speak with your health care provider."
    c. "Once your blood pressure is normal for one month, you can stop taking your medication."
    d. "Wean yourself off of the medication over a 10-day period."

35. A patient's antihypertensive drug was changed from captopril (Capoten) to nifedipine (Procardia XL) 30 mg q8h. What type of antihypertensive drug is nifedipine?
    a. Angiotensin antagonist
    b. Beta blocker
    c. Calcium channel blocker
    d. Centrally acting sympatholytic

36. What is the protein-binding power of amlodipine?
    a. Highly protein-bound
    b. Moderately to highly protein-bound
    c. Moderately protein-bound
    d. Low protein-bound

37. The nurse is assessing the patient with essential hypertension following the shift report. What might the nurse assess if the patient is experiencing side effects from his medications? *(Select all that apply.)*
    a. Dizziness
    b. Headache
    c. Increased blood pressure
    d. Nausea
    e. Paranoia

38. Aliskiren is what type of drug?
    a. ACE inhibitor
    b. Angiotensin II blocker
    c. Calcium channel blocker
    d. Direct renin inhibitor

39. What action does amlodipine (Norvasc) have in the body?
    a. Increased peripheral vascular resistance
    b. Peripheral clotting
    c. Thrombolysis
    d. Vasodilation

40. The patient, 62 years old, is taking amlodipine (Norvasc) and complains of swelling in her ankles. What is the nurse's best response to her concern?
    a. "Swelling is common when taking Norvasc. You should cut the tablet in half to reduce your dosage."
    b. "Swelling may occur with Norvasc. I will contact your health care provider to determine if the drug should be changed or if another drug should be added."
    c. "You should not be taking that drug because of your age. I will see what other antihypertensive drug you can take."
    d. "You should stop taking the drug for several days and check that the swelling has decreased."

41. What classification of drug is bisoprolol (Zebeta)?
    a. ACE inhibitor
    b. Beta blocker
    c. Calcium blocker
    d. Diuretic

42. What classification of drug is pindolol (Visken)?
    a. ACE inhibitor
    b. Beta blocker
    c. Calcium blocker
    d. Diuretic

43. What is/are the advantage(s) of using cardioselective beta-adrenergic blockers as an antihypertensive? *(Select all that apply.)*
    a. They can be abruptly discontinued without causing rebound symptoms.
    b. They help prevent bronchoconstriction.
    c. They increase serum electrolyte levels.
    d. They maintain renal blood flow.
    e. They minimize hypoglycemic effect.

44. ARBs have gained popularity for treating hypertension. Which is/are example(s) of ARB agents? *(Select all that apply.)*
    a. Irbesartan (Avapro)
    b. Losartan potassium (Cozaar)
    c. Valsartan (Diovan)
    d. Lisinopril (Prinivil)
    e. Metoprolol (Lopressor)

45. Which statement best describes the direct renin inhibitor aliskiren (Tekturna)?
    a. It is effective for treating severe hypertension.
    b. It can be combined with another antihypertensive drug such as an ARB.
    c. It can cause hypokalemia when taken as a monotherapy drug.
    d. It is more effective than calcium channel blockers in treating hypertension in African-American patients.

Case Study

Read the scenario and answer the following questions on a separate sheet of paper.

J.H., 68 years old, has a history of hypertension. She presents to her health care provider with complaints of headache, epistaxis, and dizziness. Vital signs are blood pressure 232/146 mm Hg, heart rate 62 beats/min, respiratory rate 16 breaths/min, and temperature 37.2° C oral. J.H.'s electrocardiogram reveals normal sinus rhythm with an occasional premature ventricular contraction. The health care provider calls for emergency medical services (EMS) to transport J.H. to the hospital for treatment of a hypertensive emergency. While waiting for EMS, the nurse reviews her medication list and finds that J.H. takes chlorthalidone with clonidine (Combipres) on a daily basis but "sometimes forgets a dose or two."

1. What is Combipres, and how does it work?

2. What are the options for J.H. for treatment of a hypertensive emergency?

3. What priority teaching should the nurse provide to J.H. at time of discharge from the hospital?

45 Anticoagulants, Antiplatelets, and Thrombolytics

Study Questions

Complete the following word search. Clues are given below. Circle your responses.

```
J B S J A G G R E G A T I O N U O
V M L K I N W P O F L W Y W W I L
A S I S Y L O N I R B I F Q H E D
D V T N G M X L U S P C G X Z T U
Q F S R R W A R L K C Q U U H S S
B T L K O H B P V D G H Z I H I E
Q S R A P K V W D Q C G E F S Q A
W T P N Q F E J W G L V D M I O U
T A N T I C O A G U L A N T I D U
Q F Y X K C K P Y M K H H H B A W
J F U C I T Y L O B M O R H T G Y
```

1. Clumping together of platelets to form a clot
2. Inhibits blood clot formation
3. Breakdown of fibrin for preventing clot formation
4. Lack of blood supply to tissues
5. Type of drug used to destroy blood clot formation
6. Antiplatelets are prescribed to prevent myocardial infarction and _____

Locate and circle the abbreviations for:

7. International Normalized Ratio
8. Low–molecular-weight heparin
9. Deep vein thrombosis
10. Prothrombin time

Complete the following.

11. A thrombus can form in a(n) _____ and in a(n) _____.

12. Anticoagulants are used to inhibit _____.

13. Anticoagulants and thrombolytics (have/do not have) the same action. *(Circle correct answer.)*

14. The most frequent use of heparin is to prevent _____.

15. Heparin can be given (orally/subcutaneously/intravenously). *(Circle correct answers.)*

16. The new low–molecular-weight heparins (LMWHs) are derivatives of _____. The advantage of the use of LMWHs is that they _____.

17. The International Normalized Ratio (INR) is a laboratory test to monitor the therapeutic effect of (warfarin/heparin). *(Circle correct answer.)*

18. Heparin can (decrease/increase) the platelet count, causing thrombocytopenia. *(Circle correct answer.)*

19. A thrombus disintegrates when a thrombolytic drug is administered within _____ hours following an acute myocardial infarction.

20. The action of the thrombolytic drugs streptokinase and urokinase is the conversion of _____ to _____.

21. The major complication with the use of thrombolytic drugs is _____.

22. A synthetic anticoagulant that indirectly inhibits thrombin production but is closely related in structure to heparin and LMWH is _____.

Match the drug in Column I with its drug group in Column II. Answers may be used more than once.

Column I

____ 23. Warfarin

____ 24. Aspirin

____ 25. Enoxaparin (Lovenox)

____ 26. Dalteparin sodium (Fragmin)

____ 27. Protamine sulfate

____ 28. Clopidogrel (Plavix)

____ 29. Streptokinase

____ 30. Bivalirudin (Angiomax)

____ 31. Alteplase (tissue plasminogen activator [tPA])

Column II

a. Anticoagulant: LMWH
b. Direct thrombin inhibitor (parenteral)
c. Coumarin
d. Antiplatelet
e. Anticoagulant antagonist
f. Thrombolytic

NCLEX Review Questions

Select the best response.

32. The patient has had a deep vein thrombosis in her lower leg and has been started on warfarin (Coumadin). She asks the nurse how warfarin works. What is the nurse's best response?
a. "Warfarin will help dissolve the blood clots."
b. "Warfarin is given with thrombolytics to help break up clots."
c. "Warfarin prevents new clots from forming."
d. "Warfarin dilates the veins to improve blood flow."

33. The nurse has several patients receiving warfarin. Which INR(s) should concern the nurse? *(Select all that apply.)*
a. 1.2
b. 1.4
c. 1.8
d. 2.0
e. 2.4

34. What is one of the primary reasons LMWHs are given?
a. Enhance the action of warfarin
b. Prevent cerebrovascular accidents
c. Prevention of DVTs after hip or knee surgery
d. Treatment of acute myocardial infarction

35. Which drug is not a LMWH?
    a. Enoxaparin sodium (Lovenox)
    b. Clopidogrel (Plavix)
    c. Dalteparin sodium (Fragmin)
    d. Tinzaparin sodium (Innohep)

36. The patient, 58 years old, has unstable angina and is having an emergent percutaneous transluminal coronary angioplasty (PTCA). The nurse is completing preprocedure teaching and explains that he will be receiving a medication right before the procedure and then for the next 12 hours by IV drip to prevent ischemia. What medication is the nurse teaching the patient about?
    a. Abciximab (ReoPro)
    b. Aminocaproic acid (Amicar)
    c. Protamine sulfate
    d. Warfarin (Coumadin)

37. The patient weighs 168 pounds and is going to receive abciximab (ReoPro) for unstable angina. What is the correct dosage for a continuous infusion?
    a. 9.5 mcg/min
    b. 19 mcg/min
    c. 25 mg/min
    d. 42 mg/min

38. Which statement best describes clopidogrel (Plavix)?
    a. It is the most effective anticoagulant when used with ibuprofen.
    b. It is most effective when prescribed as a single drug to prevent stroke.
    c. It is an inexpensive alternative to warfarin.
    d. It can be used together with aspirin after myocardial infarction (MI) or cerebrovascular accident (CVA) to prevent platelet aggregation.

39. The 72-year-old patient has a history of atrial fibrillation and has been discharged from the hospital on warfarin. He was taking heparin prior to being changed to warfarin for discharge. With regards to lab monitoring, what is a priority teaching intervention for the nurse?
    a. "INR and activated partial thromboplastin time (aPTT) will be monitored closely."
    b. "Periodic evaluation of your electrolytes is very important."
    c. "Your must be monitored for BUN/creatinine values to evaluate for new renal failure."
    d. "You will not need any further lab work while taking this medication."

40. Enoxaparin sodium (Lovenox) is an anticoagulant used to prevent and treat deep vein thrombosis and pulmonary embolism. To which category does this drug belong?
    a. Oral anticoagulant
    b. Low–molecular-weight heparin
    c. Standard heparin
    d. Thrombolytic

41. The 3-year-old patient has gotten into a box of rat poison under the sink. The family brings the box to the emergency department, and the main ingredient is warfarin. What priority medication will the nurse prepare to administer?
    a. Anagrelide (Agrylin)
    b. Protamine sulfate
    c. Ticlopidine (Ticlid)
    d. Vitamin K (Mephyton)

42. What is the protein-binding power of warfarin?
    a. Highly protein-bound
    b. Low protein-bound
    c. Not protein-bound at all
    d. Moderately protein-bound

43. The patient is given heparin for early treatment of deep vein thrombosis. Later, warfarin is prescribed. If the patient is also taking fluoxetine, which is highly protein-bound, what might occur?
    a. Drug displacement of the highly protein-bound drug but not displacement of warfarin
    b. Drug displacement of warfarin
    c. Drug displacement varies from patient to patient
    d. No drug displacement of either drug

44. The patient presents to the emergency department with complaints of gastrointestinal bleeding. She is currently taking fondaparinux (Arixtra) at home after having major orthopedic surgery. She has been taking 2.5 mg for the past 5 days. What does the nurse anticipate is occurring?
    a. Adverse reaction
    b. Allergic reaction
    c. Insufficient dose of fondaparinux
    d. Stevens-Johnson syndrome

45. What is one of the benefits of rivaroxaban (Xarelto)?
    a. Does not require monitoring
    b. Inexpensive
    c. Long half-life
    d. Safe to use in pregnancy

46. The patient is in the emergency department (ED) and has been diagnosed with an acute MI. The patient will be receiving streptokinase immediately while still in the ED. What might the nurse assess in a patient who is experiencing an allergic reaction to this drug? *(Select all that apply.)*
    a. Bronchospasm
    b. Dyspnea
    c. Hives
    d. Hypotension
    e. Nausea

47. The patient has received alteplase (Activase) for treatment of a CVA. The patient begins to hemorrhage. What medication does the nurse anticipate will potentially be used as treatment for this hemorrhage?
    a. Reteplase (Retavase)
    b. Aminocaproic acid (Amicar)
    c. Calcium gluconate
    d. Protamine sulfate

48. What action(s) will the nurse perform when caring for a patient who is receiving tenecteplase (TNKase)? *(Select all that apply.)*
    a. Assess for reperfusion arrhythmias.
    b. Monitor liver panel.
    c. Observe for signs and symptoms of bleeding.
    d. Obtain a type and crossmatch.
    e. Record vital signs and report changes.

49. Which patient(s) would be candidate(s) for anticoagulant use? *(Select all that apply.)*
    a. A 28-year-old with deep vein thrombosis
    b. A 35-year-old with an artificial heart valve
    c. A 45-year-old with migraines
    d. A 52-year-old who has had a knee replacement
    e. A 68-year-old with a CVA

Case Study

Read the scenario and answer the following questions on a separate sheet of paper.

R.K., 30 years old, has been diagnosed with a pulmonary embolus after having laparoscopic surgery. She is admitted to the intensive care unit and started on a heparin drip. The patient will be discharged home on warfarin and will receive therapy for 3-6 months.

1. How does heparin work in a patient who already has a pulmonary embolus?

2. How does warfarin work to prevent further development of deep vein thrombosis that may lead to pulmonary embolism?

3. What priority teaching information will the nurse need to provide for this patient prior to discharge?

46 Antihyperlipidemics and Peripheral Vasodilators

Study Questions

Match the drug in Column I with its drug group in Column II. Answers may be used more than once.

Column I

_____ 1.   Colestipol hydrochloride

_____ 2.   Gemfibrozil (Lopid)

_____ 3.   Atorvastatin (Lipitor)

_____ 4.   Simvastatin (Zocor)

_____ 5.   Cholestyramine resin (Questran)

_____ 6.   Ezetimibe (Zetia)

Column II

a.   Statins
b.   Bile-acid sequestrants
c.   Fibrates
d.   Cholesterol absorption inhibitors

NCLEX Review Questions

Select the best response.

7.   Which elevated apolipoprotein can be an indication of risk for coronary heart disease (CHD)?
   a. Apo A-1
   b. Apo A-2
   c. Apo B-100
   d. Apo C-4

8.   The patient is taking atorvastatin (Lipitor) 80 mg/day. The patient's partner calls to report that the patient is feeling weak and complaining of muscle pain. What severe side effect of statins does the nurse suspect?
   a. Stevens-Johnson syndrome
   b. Pseudomembranous colitis
   c. Gastric ulcers
   d. Rhabdomyolysis

9.   Homocysteine is a protein in the blood that has been linked to cardiovascular disease and stroke. What other negative action may it also promote?
   a. Flushing of skin
   b. Loss of blood vessel elasticity
   c. Photosensitivity and sunburn
   d. Lowering of low-density lipoprotein levels

10. The patient has intermittent claudication and complains of leg pain. He states, "I don't believe in taking all of that medicine stuff. I prefer to use only natural medicines." What herb does the nurse recognize as being used by some patients with intermittent claudication?
   a. Ginger
   b. Ginseng
   c. Ginkgo
   d. Goldenseal

11. The patient presents to the clinic for a complete physical. The patient states, "I have been doing a lot of reading, so I know what my cholesterol should be." What does the nurse know is the desired range for total cholesterol?
   a. 50-100 mg/dL
   b. 100-150 mg /dL
   c. 150-200 mg/dL
   d. 200-250 mg/dL

12. Low-density lipoproteins (LDL) are the so-called "bad" lipoproteins. Why are high levels of LDL considered unhealthy?
    a. There is an increased risk of hyperthyroidism.
    b. There is the possibility of digestive problems.
    c. There is increased risk of rhabdomyolysis.
    d. There is an increased risk of cardiovascular disease.

13. What is the standard preferred level of LDL?
    a. Less than 250 mg/dL
    b. Less than 200 mg/dL
    c. Less than 150 mg/dL
    d. Less than 100 mg/dL

14. The patient has a lipid profile drawn as part of an annual physical exam. What does the nurse know about a high-density lipoprotein (HDL) level of 22 mg/dL?
    a. This value puts the patient in a high-risk category.
    b. An HDL of 22 mg/dL places the patient in a moderate-risk category.
    c. The HDL level must be compared with all other levels before a decision can be made.
    d. This value is within the standard preferred range.

15. The patient had a total cholesterol of 228 mg/dL. After 2 months of a low-fat, low-cholesterol diet, the total cholesterol is 212 mg/dL. Why is this level not lower?
    a. The patient most likely did not adhere to the diet.
    b. Diet modification usually decreases cholesterol levels by only 10% to 30%.
    c. The patient lost less than 10 pounds on the diet.
    d. The patient's exercise program was not rigorous enough.

16. The patient is prescribed simvastatin (Zocor). She asks if she can eat whatever she wants now that she is taking Zocor. What is the nurse's best response?
    a. "Yes, you may eat whatever you want as long as you are taking Zocor."
    b. "Diet is not an important factor if you are compliant with your medications."
    c. "You should maintain a low-fat, low-cholesterol diet and exercise as well."
    d. "With Zocor, you must lose weight as well as exercise."

17. What is a usual dose of cilostazol (Pletal)?
    a. 100 mg q12h
    b. 200 mg q12h
    c. 250 mg q12h
    d. 300 mg q12h

18. What priority information should the nurse include in the health teaching plan for a patient taking cilostazol (Pletal)? *(Select all that apply.)*
    a. Take medications with meals.
    b. Avoid drinking grapefruit juice.
    c. Do not take acetaminophen.
    d. Monitor for side effects such as headache and abdominal pain.
    e. Monitor blood pressure weekly.

19. Which medication(s), other than the statins, is/are prescribed for reducing cholesterol and LDL levels? *(Select all that apply.)*
    a. Bile-acid sequestrants
    b. Alpha-adrenergic agents
    c. Direct thrombin inhibitors
    d. Nicotinic acid
    e. Antiplatelets
    f. Cholesterol absorption inhibitors

20. What type of medication is rosuvastatin (Crestor)?
    a. HMG-CoA reductase inhibitor
    b. Cholesterol absorption inhibitor
    c. Bile-acid sequestrant
    d. Combination of two antilipidemics

Case Study

Read the scenario and answer the following questions on a separate sheet of paper.

S.S., 39 years old, has a family history of coronary artery disease and has recently been having intermittent chest pains. Her cholesterol level is 267 mg/dL; her LDL level is 146 mg/dL; and her HDL is 44 mg/dL. She was initially prescribed atorvastatin (Lipitor) 10 mg/day. The dosage has now been increased to 20 mg/day. Her medical history is positive for type 2 diabetes. She has no allergies, and she tells the nurse that she is "starting to think about getting pregnant."

1. Discuss the mechanism of action for atorvastatin and the purpose of this medication.

2. What are the implications of atorvastatin and pregnancy?

3. What should be monitored during drug therapy, and how long will the drug therapy last?

4. What teaching points should be included in patient education for S.S.?

47 Drugs for Gastrointestinal Tract Disorders

Study Questions

Match the words in Column I with the description they are most associated with in Column II.

Column I

_____ 1. Adsorbents

_____ 2. Cannabinoids

_____ 3. Chemoreceptor trigger zone (CTZ)

_____ 4. Emetics

_____ 5. Opiates

_____ 6. Osmotics

_____ 7. Purgatives

Column II

a. Harsh cathartics that cause a watery stool with abdominal cramping

b. Induces vomiting (used after poisoning)

c. Hyperosmolar laxatives

d. Relieves chemotherapy-induced nausea/vomiting

e. Lies near the medulla

f. Adsorbs bacteria or toxins that cause diarrhea

g. Decreases intestinal motility, thereby decreasing peristalsis

NCLEX Review Questions

Select the best response.

8. Which area(s) in the brain cause(s) vomiting when stimulated? *(Select all that apply.)*
   a. Chemoreceptor trigger zone
   b. Nausea center
   c. Medulla
   d. Vertigo center
   e. Vomiting center

9. Of the following groups of medications, which can be used as antiemetics? *(Select all that apply.)*
   a. Anticholinergics
   b. Antihistamines
   c. Cannabinoids
   d. Opioids
   e. Phenothiazines

10. The patient has severe nausea and vomiting and has been prescribed promethazine 25 mg PO q4-6h. The patient asks how the medication works. What is the nurse's best response?
    a. "It stimulates the dopamine receptors in the brain associated with vomiting."
    b. "It blocks the histamine receptor sites and inhibits the CTZ."
    c. "It blocks the acetylcholine receptors associated with vomiting."
    d. "It prohibits the muscle contraction in the abdominal wall, preventing vomiting."

11. The 16-year-old patient has been vomiting since last night. His mother calls the health care provider for an appointment but will be unable to come in for several hours. What nonpharmacologic method(s) can the nurse suggest to decrease nausea and vomiting? *(Select all that apply.)*
    a. "Drink weak tea."
    b. "Takes sips of flat soda."
    c. "Eat small amounts of gelatin if tolerated."
    d. "Crackers may be helpful."
    e. "Breathe deeply in and out through your nose."

12. The patient has a history of seasickness but is going boating this weekend. How far in advance should the nurse advise her to apply a scopolamine patch?
    a. Immediately
    b. 1 hour
    c. 4 hours
    d. 24 hours

13. The nurse is taking care of a newly pregnant patient who is complaining of morning sickness. She asks the nurse what she can do to help stop the nausea. How will the nurse respond? *(Select all that apply.)*
    a. "Ask your health care provider for a prescription for hydroxyzine."
    b. "Take over-the-counter antiemetics like bismuth subsalicylate."
    c. "Try drinking flat soda or weak tea."
    d. "Consider some dry toast or crackers."
    e. "This will just go away in a few months. There is nothing to do."

14. Which drugs are most commonly used to treat motion sickness?
    a. Anticholinergics
    b. Antihistamines
    c. Cannibinoids
    d. Osmotics

15. The major ingredient in cannabinoids is tetrahydrocannabinol. This substance is also the main psychoactive ingredient in what other drug?
    a. Amphetamine
    b. Cocaine
    c. Heroin
    d. Marijuana

16. The patient has nausea, vomiting, and vertigo. She has been prescribed diphenidol (Vontrol). Which condition is this medication most likely to be prescribed for?
    a. Bell's palsy
    b. Ménière's disease
    c. Opiate withdrawal
    d. Stevens-Johnson syndrome

17. What is the goal behind giving activated charcoal?
    a. Absorb poison
    b. Cause diarrhea
    c. Promote vomiting
    d. Stop nausea

18. What drug(s) is/are classified as antidiarrheal? *(Select all that apply.)*
    a. Adsorbents
    b. Anticholinergics
    c. Opioids
    d. Proton pump inhibitors
    e. Selective serotonin reuptake inhibitors

19. The patient is receiving diphenoxylate with atropine (Lomotil) for treatment of diarrhea. What side effect(s) might the nurse expect to see during treatment? *(Select all that apply.)*
    a. Dilated pupils
    b. Drowsiness
    c. Hypertension
    d. Hypoglycemia
    e. Urinary retention

20. What should potentially concern the nurse caring for a patient who has been taking opiates and opiate-related drugs for an extensive period of time to treat chronic diarrhea? *(Select all that apply.)*
    a. Abuse
    b. Major side effects
    c. Misuse
    d. Potentiation
    e. Tolerance

21. The patient has recently had surgery and has been taking opioids for pain control. He has become constipated and has been prescribed a laxative. When providing health care teaching for this patient, what type of stool should the nurse tell the patient to expect?
    a. Hard and dry
    b. Liquid
    c. Soft
    d. Soft with hard pieces

22. Which is/are a type of laxative/cathartic? *(Select all that apply.)*
    a. Adsorbents
    b. Bulk-forming
    c. Emetics
    d. Emollients
    e. Stimulants

23. The patient is scheduled for a barium enema and has a prescription for bisacodyl (Dulcolax) the day before the procedure. She asks the nurse to explain how this medication works to prepare her for her test. What is the nurse's best response?
    a. "Bisacodyl increases peristalsis by irritating the sensory nerve endings in the mucosa."
    b. "By stimulating more smooth muscle contraction, bisacodyl will cause your bowel to empty."
    c. "Bisacodyl increases water in the gut."
    d. "Bisacodyl is an emetic, so you will vomit and your stomach will be empty for the test."

24. The 65-year-old patient has recently had a myocardial infarction. His health care provider has ordered docusate sodium (Colace) 200 mg daily. What is the purpose of this medication for this patient?
    a. Treat diarrhea
    b. Prevent straining with a bowel movement
    c. Stop vomiting
    d. Prevent nausea associated with arrhythmias

25. The use of saline cathartics should be questioned by the nurse for which patient?
    a. 38-year-old with diabetes
    b. 48-year-old with peripheral vascular disease
    c. 50-year-old with chronic obstructive pulmonary disease (COPD)
    d. 62-year-old with heart failure

26. Which is a bulk-forming laxative?
    a. Bisacodyl (Dulcolax)
    b. Magnesium citrate (Citroma)
    c. Psyllium (Metamucil)
    d. Sodium biphosphate (Fleet Phospho-Soda)

27. The patient is taking mineral oil as a laxative. If she continues to take mineral oil for an extended period of time, what should concern the nurse?
    a. Abdominal bloating and flatulence
    b. Decreased absorption of fat-soluble vitamins A, D, E, and K
    c. Dependence on the drug
    d. Excessive fluid loss due to diarrhea

28. What priority instructions should be given to a patient experiencing constipation? *(Select all that apply.)*
    a. Avoid use of stimulant laxatives, which may cause electrolyte imbalance.
    b. Increase water and fiber intake in your diet.
    c. Increase the amount of exercise you do regularly.
    d. Know that some laxatives may cause urine discoloration.
    e. Take a laxative every day until regularity returns.

29. With regards to the gastrointestinal system, what do opiates do?
    a. Absorb toxic materials
    b. Decrease intestinal motility
    c. Gently stimulate peristalsis
    d. Stimulate the CTZ

30. Which patient should not use a laxative/cathartic?
    a. 48-year-old patient with cirrhosis
    b. 55-year-old patient with Parkinsonism
    c. 60-year-old patient with stable angina
    d. 65-year-old patient with bowel obstruction

31. The patient has been prescribed promethazine (Phenergan) 25 mg PO for nausea that accompanies her migraines. What side effect(s) should be included in the patient teaching? *(Select all that apply.)*
    a. Blurred vision
    b. Diarrhea
    c. Drowsiness
    d. Dry mouth
    e. Hypotension

32. The patient has recently started taking prochlorperazine (Compazine) for nausea and vomiting. What priority information should be included in the health teaching plan for this patient? *(Select all that apply.)*
    a. "You may also wish to try nonpharmacologic methods to help with the nausea."
    b. "You should try to stay busy to keep your mind off the nausea."
    c. "You should avoid driving or operating heavy machinery while taking Compazine."
    d. "You should avoid alcohol while taking this medication."
    e. "You should be aware that your urine may turn dark."

33. The patient has cancer and is being treated with dronabinol (Marinol) for nausea and vomiting caused by chemotherapy. When should this drug be administered?
    a. 1-3 hours before and for 24 hours after chemotherapy
    b. 12 hours before and for 24 hours after chemotherapy
    c. 6 hours before and during chemotherapy
    d. Every 4-6 hours as needed

34. How is the dose of dronabinol (Marinol) determined?
    a. Patient age
    b. Patient size
    c. Severity of nausea
    d. Type of cancer

35. The nurse will question an order for antidiarrheal medication for which patient?
    a. 46-year-old with diabetes
    b. 36-year-old with COPD
    c. 60-year-old with heart failure
    d. 65-year-old with hepatitis C

36. The patient has severe diarrhea. What should the nurse monitor? *(Select all that apply.)*
    a. Bowel sounds
    b. Cardiac rhythm
    c. Electrolytes
    d. Vital signs
    e. White blood cell count

37. The patient is experiencing diarrhea. Which food(s) will the nurse advise the patient to avoid? *(Select all that apply.)*
    a. Bottled water
    b. Clear liquids
    c. Fried foods
    d. Milk products
    e. Raw vegetables

38. Which food(s) should the nurse encourage a patient with constipation to eat? *(Select all that apply.)*
    a. Fresh fruit
    b. Oat bran
    c. Processed cheese
    d. Water
    e. Whole grains

Case Study

Read the scenario and answer the following questions on a separate sheet of paper.

L.B., 85 years old, presents to the clinic with complaints of constipation. She lives independently in a senior living center. Approximately two months ago, L.B. fell and broke her left hip. She had her hip replaced, received physical therapy, and has returned home. She is currently taking digoxin, a calcium supplement, omeprazole (Prilosec), and hydrocodone PRN for pain. She is prescribed bisacodyl (Dulcolax) 5 mg PO.

1. What are potential causes of constipation in L.B.?

2. How does bisacodyl work to treat constipation?

3. Are there any contraindications with any of L.B.'s other medications? If so, what?

4. What priority teaching instructions are important for this patient regarding her new medication?

48 Antiulcer Drugs

Study Questions

Match the descriptor in Column I with the drug/factor in Column II. Use each term only once.

Column I

_____ 1. Risk factor for the development of peptic ulcer disease (PUD)

_____ 2. Neutralizes gastric acid

_____ 3. The first proton pump inhibitor marketed

_____ 4. Associated with recurrence of PUD

_____ 5. Used as mucoprotective in conjunction with nonsteroidal antiinflammatory drugs (NSAIDs)

_____ 6. Binds free protein in base of ulcer

_____ 7. Eradication rates require addition of this antimicrobial

_____ 8. Causes antidiarrheal effect of some antacids

_____ 9. Over-the-counter (OTC) agent used in combination to eradicate *H. pylori*

_____ 10. H_2 antagonist with multiple drug interactions

Column II

a. Pepto-Bismol
b. Magnesium hydroxide
c. *Helicobacter pylori*
d. Sucralfate
e. Cimetidine
f. Omeprazole
g. Misoprostol
h. Smoking
i. Antacids
j. Metronidazole

Match the drug in Column I with the category to which it belongs in Column II. Answers may be used more than once.

Column I

_____ 11. Rabeprazole

_____ 12. Ranitidine

_____ 13. Glycopyrrolate

_____ 14. Nizatidine

_____ 15. Esomeprazole magnesium

_____ 16. Sucralfate

_____ 17. Magaldrate

_____ 18. Famotidine

Column II

a. Anticholinergics
b. Antacid
c. Proton pump inhibitor
d. Histamine$_2$ blocker
e. Pepsin inhibitors

NCLEX Review Questions

Select the best response.

19. The patient has started taking an OTC antacid for "heartburn." He asks the nurse what is the best time to take it so it is the most effective. What is the best answer?
    a. 1 hour before meals
    b. 1-3 hours after meals and at bedtime
    c. With meals and at bedtime
    d. With meals and 1 hour after

20. With how many ounces of water should a patient take a liquid antacid for best results?
    a. 2-4
    b. 4-6
    c. 6-8
    d. 8 or more

21. Which drug(s) may be used in the treatment of ulcers? *(Select all that apply.)*
    a. Antibiotics
    b. Anticholinergics
    c. Antacids
    d. Histamine$_2$ blockers
    e. Opiates
    f. Proton pump inhibitors

22. The patient presents to the clinic with a sore throat. He tells the nurse, "I just feel like a fire-breathing dragon. It is awful when I go to bed." He has been diagnosed with gastroesophageal reflux disease (GERD). What medication(s) does the nurse know is/are used to treat GERD? *(Select all that apply.)*
    a. Antacids
    b. Anticholinergics
    c. Histamine$_2$ blockers
    d. Pepsin inhibitors
    e. Proton pump inhibitors

23. What priority information regarding nonpharmacologic treatment can the nurse provide in the health education plan to a patient who has been diagnosed with GERD? *(Select all that apply.)*
    a. Decrease or stop smoking.
    b. Elevate the head of the bed.
    c. Increase fluid intake.
    d. NSAIDs should be taken with food.
    e. Spicy foods should be avoided.

24. The patient has been diagnosed with peptic ulcer disease and has been on propantheline bromide (Pro-Banthine) 15 mg t.i.d. 30 minutes before meals and 30 mg at bedtime. How does propantheline bromide work?
    a. It blocks H$_2$ receptors.
    b. It coats the lining of the stomach.
    c. It increases gastric motility.
    d. It inhibits gastric secretions.

25. The patient has been diagnosed with an ulcer caused by *H. pylori*. Which drug(s) is/are likely to be used for treatment? *(Select all that apply.)*
    a. Amoxicillin
    b. Clarithromycin
    c. Famotidine
    d. Misoprostol
    e. Omeprazole

26. The patient presents to the clinic with complaints of gnawing abdominal pain that occurs approximately 1 hour after eating. "I have tried everything, and it just won't stop." He has been diagnosed with an ulcer. The health care provider prescribes nizatidine (Axid). What priority information should the nurse include in the teaching plan? *(Select all that apply.)*
    a. "Antacids should not be taken within 1 hour of taking your nizatidine."
    b. "Avoid alcoholic beverages and caffeine."
    c. "Eating small, frequent meals may be helpful."
    d. "This medication should be taken with meals and at bedtime."
    e. "You will need to take this for the rest of your life."

27. A patient has been diagnosed with erosive GERD. Which medication is likely to have the highest success rate?
    a. Esomeprazole (Nexium)
    b. Lansoprazole (Prevacid)
    c. Omeprazole (Prilosec)
    d. Rabeprazole (Aciphex)

28. Which side effect(s) of ranitidine (Zantac) will the nurse monitor for in the patient? *(Select all that apply.)*
    a. Confusion
    b. Headache
    c. Hypertension
    d. Loss of libido
    e. Nausea

29. Which medication(s) will concern the nurse if prescribed for a patient who is taking esomeprazole (Nexium)? *(Select all that apply.)*

    a. Ampicillin
    b. Digoxin
    c. Ketoconazole
    d. Lisinopril
    e. Propranolol

30. The patient is taking high-dose NSAID therapy for arthritis. She is also taking sucralfate. What laboratory value would concern the nurse?
    a. Hgb 14.1 gm/dL
    b. Potassium 4.2 mEq/L
    c. Blood glucose 185 mg/dL
    d. INR 1.1

Case Study

Read the scenario and answer the following questions on a separate sheet of paper.

S.S., 63 years old, has a high-stress job as a county judge. She complains of abdominal distress after eating. She is currently taking aluminum hydroxide (Amphojel) 30 mL with meals and at bedtime. She has been diagnosed with an ulcer.

1. What are the various classes of drugs that can be used to treat ulcers?

2. What drug class does aluminum hydroxide belong to and how does it work?

3. Is this the proper dose for S.S.?

4. What priority health teaching should the nurse also provide for S.S.?

49 Drugs for Eye and Ear Disorders

Study Questions

Complete the following word search. Clues are given in questions 1-12. Circle your responses.

```
C X C P I A I R U N A L K L W G Z C G M G P A A U N D Z Q Z F R
L N F E A I S X L A G O G D K K Y X P K V N P V S O P R Z D R I
S R O T I B I H N I E S A R D Y H N A C I N O B R A C L T E M Z
U E A S M S T V R P Z P D S D E U E I X X W A N E T L Q Q H L W
A Y D L F O I J C W D U S Z V H B Z T D N Y E M M J V L B Y N Y
K R E N M X N T E A R S B Q U P T E P C P R T G L G O L K D S P
L R S I E C T C I N C R E A S E T O B Z D V P B T O Q K D R N O
T S F L S I R M S V A M O C U A L G V L E T C J S U I J G A Q M
S B K U A I A J H C I Y O B B L J Z I J O Z H M I L W F X T Y T
N T J W E J O T W Z I T D Y K T M H F D O O O C C V Y P C I H K
I U X A R Z C W Y R D T C O B H C F D S S T D V Z W H Y U O S U
Q W V A C C U T O I S V E N B B U N C E I S E S T C X A M N B H
N J Z V N Z L M I N B C V R U N N R S C C J B J U C L E P C P P
R D V Y I D A M A S W W E W U J G W S H C R H M K G C N F F Y I
L N P O E P R Y V B V N C A R I N I I B U N E L A Y A S Y R V Y
X L T Q S S B R R J A Q P I P K D O E I F O H A P X K R I D R O
E E B T B M F X G K L S E V S Y W E C R E Y W U S X Z T G Y D Q
Z C L R T W I P Z Q E A Y J X P D R J R O W F B I E R S P J O S
O B U L Q L B Z V N B D T U Y X D A Q Z Y F V X P L W G I Y V W
L Q X E W H C E A C Y C L O P L E G I C S K T O N U W I X W T F
```

1. Topical anesthetics are used during an eye exam and before removal of a(n) _____ from the eye.

2. Lubricants are used to moisten contact lenses and/or to replace _____.

3. Miotics are used to lower _____ pressure.

4. Carbonic anhydrase inhibitors were developed as _____. They are effective in treating _____.

5. Osmotic drugs are used to (decrease/increase) the vitreous humor volume. *(Circle correct answer.)*

6. Mannitol is contraindicated for clients with the condition of _____ or _____.

7. The drug group used to paralyze the muscles of accommodation is _____.

8. Acute otitis media occurs most frequently in _____.

9. Instruct patients with glaucoma to avoid atropine-like drugs because they (decrease/increase) intraocular pressure. *(Circle correct answer.)*

10. Antiinfectives are used to treat infections of the eye, including inflammation of the membrane covering the eyeball and lining the eyelid known as _____.

11. Drugs that interfere with production of carbonic acid, leading to decreased aqueous humor formation and decreased intraocular pressure, belong to the group _____.

12. The group of drugs used in the emergency treatment of acute closed-angle glaucoma because of the ability to rapidly decrease intraocular pressure is the _____.

Match the term in Column I with its definition in Column II.

Column I

_____ 13. Conjunctivitis

_____ 14. Optic

_____ 15. Cerumen

_____ 16. Lacrimal duct

_____ 17. Miosis

_____ 18. Otic

Column II

a. Passage that carries tears into the nose
b. Contraction of the pupil
c. Ear
d. Eye
e. Inflammation of the membrane covering the eyeball
f. Earwax

NCLEX Review Questions

Select the best response.

19. The patient presents to her ophthalmologist for a routine eye examination. Prior to the exam, eye-drops are used to dilate her eyes. Such medication belongs to which group of drugs?
   a. Carbonic anhydrase inhibitors
   b. Cerumenolytics
   c. Mydriatics
   d. Osmotics

20. A patient is taking acetazolamide (Diamox) for acute closed-angle glaucoma. The nurse will assess for which side effect associated with drugs in the group?
   a. Agitation
   b. Constipation
   c. Electrolyte imbalances
   d. Urinary retention

21. The African-American patient has open-angle glaucoma. The nurse knows that which glaucoma medication is more effective in African-American patients?
   a. Bimatoprost (Lumigan)
   b. Latanoprost (Xalatan)
   c. Travoprost (Travatan Z)
   d. Tafluprost (Zioptan)

22. The patient has open-angle glaucoma and is being treated with latanoprost (Xalatan). What is/are priority teaching point(s) for this patient? *(Select all that apply.)*
   a. Permanent brown pigmentation of the iris may occur.
   b. Eyelids may darken.
   c. Blurred vision may occur.
   d. Eyes may feel itchy.
   e. Pupils may get very small.

23. A patient who has frequent cerumen impaction has had his ears irrigated at the clinic. To determine the results of the irrigation, what structure must be visualized?
   a. Auricle
   b. External auditory canal
   c. Semicircular canals
   d. Tympanic membrane

24. The patient has frequent cerumen buildup. Which medication does the nurse anticipate the health care provider will suggest for this patient?
   a. Bimatoprost (Lumigan)
   b. Carbamide peroxide (Debrox)
   c. Echothiphate (Phospholine Iodide)
   d. Proparacaine (Alcaine)

25. The patient is receiving pilocarpine (Isopto Carpine) eyedrops for treatment of glaucoma. Which side effect(s) is/are most likely to occur? *(Select all that apply.)*
   a. Blurred vision
   b. Brow ache
   c. Dry mouth
   d. Headache
   e. Nausea
   f. Vomiting

26. The patient has a severe increase in intraocular pressure and requires mannitol (Osmitrol). What is/are side effect(s) that the nurse must be aware of? *(Select all that apply.)*
   a. Constipation
   b. Dizziness
   c. Electrolyte imbalance
   d. Headache
   e. Nausea

27. A baby is born vaginally to a mother with gonorrhea and has ophthalmia neonatorum. What is the
medication of choice for treatment?
   a. Gentamicin sulfate
   b. Silver nitrate 1%
   c. Sulfacetamide
   d. Tetracycline HCl

28. Which solution(s) is/are commonly used to irrigate
the ear? *(Select all that apply.)*
   a. Acetic acid
   b. Boric acid
   c. Cyclopentolate HCl
   d. Hydrogen peroxide 3%
   e. Hypotonic HCl solution 10%

29. The patient has been diagnosed with dry age-
related macular degeneration (ARMD). What
medication(s) is/are available for treatment? *(Select
all that apply.)*
   a. Aflibercept (Eylea)
   b. Bevacizumab (Avastin)
   c. Pegaptanib (Macugen)
   d. Ranibizumab (Lucentis)
   e. There is no treatment for dry ARMD.

30. A patient presents to his ophthalmologist with complaints of dry, itching eyes. He works as a land-
scaper. What option(s) does he have for treatment?
(Select all that apply.)
   a. Naphazoline (Clear Eyes)
   b. Olopatadine (Patanol)
   c. Oxymetazoline (Ocuclear)
   d. Tetrahydrozoline (Opti-Clear)
   e. Tetracaine HCl (Pontocaine)

Case Study

**Read the scenario and answer the following questions
on a separate sheet of paper.**

Y.G., 80 years old, has chronic open-angle glaucoma and
ocular hypertension. She presents to her health care provider for a follow-up appointment. Her medical history
is also positive for hypertension, depression, arthritis,
and atrial fibrillation. She states that she has been "doing
pretty good, I guess." She denies any specific complaints
except some blurred vision. She self-administers timolol
(Timoptic) 2 gtt q8h.

1. What is open-angle glaucoma?

2. What kind of a medication is timolol, and how does
it work?

3. How are these eyedrops administered?

4. Is this the appropriate dose for this patient? Why or
why not?

50 Drugs for Dermatologic Disorders

Study Questions

Match the term in Column I with the correct description in Column II.

Column I

_____ 1. Macule

_____ 2. Vesicle

_____ 3. Plaque

_____ 4. Papule

Column II

a. Raised, palpable lesion <1 cm in diameter
b. Hard, rough, raised lesion; flat on top
c. Flat lesion with varying color
d. Raised lesion filled with fluid and <1 cm in diameter

Match the condition in Column I to the drug that treats it in Column II. Multiple drugs may be used for a condition.

Column I

_____ 5. Psoriasis

_____ 6. Burns

_____ 7. Acne

Column II

a. Tetracycline
b. Isotretinoin (Amnesteem)
c. Azelaic acid (Azelex)
d. Estrostep
e. Alefacept (Amevive)
f. Silver sulfadiazine

NCLEX Review Questions

Select the best response.

8. The 18-year-old patient has acne. Which type(s) of drugs is/are used to treat this condition? *(Select all that apply.)*
   a. Antibiotics
   b. Antifungals
   c. Glucocorticoids
   d. Keratolytics
   e. Nonsteroidal antiinflammatories
   f. T-cell antagonists

9. Psoriasis affects what percentage of the population in the United States?
   a. Less than 1%
   b. 2% to 4%
   c. 5% to 7%
   d. 8% to 10%

10. The patient has psoriasis and presents to her health care provider for treatment. She states that her "lizard skin" is really embarrassing. The health care provider orders calcipotriene (Dovonex). When the patient asks how this medication will work, what is the nurse's best answer?
    a. "This medication will help stop the proliferation of cells."
    b. "It will be very effective against the itching that goes with psoriasis."
    c. "Calcipotriene will cure psoriasis."
    d. "It can be used like makeup to cover up the scales."

11. The patient has psoriasis and is going to be started on a course of infliximab (Remicade). What does the nurse tell the patient about the dosing regimen he will be following?
    a. "Infliximab is a gel that you will use after bathing."
    b. "Infliximab is a medication that is administered by IV at prescribed intervals."
    c. "You will be able to give yourself an injection once per week."
    d. "This is an oral medicine that you will be on for the rest of your life."

12. Which is/are common cause(s) of contact dermatitis? *(Select all that apply.)*
    a. Anesthetics
    b. Cosmetics
    c. Dyes
    d. Peanuts
    e. Sumac

13. The patient has been prescribed tetracycline for acne. What is the standard dose?
    a. 125-250 mg b.i.d.
    b. 250-500 mg b.i.d.
    c. 500-750 mg b.i.d.
    d. 750-1000 mg b.i.d.

14. What is a major side effect of tetracycline?

    a. Cardiac arrhythmias
    b. Glucose intolerance
    c. Hemorrhagic shock
    d. Photosensitivity

15. What priority information should be provided to the patient taking tetracycline for acne? *(Select all that apply.)*
    a. Alert the health care provider if pregnant or possibly pregnant.
    b. Avoid the use of harsh cleansers.
    c. Eat a high-fiber diet.
    d. It should not be used with isotretinoin.
    e. Use a sunscreen with SPF 2.

16. The patient has male pattern baldness. What medication can be utilized to treat male pattern baldness?
    a. Acitretin
    b. Methotrexate
    c. Minoxidil
    d. Tretinoin

17. The patient, 3 years old, is sent home from daycare with a large sore at the corner of his nostril. He has been diagnosed with impetigo. What is a causative agent?
    a. Herpes simplex virus
    b. *Klebsiella pneumoniae*
    c. *Neisseria gonorrhoeae*
    d. *Staphylococcus aureus*

18. The patient presents to his health care provider's office with complaints of severe rash and itching after a hunting trip. He has been diagnosed with contact dermatitis from poison ivy. What antipruritic agent(s) can be utilized for this patient? *(Select all that apply.)*
    a. Triamcinolone (Aristocort)
    b. Dexamethasone (Decadron)
    c. Diphenhydramine (Benadryl)
    d. Fluconazole (Diflucan)
    e. Salicylic acid (Sebulex)

19. What drug(s) is/are known to cause alopecia? *(Select all that apply.)*
    a. Antineoplastic agents
    b. Antiarrhythmics
    c. Cephalosporins
    d. Oral contraceptives
    e. Sulfonamides

Case Study

Read the scenario and answer the following questions on a separate sheet of paper.

C.S., 24 years old, has sustained full-thickness burns over his anterior chest and partial-thickness burns over his forearms bilaterally. Mafenide acetate (Sulfamylon Cream) is ordered to be applied to his burns.

1. What is the difference between full- and partial-thickness burns?

2. What type of drug is mafenide acetate?

3. What other options are available for a topical burn preparation?

4. What are priority nursing interventions for this patient?

51 Endocrine Drugs: Pituitary, Thyroid, Parathyroid, and Adrenal Disorders

Study Questions

Match the information in Column I with the correct term in Column II.

Column I

_____ 1. Growth hormone hypersecretion after puberty

_____ 2. Anterior pituitary gland

_____ 3. Initials for adrenocorticotropic hormone

_____ 4. Initials for antidiuretic hormone

_____ 5. Severe hypothyroidism in children

_____ 6. Ductless glands that produce hormones

_____ 7. Growth hormone hypersecretion during childhood

_____ 8. Cortisol hormone secreted from the adrenal cortex

_____ 9. Pituitary gland

_____ 10. Aldosterone hormone secreted from the adrenal cortex

_____ 11. Severe hypothyroidism in adults

_____ 12. Posterior pituitary gland

_____ 13. Toxic hyperthyroidism because of hyperfunction of the thyroid gland

_____ 14. T_4 hormone secreted by the thyroid gland

_____ 15. T_3 hormone secreted by the thyroid gland

Column II

a. ADH

b. Gigantism

c. Mineralocorticoid

d. Neurohypophysis

e. Triiodothyronine

f. Acromegaly

g. Myxedema

h. Endocrine

i. Adenohypophysis

j. ACTH

k. Thyrotoxicosis

l. Thyroxine

m. Glucocorticoid

n. Cretinism

o. Hypophysis

Match the condition in Column I with the cause in Column II. Answers may be used more than once.

Column I

_____ 16.   Hyperglycemia

_____ 17.   Buffalo hump

_____ 18.   Hypoglycemia

_____ 19.   Seizures

_____ 20.   Fatigue

_____ 21.   Impaired clotting

_____ 22.   Cataract formation

_____ 23.   Hypotension

_____ 24.   Hypervolemia

_____ 25.   Peptic ulcer

Column II

a.   Adrenal hyposecretion

b.   Adrenal hypersecretion

Match the nursing intervention in Column I with the correct rationale related to glucocorticoid drug administration in Column II.

Column I

_____ 26.   Monitor vital signs.

_____ 27.   Monitor weight after taking a cortisone preparation for more than 10 days.

_____ 28.   Monitor laboratory values, especially blood glucose and electrolytes.

_____ 29.   Instruct the patient to take the cortisone with food.

_____ 30.   Advise the patient to eat foods rich in potassium.

_____ 31.   Instruct the patient not to abruptly discontinue the cortisone preparation.

_____ 32.   Report changes in muscle strength and signs of osteoporosis.

_____ 33.   Teach the patient to report signs and symptoms of drug overdose.

Column II

a.   Cortisone increases sodium retention and increases blood pressure.

b.   Adrenal crisis may occur if cortisone is abruptly stopped.

c.   Glucocorticoid drugs promote loss of potassium.

d.   Weight gain occurs with cortisone use as a result of water retention.

e.   Glucocorticoid drugs promote sodium retention, potassium loss, and increased blood glucose.

f.   Cortisone promotes loss of muscle tone and loss of calcium from bone.

g.   Glucocorticoid drugs may cause moon face, puffy eyelids, edema in the feet, dizziness, and menstrual irregularity at high doses.

h.   Glucocorticoid drugs can irritate the gastric mucosa and may cause peptic ulcer.

NCLEX Review Questions

Select the best response.

34. 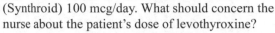 A 65-year-old patient is being treated for hypothyroidism. The patient is taking levothyroxine (Synthroid) 100 mcg/day. What should concern the nurse about the patient's dose of levothyroxine?
    a. It is too low for the patient's age.
    b. It is too high a dose for the patient's age.
    c. Nothing; it is within the normal maintenance dose.
    d. Nothing; someone the patient's age should start at a low dose.

35. How soon after starting levothyroxine (Synthroid) should the patient report feeling its effects?
    a. 3-4 days
    b. 4-7 days
    c. 1-2 weeks
    d. 2-4 weeks

36. The nurse assesses the patient for symptoms of hyperthyroidism. Which is/are symptom(s) of hyperthyroidism? *(Select all that apply.)*
    a. Chest pain
    b. Constipation
    c. Excessive sweating
    d. Tachycardia
    e. Tinnitus

37. The nurse is speaking to the patient with hypothyroidism about avoiding foods that can inhibit thyroid secretion. Which statement(s) indicate(s) that the patient understands the teaching? *(Select all that apply.)*
    a. "I don't eat string beans as they give me gas, so I won't miss them."
    b. "I hate to give up strawberries, but I want to feel better."
    c. "Radishes burn my tongue, so no great loss if I should avoid them."
    d. "Really? I have to give up potatoes?"
    e. "I won't eat any peas anymore."

38. What time of day should the nurse teach the patient to take levothyroxine?
    a. Before breakfast
    b. With breakfast
    c. After breakfast
    d. With lunch

39. What is priority information to include in the health teaching plan for the patient with hypothyroidism? *(Select all that apply.)*
    a. Avoid over-the-counter (OTC) drugs.
    b. Report numbness and tingling of the hands to the health care provider.
    c. Increase food and fluid intake.
    d. Take medication with food.
    e. Wear a Medic-Alert information device.

40. A patient is taking prednisone for an exacerbation of arthritic knee pain. What is the usual dose of prednisone?
    a. 0.5-6 mg/day
    b. 5-60 mg/day
    c. 60-100 mg/day
    d. 100-125 mg/day

41. While a patient is taking prednisone, which laboratory value should be closely monitored?
    a. Hematocrit
    b. Hemoglobin
    c. Magnesium
    d. Potassium

42. The patient has been started on prednisone for bronchitis to decrease inflammation. When is the best time to take prednisone?
    a. Before meals
    b. With meals
    c. 1 hour after meals
    d. At bedtime

43. Which drug(s) should be used with caution when taking a glucocorticoid? *(Select all that apply.)*
    a. Acetaminophen
    b. Nonsteroidal antiinflammatory drugs (NSAIDs), including aspirin
    c. Oral anticoagulants
    d. Phenytoin
    e. Potassium-wasting diuretics

44. What is/are priority nursing intervention(s) to implement in the care of a patient taking prednisone? *(Select all that apply.)*
    a. Follow the physical therapy regimen.
    b. Monitor for signs and symptoms of hyponatremia.
    c. Monitor vital signs.
    d. Obtain a complete medication history.
    e. Record daily weight.

45. Which statement by a patient taking prednisone indicates that she needs more education about her medications?
    a. "I should wear a Medic-Alert device or carry a card."
    b. "I will make sure I force fluids daily."
    c. "I will not abruptly stop taking my medication."
    d. "I will take glucocorticoids only as ordered."

46. When an herbal laxative such as cascara or senna and herbal diuretics such as celery seed or juniper are taken with a corticosteroid, what imbalance may occur?
    a. Hypoglycemia
    b. Hypokalemia
    c. Hyponatremia
    d. Hypophosphatemia

47. What changes can occur when ginseng is taken with a corticosteroid?
    a. Central nervous system (CNS) depression
    b. CNS stimulation and insomnia
    c. Counteraction of the effects of the corticosteroid
    d. Electrolyte imbalance

48. Which drug would the nurse anticipate using for a procedure to diagnose adrenal gland dysfunction?
    a. Corticotropin (Acthar)
    b. Ketoconazole (Nizoral)
    c. Metyrapone (Metopirone)
    d. Prednisolone (Delta-Cortef)

49. The nurse advises a patient to avoid potassium loss by eating which food(s)? *(Select all that apply.)*
    a. Nuts
    b. Meats
    c. Vegetables
    d. Dried fruits
    e. Applesauce

50. Which drug(s) is/are known to interact with levothyroxine (Synthroid)? *(Select all that apply.)*
    a. Anticoagulants
    b. Digitalis
    c. Diuretics
    d. NSAIDs
    e. Oral antidiabetics

51. The nurse assesses a patient for the side effects of prednisone. What assessment finding(s) may be present? *(Select all that apply.)*
    a. Anorexia
    b. Edema
    c. Hypertension
    d. Increased blood sugar
    e. Mood changes

Case Study

Read the scenario and answer the following questions on a separate sheet of paper.

R.K., 48 years old, has been diagnosed with adrenal insufficiency and is scheduled to start treatment with hydrocortisone.

1. What signs and symptoms are associated with adrenal insufficiency?

2. What is the dosage of hydrocortisone and how is it administered?

3. What priority teaching is important for this patient?

52 Antidiabetics

Study Questions

Match the term in Column I with its definition in Column II.

Column I

_____ 1. Diabetes mellitus

_____ 2. Insulin

_____ 3. Hypoglycemic reaction

_____ 4. Type 1 diabetes

_____ 5. Type 2 diabetes

_____ 6. Ketoacidosis

_____ 7. Lipodystrophy

_____ 8. Polydipsia

_____ 9. Polyphagia

_____ 10. Polyuria

_____ 11. Dawn phenomenon

Column II

a. Increased hunger

b. Type of diabetes with some beta cell function

c. Increased urine output

d. Hyperglycemia on awakening

e. Diabetic acidosis

f. Disease resulting from deficient glucose metabolism

g. Increased thirst

h. Protein secreted from the beta cells of the pancreas

i. Tissue atrophy

j. Type of diabetes with no beta cell function

k. Reaction to low blood glucose

Match the terms in Column I with their definitions in Column II.

Column I

_____ 12. NPH insulin

_____ 13. Lipoatrophy

_____ 14. Sulfonylureas

_____ 15. Glucagon

_____ 16. Lispro insulin

Column II

a. Oral hypoglycemic drug group

b. Hyperglycemic hormone that stimulates glycogenolysis

c. Intermediate-acting insulin

d. Long-acting insulin

e. Tissue atrophy

f. Rapid-acting insulin

Match the nursing intervention in Column I with its rationale in Column II.

Column I

_____ 17. Monitor blood glucose levels.

_____ 18. Instruct the patient to report signs and symptoms of "insulin shock" (hypoglycemic reaction).

_____ 19. Inform the patient to have orange juice or a sugar-containing drink available if a hypoglycemic reaction occurs.

_____ 20. Instruct the patient to check the blood sugar daily.

_____ 21. Instruct the patient to adhere to the prescribed diet.

_____ 22. Instruct family members on how to administer glucagon by injection for a hypoglycemic reaction.

_____ 23. Advise the patient to obtain a Medic-Alert card or tag.

Column II

a. Done to make sure it is within normal levels.

b. Orange juice or a sweetened beverage adds sugar to the body for insulin utilization.

c. Diet is prescribed according to amount of insulin given per day.

d. Signs and symptoms include nervousness, tremors, cold and clammy skin, and slurred speech.

e. Patient may be unable to swallow orange juice.

f. Needed in case of a severe hypoglycemic reaction where the patient may be unconscious.

g. Prevents incidences of hyper- and hypoglycemia.

NCLEX Review Questions

Select the best response.

24. What is/are the major symptom(s) that characterize diabetes? *(Select all that apply.)*
   a. Polydipsia
   b. Polyphagia
   c. Polyposia
   d. Polyrrhea
   e. Polyuria

25. Which drug(s) may cause hyperglycemia? *(Select all that apply.)*
   a. Epinephrine
   b. Hydrochlorothiazide
   c. Levothyroxine
   d. Prednisone
   e. Thiazolidinediones

26. What is the rationale for rotation of insulin injection sites?
   a. It prevents an allergic reaction.
   b. It prevents lipodystrophy.
   c. It prevents polyuria.
   d. It prevents rejection of insulin.

27. What is the only type of insulin that may be administered IV?
   a. Detemir
   b. Lantus
   c. NPH
   d. Regular

28. Which clinical manifestation(s) may be seen in a patient experiencing a hypoglycemic (insulin) reaction? *(Select all that apply.)*
   a. Abdominal pain
   b. Headache
   c. Excessive perspiration
   d. Nervousness
   e. Tremor
   f. Vomiting

29. Which clinical manifestation(s) may be seen in a patient experiencing diabetic ketoacidosis (hyperglycemia)? *(Select all that apply.)*
   a. Bradycardia
   b. Dry mucous membranes
   c. Fruity breath odor
   d. Kussmaul's respirations
   e. Polyuria
   f. Thirst

30. The patient has type 1 diabetes. Which medication should the patient not use to control his diabetes?
    a. Insulin glulisine (Apidra)
    b. Insulin lispro (Humalog)
    c. Insulin aspart (NovoLog)
    d. Tolazamide (Tolinase)

31. Which information should be included in health teaching for patients taking insulin? *(Select all that apply.)*
    a. Adhere to the prescribed diet.
    b. Alter insulin dose based on how you're feeling.
    c. Be sure to exercise.
    d. Monitor blood glucose level.
    e. Recognize signs of hypoglycemic reaction.
    f. Take insulin as prescribed.

32. Which information should be included in health teaching for patients taking oral antidiabetic (hypoglycemic) drugs? *(Select all that apply.)*
    a. Adhere to prescribed diet.
    b. Monitor blood glucose levels.
    c. Monitor weight.
    d. Participate in regular exercise.
    e. Take medications based on blood glucose.

33. Lipoatrophy is a complication that occurs when insulin is injected repeatedly in one site. What is the physiologic effect that occurs?
    a. Depression under the skin surface
    b. Bruising under the skin
    c. Raised lump or knot on the skin surface
    d. Rash at a raised area on the skin surface

34. Where should the patient who takes insulin daily be taught to store the opened insulin?
    a. In a cool place
    b. In the light
    c. In the freezer
    d. Wrapped in aluminum

35. How should the nurse or patient prepare insulin prior to administration?
    a. Add diluent to the bottle.
    b. Allow air to escape from the bottle.
    c. Roll the bottle in the hands.
    d. Shake the bottle well.

36. The nurse is preparing to give a patient his daily insulin. The patient receives both NPH and regular insulin. What is the best action by the nurse?
    a. Prepare one injection; draw up both simultaneously and mix well.
    b. Prepare one injection; draw up NPH insulin first.
    c. Prepare one injection; draw up regular insulin first.
    d. Prepare two separate injections.

37. Which type of syringe should be used to administer a patient's daily insulin dose of 6 units of U100 regular and 14 units of U100 NPH?
    a. 2-mL syringe
    b. 5-mL syringe
    c. U40 insulin syringe
    d. U100 insulin syringe

38. The patient needs to develop a "site rotation pattern" for insulin injections. The American Diabetes Association suggests which action(s)? *(Select all that apply.)*
    a. Choose an injection site for a week.
    b. Change the injection area of the body every day.
    c. Inject insulin each day at the injection site at 1½ inches apart.
    d. Inject insulin IM in the morning and SQ at night.
    e. With two daily injection times, use the right side in the morning and the left side in the evening.

39. When should the nurse expect that the patient may experience a hypoglycemic reaction to regular insulin if administration occurs at 0700 and the patient does not eat?
    a. 0800-0900
    b. 0900-1300
    c. 1300-1500
    d. 1500-1700

40. How long after NPH administration would the nurse expect the patient's insulin to peak?
    a. 1-2 hours
    b. 2-6 hours
    c. 6-12 hours
    d. 12-15 hours

41. Lantus is a long-acting insulin. Which statement(s) best describe(s) Lantus? *(Select all that apply.)*
    a. Always combine it with regular insulin for good coverage.
    b. It is given in the evening.
    c. It is safe because hypoglycemia cannot occur.
    d. It is available in a 3-mL cartridge insulin pen.
    e. Some patients complain of pain at the injection site.

42. What is a method to determine if the patient has developed an allergy to insulin?
    a. Chemistry laboratory tests
    b. History of other allergies
    c. Skin test with different insulin preparations
    d. Urinalysis to check for glucose

43. The insulin pump, though expensive, has become popular in the management of insulin. What does the nurse know about this method of insulin delivery?
    a. It can be used with modified insulins (NPH) as well as regular insulin.
    b. It can be used with the needle inserted at the same site for weeks.
    c. It is more effective in decreasing the number of hypoglycemic reactions.
    d. It is more effective for use by the type 2 diabetic patient.

44. What is an action of an oral hypoglycemic agent?
    a. It increases the number of insulin cell receptors.
    b. It increases the number of insulin-producing cells.
    c. It replaces receptor sites.
    d. It replaces insulin.

45. The patient asks if Prandin is oral insulin. What is the nurse's best response?
    a. "No, it is not the same as insulin, and Prandin can be taken even when the blood sugar remains greater than 250 mg/dL."
    b. "No, it is not the same as insulin. Prandin can be used only when there is some beta cell function."
    c. "Yes, it is the same as injected insulin, except it is taken orally."
    d. "Yes, it is similar, but hypoglycemic reactions (insulin shock) do not occur with Prandin."

46. Which effect(s) is/are representative of second-generation sulfonylureas? *(Select all that apply.)*
    a. Effective doses are less than with first-generation sulfonylureas.
    b. They increase tissue response and decrease glucose production by the liver.
    c. They have less displacement from protein-binding sites by other highly protein-bound drugs.
    d. They have more hypoglycemic potency than first-generation sulfonylureas.

47. The nonsulfonylureas are used to control serum glucose levels after a meal. What best describes their action?
    a. They cause a hypoglycemic reaction.
    b. They decrease hepatic production of glucose from stored glycogen.
    c. They increase the absorption of glucose from the small intestine.
    d. They raise the serum glucose level following a meal.

48. A patient newly diagnosed with type 2 diabetes has been prescribed acarbose (Precose), and he asks the nurse how the medication works if it is not insulin. What is the nurse's best response?
    a. "It works by increasing insulin production; thus it can cause a hypoglycemic reaction."
    b. "It works by stimulating the beta cells to produce insulin."
    c. "It works through increasing glucose metabolism."
    d. "It works through inhibiting digestive enzymes in the small intestine, which releases glucose from the complex carbohydrates in the diet (less sugar is available)."

49. The patient has type 2 diabetes and has just been prescribed pioglitazone HCl (Actos). This medication is in the thiazolidinedione group of nonsulfonylureas. How does this group of oral antidiabetics work?
    a. They decrease glucose utilization.
    b. They increase insulin sensitivity for improving blood glucose control.
    c. They increase the uptake of glucose in the liver and small intestine.
    d. They promote absorption of glucose from the large intestine.

50. In 2007 the FDA added a warning to rosiglitazone (Avandia). What was the warning regarding?
    a. Blood dyscrasias
    b. Increased risk of heart attack
    c. Increased risk of kidney failure
    d. Potential for severe liver dysfunction

51. Patients taking thiazolidinedione drugs such as pioglitazone (Actos) and rosiglitazone (Avandia) should have which laboratory test(s) monitored?
    a. BUN
    b. Cardiac enzymes
    c. Hemoglobin and hematocrit
    d. Liver enzymes

52. Herb-drug interaction must be assessed in patients taking herbs and antidiabetic agents. How do ginseng and garlic affect insulin or oral antidiabetic drugs?
    a. They can be taken with insulin without any effect, but can cause a hypoglycemic reaction with oral antidiabetic drugs.
    b. They can lower the blood glucose level, thus causing a hypoglycemic effect.
    c. They decrease the effect of insulin and antidiabetic drugs, causing a hyperglycemic effect.
    d. They may decrease insulin requirements.

53. What is/are the recommended guideline(s) for use of oral antidiabetics in patients with diabetes? *(Select all that apply.)*
    a. Diagnosis of diabetes mellitus for <10 years
    b. Fasting blood sugar <200 mg/dL
    c. Normal renal and hepatic function
    d. Onset at age 40 years or older
    e. Underweight patient

54. Which drug(s) or category(ies) of drugs will inter- act with a sulfonylurea? *(Select all that apply.)*
    a. Antacids
    b. Anticoagulants
    c. Anticonvulsants
    d. Aspirin
    e. Sulfonamides

55. What is/are contraindication(s) for the use of oral antidiabetic drugs? *(Select all that apply.)*
    a. Breastfeeding
    b. Pregnancy
    c. Renal dysfunction
    d. Severe infection
    e. Type 2 diabetes

Case Study

Read the scenario and answer the following questions on a separate sheet of paper.

K.C., 25 years old, has type 1 diabetes, which is normally well-controlled with daily insulin. He has been under increased stress recently due to preparing for defense of his thesis. His friends bring him into the emergency department because "he is acting funny." Before the triage nurse can ask his friends any further questions, they leave. Initially, K.C. is confused, complaining of a headache and has slurred speech. His glucose in triage reads "low" on the glucometer. While waiting to be taken to a treatment room, he becomes unresponsive.

1. What is a possible cause of his symptoms?

2. How will this be treated before he becomes unconscious?

3. What are treatment options after he loses consciousness?

53 Female Reproductive Cycle I: Pregnancy and Preterm Labor Drugs

Study Questions

Match the terms in Column I with the definitions in Column II.

Column I

_____ 1. Preeclampsia

_____ 2. Gestational hypertension

_____ 3. HELLP

_____ 4. L/S (lecithin/sphingomyelin) ratio

_____ 5. Eclampsia

_____ 6. Preterm delivery

_____ 7. Progesterone

_____ 8. Surfactant

_____ 9. Teratogens

_____ 10. Tocolytic therapy

Column II

a. New onset of seizures with preeclampsia

b. Prior to 37 gestational weeks

c. Drug therapy to decrease uterine muscle contractions

d. Maintains the uterine environment to nourish the blastocyst

e. Decreases the incidence of respiratory distress syndrome (RDS)

f. Hypertension during pregnancy

g. Gestational hypertension with proteinuria

h. Substances that cause developmental abnormalities

i. Predictor of fetal lung maturity and risk for neonatal RDS

j. *H*emolysis, *E*levated *L*iver enzymes, and *L*ow *P*latelet count

Match the letters of the substance in Column II with the associated adverse effects in Column I. Some substances may have more than one adverse effect.

Column I

_____ 11. Increased risk of spontaneous abortion

_____ 12. Smaller head circumference without catch-up

_____ 13. Hypertonicity, tremulousness in baby

_____ 14. Abruptio placentae and premature delivery

_____ 15. Degenerative placental lesions

_____ 16. Heavy use leads to shortened gestation

_____ 17. Decreased sucking reflex

_____ 18. Ataxia, syncope, vertigo

_____ 19. Altered facial features, mild to moderate mental retardation

Column II

a. Alcohol

b. Caffeine

c. Cocaine

d. Heroin

e. Marijuana

f. Barbiturates

g. Tobacco/nicotine

h. Tranquilizer

NCLEX Review Questions

Select the best response.

20. What maternal physiologic change(s) is/are seen during pregnancy that affect(s) drug dosing? *(Select all that apply.)*
    a. Decreased urine output
    b. Gastric motility is more rapid, resulting in faster absorption
    c. Increased fluid volume
    d. Increased glomerular filtration rate and rapid elimination of drugs
    e. Increased liver metabolism of drugs

21. The mechanism by which drugs cross the placenta is similar to the way drugs infiltrate which type of body tissue?
    a. Breast
    b. Liver
    c. Subcutaneous
    d. Uterine

22. What is/are the important factor(s) that determine(s) the teratogenicity of any drug ingested during pregnancy? *(Select all that apply.)*
    a. Dosage
    b. Duration of exposure
    c. Gastric motility
    d. Timing
    e. Urinary clearance

23. Surfactant is produced by type II alveolar cells in the lungs. Its purpose is to decrease surface tension and keep the alveoli open. What is the composition of surfactant? *(Select all that apply.)*
    a. Albumin
    b. Lecithin
    c. Progesterone
    d. Sphingomyelin
    e. Thiamine

24. What is the purpose of determining the L/S ratio?
    a. Determines the date of delivery
    b. Determines the maturity of the fetal lungs
    c. Determines the ratio of urine output/glomerular filtration rate
    d. Predictor of premature labor

25. The patient is in preterm labor at 28 weeks. The health care provider prescribes betamethasone 12 mg IM q24h × 2. The patient wants to know why she has to receive the medication. What is the nurse's best response?
    a. "Betamethasone will stop your labor."
    b. "It will help the fetus' lungs mature more quickly."
    c. "It will promote closure of a patent ductus arteriosus."
    d. "This medication will promote fetal adrenal maturity."

26. The patient has been diagnosed with gestational hypertension. What is/are the treatment goal(s) for this patient? *(Select all that apply.)*
    a. Decrease the incidence of preterm labor (PTL)
    b. Delivery of an uncompromised infant
    c. Ensure future ability to conceive
    d. Prevention of HELLP syndrome
    e. Prevention of seizures

27. The nurse works in a prenatal clinic. What is/are the most common complaint(s) she will see that will generate a request for medication? *(Select all that apply.)*
    a. Gastric acidity
    b. Headaches
    c. Nausea
    d. Vomiting
    e. Weakness

28. The patient has iron-deficiency anemia and is pregnant with her first child. Her health care provider has prescribed ferrous sulfate 325 mg b.i.d. Which laboratory value will show the first indication that she is responding to the iron supplement?
    a. Increased BUN
    b. Increased hemoglobin and hematocrit
    c. Increased reticulocyte count
    d. Increased INR

29. The patient is 16 weeks pregnant. She presents to her health care provider with nasal congestion, cough, and headache. She states, "I guess I just have a cold. What can I take for my cold to feel better?" What is the nurse's best response?
    a. "A combination of pseudoephedrine, aspirin, and diphenhydramine will work."
    b. "Acetaminophen should be safe to take for your headache."
    c. "Taking 1000 mg of vitamin C will shorten your symptoms."
    d. "Echinacea and garlic should help."

30. The patient presents to the clinic for her first prenatal visit with her entire family. She is a recent immigrant from Mexico and does not speak English. What priority action(s) will the nurse take to ensure culturally competent care? *(Select all that apply.)*
    a. Obtain a translator for her visit.
    b. Explain the importance of prenatal vitamins and their safety.
    c. Use a family member to translate.
    d. Hurry through the exam to stay on schedule.
    e. Provide extensive discharge instructions.

31. The patient presents to her health care provider with complaints of morning sickness. "I didn't have it with my first. I'm just not sure what to do." What nonpharmacologic measure(s) can the nurse suggest? *(Select all that apply.)*
    a. Avoid fatty or spicy foods.
    b. Avoid fluids before arising.
    c. Drink flat soda between meals.
    d. Eat crackers, dry toast, cereal, or complex carbohydrates.
    e. Eat a high-protein snack at bedtime.

32. The patient is in her third trimester and presents to her health care provider complaining of severe heartburn. What is/are some nonpharmacologic method(s) the nurse can suggest to help with her symptoms? *(Select all that apply.)*
    a. Avoid citrus juices.
    b. Avoid spicy foods.
    c. Do not lie down immediately after eating.
    d. Drink carbonated beverages.
    e. Eat smaller meals.

33. What is/are priority teaching goal(s) for a patient with gestational hypertension? *(Select all that apply.)*
    a. Discuss important symptoms to report to the health care provider.
    b. Explain to the patient the importance of weighing herself daily.
    c. Instruct the patient to lie on her right side.
    d. Stress the importance of adequate fluid intake.

34. The patient is in her first trimester of pregnancy. She has been started on a prenatal vitamin with iron. What priority teaching will the nurse provide for this patient? *(Select all that apply.)*
    a. Antacids can be taken with the iron tablet to help with epigastric discomfort.
    b. Ensure adequate fluid and fiber intake to assist with constipation.
    c. Iron can be taken with food if necessary to prevent nausea.
    d. Jaundice is a common side effect of iron supplements.
    e. Organ meats like liver are a good source of iron.

35. Which food(s) should the nurse recommend a pregnant woman eat to increase her iron intake? *(Select all that apply.)*
    a. Broccoli
    b. Cabbage
    c. Apples
    d. Potatoes
    e. Salmon

36. What is the recommended daily allowance of folic acid for a pregnant woman?
    a. 100-400 mcg
    b. 400-800 mcg
    c. 800-1200 mcg
    d. 1200-1600 mcg

37. Which is the most commonly ingested nonprescription drug during pregnancy?
    a. Acetaminophen
    b. Aspirin
    c. Diphenhydramine
    d. Ibuprofen

38. Which priority intervention(s) should the nurse implement for the patient receiving a beta-sympathomimetic drug? *(Select all that apply.)*
    a. Auscultate breath sounds every 4 hours.
    b. Encourage patient to sleep on her back.
    c. Have atropine available as a reversal agent.
    d. Monitor maternal vital signs every 5 minutes when receiving IV dose.
    e. Restrict all fluid.

39. Which nursing intervention(s) should a patient receiving magnesium sulfate for preeclampsia require? *(Select all that apply.)*
   a. Administer the loading dose as a bolus given IVP.
   b. Continuously monitor vital signs and fetal monitor.
   c. Encourage patient to ambulate in room to prevent blood clots.
   d. Have calcium gluconate available at the bedside.
   e. Monitor deep tendon reflexes (DTR).

40. What clinical manifestation(s) would the nurse assess in someone experiencing magnesium toxicity? *(Select all that apply.)*
   a. Absent DTRs
   b. Fever
   c. Muscle pain
   d. Rapid decrease in respiratory rate
   e. Tachycardia
   f. Weight gain

41. The patient is in labor and is receiving magnesium sulfate. She asks how long she will be on the medication. What is the nurse's best response?
   a. Until the time of delivery
   b. 4 hours postpartum
   c. 12 hours postpartum
   d. 24 hours postpartum

42. The patient is 38 weeks pregnant and is complaining of a sinus headache. Her blood pressure is 114/62 mm Hg, heart rate 88 beats/min, and respiratory rate 18 breaths/min. She has no edema and no protein in her urine. She tells the nurse that she always takes a combination medication when she gets headaches that contains aspirin, acetaminophen, and caffeine. What may occur with the use of aspirin late in pregnancy? *(Select all that apply.)*
   a. Decreased hemostasis in the newborn
   b. Increased maternal blood loss at delivery
   c. Increased risk of anemia
   d. Low–birth-weight infant
   e. Precipitous delivery

43. The patient is receiving magnesium sulfate for gestational hypertension. Which side effect(s) of this medication may be expected? *(Select all that apply.)*
   a. Dizziness
   b. Flushing
   c. Hyperreflexia
   d. Slurred speech
   e. Urinary incontinence

44. What is HELLP?
   a. A form of gestational diabetes
   b. Another acronym for premature rupture of membranes
   c. Disease process that occurs in mothers of multiples
   d. Severe sequela of preeclampsia

45. Which medication(s) may be beneficial in the treatment of gestational hypertension? *(Select all that apply.)*
   a. Furosemide
   b. Hydralazine
   c. Lisinopril
   d. Methyldopa
   e. Nifedipine

Case Study

Read the scenario and answer the following questions on a separate sheet of paper.

K.R., 40 years old, is pregnant with her fourth child. She is at 33 weeks gestation. She has had one miscarriage and has two living children, ages 15 and 9 years. It is 2100 on Friday night and her health care provider's office is closed, so she has left a message with the answering service. She contacts OB triage and states, "I think I may be having contractions, but I know I'm too early. My 15-year-old was born at 30 weeks, and I am so scared that this is happening again." She complains of lower abdominal tightening and back discomfort that comes and goes about every 8 minutes.

1. What are some priority questions for the nurse to ask?

2. What puts K.R. at high risk for PTL?

3. What are some nonpharmacologic measures to treat PTL? What are some pharmacologic options to treat PTL?

4. What needs to be done for the fetus at 33 weeks gestation?

54 Female Reproductive Cycle II: Labor, Delivery, and Preterm Neonatal Drugs

Study Questions

Crossword puzzle: Use the definitions to determine the correct terms.

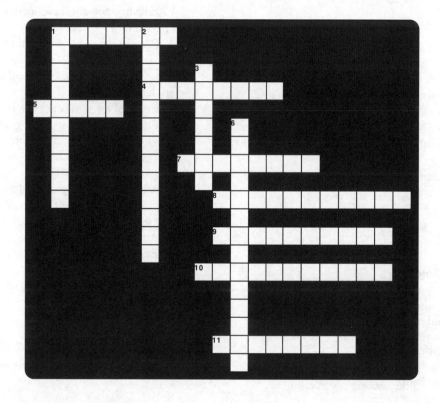

Across

1. Type of pain caused by pressure of the presenting part and stretching of the perineum and vagina
4. Type of anesthesia that achieves pain relief during labor and delivery without loss of consciousness
5. Receptors activated by morphine
7. Softening of the cervix
8. Scoring system to assist in predicting whether labor induction may be successful (2 words)
9. Commonly prescribed synthetic opioid for pain control during labor
10. Tightening and shortening of uterine muscles
11. Type of pain carried by sympathetic fibers from the cervix and uterus

Down

1. A lipoprotein in the alveoli that works to keep the alveoli open during expiration
2. Route of administration of surfactant used for rescue
3. Trade name of a drug used for labor augmentation
6. Uterine inactivity or hypotonic contractions (2 words)

NCLEX Review Questions

Select the best response.

12. The primary advantage of butorphanol tartrate (Stadol) and nalbuphine (Nubain) is their *dose ceiling effect*. What does this mean?
    a. Additional doses of the medication do not increase the degree of respiratory depression.
    b. Both of these medications must be given together to get the dose ceiling effect.
    c. Only one dose is administered to obtain the desired effect.
    d. This means that there is no limit as to how much of the drug can be used to obtain the desired effect.

13. The patient has received spinal anesthesia for delivery. What should the nurse monitor in this patient?
    a. Hemoglobin and hematocrit
    b. Palpitations
    c. Pedal edema
    d. Postdural headache

14. What is/are treatment(s) for postdural headaches? *(Select all that apply.)*
    a. Analgesics
    b. Bedrest
    c. Blood patch
    d. Caffeine
    e. Decreased fluids

15. When should pain medication be administered to the laboring patient using the IV route?
    a. At the beginning of the uterine contraction
    b. At the end of the uterine contraction
    c. Between uterine contractions
    d. In the middle of the uterine contraction

16. The patient has a history of heroin abuse and is in labor. Which medication is absolutely contraindicated for this patient?
    a. Hydroxyzine (Atarax)
    b. Meperidine (Demerol)
    c. Pentobarbital (Nembutal)
    d. Butorphanol tartrate (Stadol)

17. A baby was born within 15 minutes after his mother received pain medication and now has respiratory depression. Which medication is the best to provide reversal of neonatal respiratory depression?
    a. Calcium gluconate
    b. Calcium carbonate
    c. Flumazenil (Romazicon)
    d. Naloxone (Narcan)

18. Before administration of general anesthesia, a laboring woman is administered 30 mL of citric acid/sodium citrate (Bicitra). What is the purpose of giving this medication?
    a. Decrease gastric acidity
    b. Enhance anesthesia induction
    c. Maintain a patent airway
    d. Prevent nausea and vomiting

19. What should be done before administration of an epidural?
    a. Bolus of crystalloids, 500-1000 mL IV
    b. Preprocedural echocardiogram
    c. The patient's verbal consent to the procedure
    d. Type and crossmatch for blood administration

20. A patient is receiving an epidural, and her blood pressure is beginning to drop. What is the first action the nurse should take?
    a. Administer oxygen.
    b. Expect an order to administer 5-15 mg ephedrine IV.
    c. Expect an order to transfuse with 1 unit of packed red cells.
    d. Turn her on her left side.

21. Which value or greater on the Bishop score are associated with successful labor induction?
    a. 5
    b. 6
    c. 8
    d. 10

22. During which stage of labor do women commonly receive ergot alkaloids?
    a. First
    b. Second
    c. Third
    d. Fourth

23. Before administering methylergonovine

(Methergine), which baseline value should be
measured?
    a. Blood pressure
    b. Fetal heart rate
    c. Maternal hourly urinary output
    d. Respiratory rate

24. If a patient has received meperidine (Demerol) and
then receives a dose of naloxone, what will the
woman in labor experience?
    a. Increased pain relief
    b. Increased pain
    c. Increased fetal heart rate decelerations
    d. Increased fetal heart rate variability

25. The nurse is aware that many factors influence the
choice of pain control. What is the most important
factor?
    a. Amount of time likely until delivery
    b. Frequency of contractions
    c. Intensity of contractions
    d. Patient preference

26. What should the nurse know about the use of barbiturates in labor?
    a. Active labor is the most appropriate time for
    their use.
    b. Barbiturates make the delivery time
    unpredictable.
    c. The narcotic antagonists will counteract respira-
    tory depression.
    d. Narcotics offer more complete pain relief.

27. Which priority information should be included in
patient teaching about an analgesic during labor?
(Select all that apply.)
    a. Effects on labor
    b. Effects on newborn
    c. Expected time delivery will occur
    d. Methods of administration
    e. Restrictions placed on mobility

28. Which statement about the patient who receives
continuous lumbar epidural block anesthesia in repeated doses is accurate?
    a. Before 8-cm dilation, there is a risk of arresting
    the first stage of labor.
    b. Each time the injection procedure occurs, docu-
    mentation must be complete.
    c. Following injection, the patient needs to be
    placed flat immediately to ensure dispersion of
    the local anesthetic.
    d. The method is suitable for vaginal delivery, but
    not for a cesarean delivery, because the density
    of the block cannot be manipulated.

29. In relation to uterine contractions, how should spinal anesthesia be administered?
    a. Before
    b. During
    c. Immediately after
    d. 1-2 minutes after

30. The nurse assesses a patient receiving a local anesthetic for side effects. What should the nurse monitor for in this patient? *(Select all that apply.)*
    a. Dizziness
    b. Hypertension
    c. Metallic taste in mouth
    d. Nausea
    e. Palpitations

31. Which baseline data should the nurse collect on
a patient having an IV oxytocin induction at 41+
weeks gestation? *(Select all that apply.)*
    a. Deep tendon reflexes
    b. Fetal heart rate
    c. Pulse rate and blood pressure
    d. Type and crossmatch for blood
    e. Uterine activity

32. The nurse monitors a patient having an IV oxytocin
induction at 41+ weeks gestation for signs of uterine rupture. What would the nurse assess in a patient who has experienced uterine rupture? *(Select
all that apply.)*
    a. Hemorrhage
    b. Hypertension
    c. Loss of fetal heart rate
    d. Projectile vomiting
    e. Sudden increased pain

33. Which type(s) of systemic drug groups is/are used
during labor? *(Select all that apply.)*
    a. Antiepileptics
    b. Mixed narcotic agonists-antagonists
    c. NSAIDs
    d. Narcotic agonists
    e. Tranquilizers

34. The patient has received a sedative-hypnotic drug
and antiemetic/antihistamine for analgesia during
labor. This has placed the neonate at risk for which
alteration(s)? *(Select all that apply.)*
    a. CNS depression
    b. Decreased fetal heart rate variability
    c. Hypotonia
    d. Hypothermia
    e. Urinary retention

35. The patient is complaining of labor pain. This somatic pain is caused by pressure of the presenting part and stretching of the perineum and vagina. This pain is experienced in which stage(s) of labor? *(Select all that apply.)*
    a. First
    b. Latent
    c. Second
    d. Transition
    e. Third

36. Which type(s) of anesthesia may be used for cesarean deliveries? *(Select all that apply.)*
    a. Caudal block
    b. Epidural anesthesia
    c. General anesthesia
    d. Pudendal anesthesia
    e. Spinal anesthesia

37. A baby is born at 30 weeks gestation and is having respiratory distress. What type of medication will be given to help the baby's lungs?
    a. Antibiotics
    b. Benzodiazepines
    c. Calcium chloride
    d. Surfactant replacement

Case Study

Read the scenario and answer the following questions on a separate sheet of paper.

K.E., 22 years old, is at 38 weeks gestation and has intrauterine growth retardation (IUGR). She is scheduled for an induction.

1. What medications are used as induction agents, and what other methods may be used to induce labor?

2. What priority teaching instructions will the nurse provide on arrival to the hospital?

3. What analgesic options are available to K.E.?

55 Postpartum and Newborn Drugs

Study Questions

Crossword puzzle: Use the definitions to determine the correct terms.

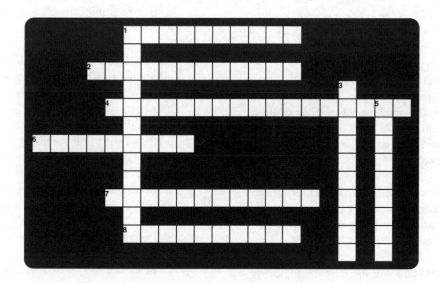

Across

1. The period from delivery until 6 weeks postpartum
2. Provides prophylaxis against eye infections
4. Syndrome where there is transmission of the rubella virus to the fetus via the placenta (2 words)
6. Skin rash caused by an allergic reaction
7. Skin inflammation resulting from contact with an irritating substance or allergen
8. Incision made to enlarge the vaginal opening to facilitate delivery

Down

1. Prevents hemorrhagic disease of the newborn
3. Local anesthetic that can be used for an episiotomy
5. Production and release of milk by mammary glands

NCLEX Review Questions

Select the best response.

9. Which is/are the most commonly used medication(s) for the relief of perineal pain resulting from episiotomy or laceration? *(Select all that apply.)*
   a. Benzocaine
   b. Erythromycin
   c. Mineral oil
   d. Tucks
   e. Witch hazel compresses

10. The nurse is administering a stool softener to a postpartum patient. The patient asks what the purpose/action of this medication is. What is the nurse's best response?
    a. "To decrease perineal discomfort and facilitate stool passage postdelivery."
    b. "To decrease the incidence of gas, thus decreasing perineal pain."
    c. "To decrease the need for eating fiber while in the postpartum period."
    d. "To make sure you have a bowel movement before discharge."

11. A postpartum patient with a repaired fourth-degree laceration has benzocaine topical spray. She asks if she can also use a heat lamp on her perineum for additional comfort. What is the nurse's best answer?
    a. "No, the heat lamp will increase the incidence of bacteria growth."
    b. "No, use of a heat lamp with benzocaine may cause tissue burns."
    c. "What a good idea; it will decrease pain while improving healing."
    d. "Yes, you can use a heat lamp to augment the action of benzocaine."

12. Relief of afterbirth pains may be a concern for the postpartum patient. Which factor(s) is/are associated with an increased risk of afterbirth pains? *(Select all that apply.)*
    a. Breastfeeding
    b. Multiparity
    c. Precipitous delivery
    d. Preeclampsia
    e. Primigravida

13. The patient has decided that she does not want to breastfeed and has asked the nurse for suggestions. What intervention(s) can the nurse implement to suppress lactation? *(Select all that apply.)*
    a. Have the patient drink sage tea every 6 hours
    b. Ice packs to breasts and axillae
    c. Tight, supportive bra
    d. Warm compresses
    e. Warm shower water directed to the breasts

14. When is the best time to administer the standard dose of Rh immune globulin D?
    a. After chorionic villus sampling and at 38 weeks gestation
    b. At 28 weeks gestation and again within 72 hours after delivery
    c. Before amniocentesis and at 38 weeks gestation
    d. Only at 28 weeks gestation

15. After which procedure should the patient receive a microdose of Rh immune globulin D?
    a. Abortion before 13 weeks
    b. Abortion after 16 weeks
    c. Amniocentesis
    d. Chorionic villus sampling

16. Which clinical manifestation(s) is/are commonly reported side effect(s) of the "-caine" drugs used in local or topical agents ordered for postpartum patients? *(Select all that apply.)*
    a. Burning
    b. Itching
    c. Petechiae
    d. Sloughing of tissue
    e. Stinging

17. Which clinical manifestation(s) is/are commonly reported side effect(s) of the hydrocortisone local or topical drugs used in products ordered with occlusive dressings for postpartum patients? *(Select all that apply.)*
    a. Alopecia
    b. Burning
    c. Folliculitis
    d. Itching
    e. Swelling

18. Which ophthalmic ointment is administered to the newborn immediately after birth?
    a. Bacitracin
    b. Erythromycin
    c. Gentamicin
    d. Penicillin

19. Which priority information should be included in patient teaching regarding ophthalmic and parenteral drugs administered to the neonate immediately after birth?
    a. Swelling of eyes usually disappears in the first 24-48 hours.
    b. All parenteral medications can be administered in one injection.
    c. The injection is not painful for the baby.
    d. If the mother has had hepatitis immunizations, the newborn will not receive the hepatitis B immunization.

Case Study

Read the scenario and answer the following question on a separate sheet of paper.

J.G., 32 years old, is 5 days postpartum from a vaginal delivery. She did not have an episiotomy but has a third-degree tear. She calls her obstetrics clinic and tells the nurse, "I just feel so overwhelmed. I hurt. I'm tired. I want to breastfeed, but I'm sore. I just don't know what to do."

1. What is the nurse's best response to these questions, and what interventions may the nurse suggest?

56 Drugs for Women's Reproductive Health and Menopause

Study Questions

Crossword puzzle: Use the definitions to determine the correct terms.

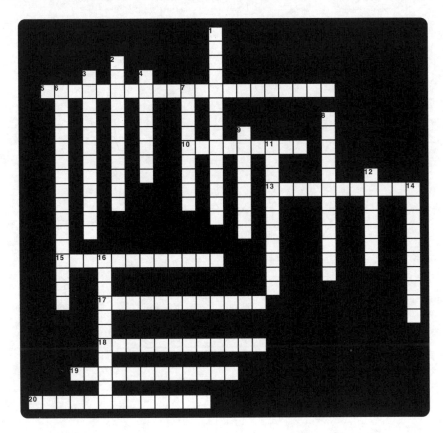

Across

5. Higher dose of estrogen increases the risk of this occurring (2 words)
10. Derivative of the steroid testosterone
13. Heavy periods
15. Painful periods
17. Loss of bone mass predisposing patient to fractures
18. Surgical removal of the ovaries
19. Medication that stops pregnancy in the uterus
20. Midcycle pain usually associated with ovulation

Down

1. Infrequent or very light menstruation
2. Painful sexual intercourse
3. Another name for emergency contraception (2 words)
4. Hyperpigmentation of the skin
6. The most commonly used synthetic estrogen (2 words)
7. The permanent cessation of menstruation
8. First marketed as RU486
9. The start of spontaneous menstruation
11. Another name for the progestin-only oral contraceptive pill (2 words)
12. Yeast microbe that causes vaginitis
14. Absence of periods
16. Drug given to cause the uterus to contract and expel the products of conception

NCLEX Review Questions

Select the best response.

21. The patient presents to her health care provider for an evaluation for contraception. She states, "My schedule is such a mess, and I get so busy. I don't know what would be the best method for me." Which contraceptive method(s) would be a good choice for this patient? *(Select all that apply.)*
    a. Depo-Provera injection
    b. Nexplanon
    c. NuvaRing
    d. Ortho-Evra patch
    e. Ortho-Novum 10/11

22. Which mode(s) of action is/are correct for emergency contraception? *(Select all that apply.)*
    a. Causes an abortion
    b. Delays ovulation
    c. Interferes with hormones for implantation
    d. Interferes with tubal transport of embryo
    e. Menstruation starts immediately to remove any products of conception

23. The patient wants to start oral contraceptives and want to know why she should use an oral contraceptive instead of another method. What does the nurse list as the advantage(s) of using oral contraceptives? *(Select all that apply.)*
    a. Ease of use
    b. High degree of effectiveness
    c. Low cost
    d. Relative safety
    e. You can't be allergic to oral contraceptives

24. Which individual should not take oral contraceptives?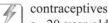
    a. 20-year-old who is not sexually active
    b. 40-year-old with diabetes
    c. 38-year-old with breast cancer
    d. 48-year-old with emphysema

25. In which patient(s) should combined hormone contraceptives (CHCs) be used with caution? *(Select all that apply.)*
    a. 37-year-old who smokes
    b. 45-year-old who does not exercise
    c. 38-year old with diabetes
    d. 28-year-old with epilepsy
    e. 18-year-old with depression

26. The patient works the night shift and realizes when she wakes up for work that she has missed a dose of her CHC. She calls the on-call nurse and asks what she should do. What is the nurse's best response?
    a. "It isn't a big deal. Just take one tomorrow."
    b. "Stop this pack and use alternative birth control for the next month."
    c. "Take your dose now, and then get back on schedule with the next one."
    d. "Take two now and use an alternative method of birth control."

27. A patient who has been taking Tri-Levlen for contraception reports a variety of side effects. Which clinical manifestation(s) is/are due primarily to an excess of estrogen? *(Select all that apply.)*
    a. Acne
    b. Breast tenderness
    c. Fluid retention
    d. Leg cramps
    e. Nausea

28. A patient who has been taking Tri-Levlen for contraception reports her current drug history. Which drug(s) will interact with her oral contraceptive? *(Select all that apply.)*
    a. Aspirin
    b. Fluoxetine
    c. Folic acid
    d. Phenobarbital
    e. Topiramate

29. Which laboratory value should be monitored closely in a patient who has been taking drospirenone (Yasmin) for contraception?
    a. Blood glucose
    b. Hemoglobin
    c. Potassium
    d. Thyroid-stimulating hormone

30. A patient who has been using NuvaRing for contraception calls and reports that the device fell out. What is the nurse's best advice?
    a. "Discard the current pill pack and start a new package of pills."
    b. "Do a home pregnancy test and report the results."
    c. "Rinse it off if it has been less than 3 hours and reinsert."
    d. "Throw it away and get a new one."

31. The family planning nurse would be correct to tell a patient to stop taking her combined oral contraceptive and notify her health care provider if she experiences which alteration?
    a. Increased vaginal discharge
    b. Severe headaches
    c. Lighter/shorter periods
    d. Menstrual cramping

32. The patient presents to her health care provider for contraceptive advice. She tells the nurse she does not like to take pills but does not want to get pregnant. What other option(s) can the nurse discuss with the patient? *(Select all that apply.)*
    a. Bioidentical therapy
    b. Condoms
    c. Diaphragm
    d. An intrauterine device (IUD)
    e. Nexplanon

33. What risk factor decreases with the use of progestin in hormone therapy (HT)?
    a Breast cancer
    b. Cervical cancer
    c. Endometrial cancer
    d. Endometrial hyperplasia

34. The patient is having complaints associated with menopause and presents to her health care provider to discuss HT. She states, "I just want to enjoy everything now and travel. I have too much to do to slow down with hot flashes and mood swings and taking a pill every day." The health care provider prescribes an estrogen patch (Estraderm transdermal system). What is an advantage of this system?
    a. It is absorbed directly into bloodstream.
    b. It is applied five times per week for 2 weeks using rotation of sites.
    c. It is less expensive than tablets.
    d. It results in fewer headaches.

35. Which medication(s) is/are used to treat osteoporosis? *(Select all that apply.)*
    a. Beta blockers
    b. Bisphosphonates
    c. Estrogen
    d. Progestins
    e. Selective estrogen receptor modulators (SERMs)

36. Which medication(s) is/are used in a medical abortion? *(Select all that apply.)*
    a. Ella
    b. Levonorgestrel
    c. Methotrexate
    d. Mifepristone
    e. Ovral

Case Study

Read the scenario and answer the following questions on a separate sheet of paper.

During her gynecology intake interview with the nurse practitioner at her company's new health care clinic, C.W., age 55 years, states, "I seem to be having more discomfort when I have intercourse. I don't lubricate when I want and need to; if my husband hurries me, it is downright painful. This is probably my problem, but my husband thinks that after a 35-year marriage, I just don't really want to have sex anymore."

The nurse compiles a few more facts about C.W. for review and consideration. In addition to her dyspareunia, C.W. has urinary frequency and urgency, itching, thinning vaginal epithelium with a glazed-looking appearance, and minimal elasticity upon speculum examination.

C.W. is Caucasian, is very thin, and reports no periods for nearly 2 years. She has no history of vaginal infections, and her hygiene is excellent.

1. Given this history, what does the nurse suspect is occurring, and what other history would be important to obtain regarding symptoms?

2. What treatment options can be offered to this patient?

3. What other health concerns should be discussed?

57 Drugs for Men's Health and Reproductive Disorders

Study Questions

Match the terms in Column I with the definitions in Column II.

Column I

_____ 1. Anabolic steroids

_____ 2. Androgen

_____ 3. Hirsutism

_____ 4. Spermatogenesis

_____ 5. Virilization

_____ 6. Antiandrogens

_____ 7. Cryptorchidism

_____ 8. Gynecomastia

_____ 9. Oligospermia

_____ 10. Priapism

Column II

a. Low sperm count

b. Undescended testis

c. Breast swelling or soreness

d. Ongoing painful erection

e. Growth of facial hair and vocal huskiness in women

f. Formation of spermatozoa

g. Steroid hormones related to the hormone testosterone

h. Testosterone

i. Blocks the synthesis or action of androgens

j. Increased hair growth

NCLEX Review Questions

Select the best response.

11. Of the following patients, which one should not receive sildenafil (Viagra)?
    a. 56-year-old with hepatitis
    b. 58-year-old with seizure disorder
    c. 62-year-old with renal insufficiency
    d. 68-year-old with unstable angina

12. The 17-year-old patient is receiving androgen therapy for hypogonadism. He asks the nurse what androgen therapy does. What is the nurse's best response?
    a. "It ensures the ability to respond sexually."
    b. "It ensures adequate sperm production."
    c. "It promotes larger stature through protein deposition."
    d. "It stimulates the development of secondary sex characteristics."

13. A 16-year-old wrestler at local high school tells the nurse during his annual sports physical that some of the athletes at his school use hormones to "bulk up" during the season. He wants to know if this is something he could do and if it is safe. What is the nurse's best response?
    a. "A safer way to bulk up is to eat an all-protein diet."
    b. "As long as they don't use other street drugs, this is probably safe."
    c. "This can cause serious, often irreversible, health problems even years later."
    d. "This is a safe practice as long as a health care provider adjusts the dose."

14. The patient is receiving androgen therapy. He has a history of cardiovascular disease, diabetes, and chronic obstructive pulmonary disease. What should the nurse be aware of with regards to his medications and his history?
    a. Androgens may decrease blood glucose levels, and insulin doses must be adjusted.
    b. Androgens decrease the effect of anticoagulants.
    c. Phenytoin potentiates the action of androgens.
    d. There are no interactions with steroids.

15. What is/are the indication(s) for androgen therapy in women? *(Select all that apply.)*
    a. Advanced carcinoma of the breast
    b. Delayed development of sexual characteristics
    c. Endometriosis
    d. Infertility
    e. Severe premenstrual syndrome

16. A teenaged male patient is receiving androgen therapy for hypogonadism. What side effect(s) might this patient experience? *(Select all that apply.)*
    a. Gynecomastia
    b. Continuous erection
    c. Deepening of voice
    d. Urinary urgency
    e. Visual disturbances

17. What is/are the indication(s) for antiandrogen medications? *(Select all that apply.)*
    a. Advanced prostatic cancer
    b. Erectile dysfunction
    c. Male pattern baldness
    d. Menopausal symptoms
    e. Benign prostatic hypertrophy (BPH)

Case Study

Read the scenario and answer the following questions on a separate sheet of paper.

H.H., 60 years old, has a history of diabetes and hypertension and presents to his health care provider. He states, "I'm really kind of embarrassed about this, but I can't satisfy my partner anymore. Could I get some of that medicine so I can keep an erection?"

1. What is erectile dysfunction, and how does it relate to the patient's history?

2. What class of medications is the patient referring to, and how does it work?

3. What are common side effects associated with this class of drugs?

4. What health teaching should the nurse provide for the patient regarding erectile dysfunction?

58 Drugs for Disorders in Women's Health, Infertility, and Sexually Transmitted Infections

Study Questions

Crossword puzzle: Use the definitions to determine the correct terms.

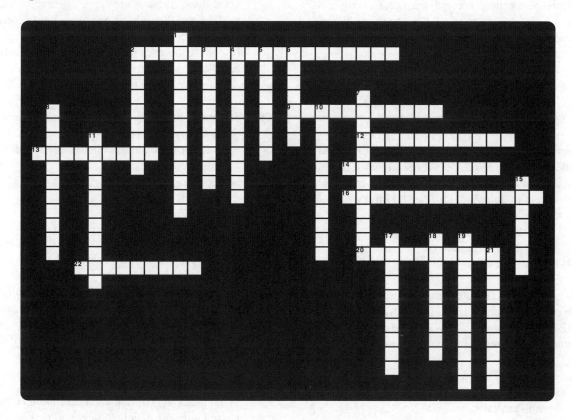

Across

2. Increased pigmentation and thickening of the skin (2 words)
9. Benign tumors in the uterus
12. Uterine bleeding greater than 80 mL or for more than 7 days occurring at regular intervals
13. What is in micronized progesterone that makes it contraindicated in some individuals (2 words)
14. Absence of ovulation
16. This type of drug suppresses ovulation and causes long-term endometrial atrophy
20. Absence of menses
22. A sexually transmitted infection (STI) that is treated with ceftriaxone plus either azithromycin or doxycycline

Down

1. Abnormal location of endometrial tissue outside the uterus
2. Drug used as primary therapy in the treatment of genital herpes
3. An STI for which a vaccine exists (2 words)
4. Herb taken to relieve depression (3 words)
5. A disease that is transmitted transplacentally
6. Resistance to this hormone is a hallmark of polycystic ovary syndrome (PCOS)
7. Pelvic pain that is associated with the menstrual cycle
8. Type of underwear men should use to improve male fertility (2 words)

(Continued next page)

10. Inability to conceive a child after 12 months of unprotected sex

11. A trade name for the gonadotropin-releasing hormone (Gn-RH) agonist leuprolide (2 words)

15. A drug that may be used to treat endometriosis

17. Drug of choice for the treatment of syphilis

18. Used in combination with estrogen to treat dysfunctional uterine bleeding

19. Herb that prevents progesterone overproduction and inhibits prolactin release

21. Most effective risk-reducing behavior for avoidance of STIs

NCLEX Review Questions

Select the best response.

23. The patient presents to the clinic complaining of dysuria and yellow-green discharge. Culture confirms *Neisseria gonorrhoeae*. Since this patient has presented with an STI, what other test should the patient be counseled to consider?
    a. Fasting blood sugar
    b. Fertility workup
    c. Human immunodeficiency virus (HIV) testing
    d. Liver panel

24. All recent sexual partners need to be informed of a patient's diagnosis of gonorrhea, and until reculturing demonstrates a cure, what will the nurse advise the patient to do prevent further STI transmission?
    a. Abstain or use condoms during sex.
    b. Ask partners to take antibiotics.
    c. Douche before intercourse.
    d. Only engage in anal intercourse.

25. The patient has repeatedly tested positive for gonorrhea, chlamydia, and human papillomavirus (HPV) and is being followed at the county health clinic. In teaching her about the transmission of STIs, the nurse is aware that which sexual activity can cause the most trauma?
    a. Genital-anal
    b. Genital-genital
    c. Oral-genital
    d. Mouth-to-mouth

26. The patient who has a history of repeated gonorrhea, chlamydia, and HPV asks how long she has to abstain from sex. What is the nurse's best response?
    a. "For at least two months."
    b. "Until the medications are finished"
    c. "Until your partner finishes his treatment."
    d. "You may have sex using condoms."

27. The patient asks if gonorrhea and syphilis are the same thing. What is the nurse's best response?
    a. "No, but if you have one, you should consider being tested for the other."
    b. "No, gonorrhea has no serious side effects."
    c. "No, only women get gonorrhea."
    d. "No, syphilis cannot be cured."

28. The patient is being treated for recurrent gonorrhea. She has just had a positive pregnancy test. Of the following medications, which is contraindicated?
    a. Amoxicillin
    b. Ciprofloxacin
    c. Duracef
    d. Zithromax

29. The patient wonders if her HPV will be cured. What is the nurse's best response?
    a. "Cryotherapy will cure your HPV."
    b. "HPV will go away on its own eventually with or without treatment."
    c. "Medications can eliminate recurrences."
    d. "The lesion can be removed, but the HPV cannot be cured."

30. The patient would like to know how HIV is spread. What method(s) of transmission should be discussed with the patient? *(Select all that apply.)*
    a. Breast milk
    b. Contact with infected blood
    c. Saliva
    d. Sexual contact
    e. Urine

31. What reason(s) is/are the most appropriate to justify the nurse asking a patient with repeated gonorrhea, chlamydia, and HPV if she would like to be tested for HIV? *(Select all that apply.)*
    a. Early detection is the best hope for cure.
    b. Repeated infections suggest immunocompromise.
    c. The nurse is required by law to do so.
    d. STIs indicate possible risky behavior.
    e. Treatment will prevent her from passing it on.

32. A married couple has a fertility workup, and the wife has been prescribed clomiphene citrate (Clomid). The nurse explains clomiphene citrate's action. How does the medication work to improve fertility?
    a. It normalizes prolactin levels.
    b. It replaces follicle-stimulating hormone (FSH).
    c. It stimulates luteinizing hormone (LH).
    d. It stimulates ovulation.

33. The patient has started taking clomiphene citrate (Clomid) for infertility. She inquires about the side effects of the medication. What is the nurse's best answer?
    a. "It can cause decreased appetite."
    b. "Mild insomnia may occur while taking this drug."
    c. "You will experience breast tenderness."
    d. "You will need to drink more fluid, as this drug will cause dehydration."

34. Which patient(s) should not be placed on clomiphene citrate? *(Select all that apply.)*
    a. 26-year-old with fibroids
    b. 28-year-old with depression
    c. 33-year-old who is pregnant
    d. 35-year-old with gastroesophageal reflux disease (GERD)
    e. 37-year-old with ovarian failure

35. What is the drug leuprolide (Lupron Depot) used to treat?
    a. Dysmenorrhea
    b. Endometriosis
    c. HIV
    d. Infertility

36. When teaching a patient about the correct use of nafarelin (Synarel Nasal Spray), which priority information should be provided? *(Select all that apply.)*
    a. Administer one spray in both nostrils b.i.d.
    b. Epistaxis is to be expected.
    c. Precise guidelines must be followed.
    d. The medication will be taken for 1 year.
    e. Use a nasal decongestant to increase absorption.

37. The patient has been sexually assaulted and presents to the emergency department for treatment. What antibiotic(s) will be prescribed as prophylaxis? *(Select all that apply.)*
    a. Cephazolin
    b. Ceftriaxone
    c. Doxycycline
    d. Erythromycin
    e. Metronidazole

Case Study

Read the scenario and answer the following questions on a separate sheet of paper.

K.E., 21 years old, presents to her health care provider with complaints of depression, weight gain, and headaches that appear to coincide with her menstrual cycle. She has been diagnosed with premenstsrual syndrome (PMS).

1. What is the difference between PMS and premenstrual dysphoric disorder (PMDD)?

2. What nonpharmacologic methods can be offered to the patient?

3. What medications might be beneficial, and why?

59 Adult and Pediatric Emergency Drugs

Study Questions

Match the condition in Column I with the drug that treats it in Column II.

Column I

___ 1. Anaphylactic shock

___ 2. Angina pectoris

___ 3. Opioid overdose

___ 4. Extravasation of dopamine

___ 5. Hypoxemia

___ 6. Torsades de pointes

___ 7. Premature ventricular contractions (PVCs)

___ 8. Atrial fibrillation

___ 9. Increased intracranial pressure

___ 10. Profound bradycardia with hypotension

___ 11. Paroxysmal supraventricular tachycardia (PSVT)

Column II

a. Magnesium sulfate

b. Diltiazem

c. Atropine sulfate

d. Mannitol

e. Phentolamine

f. Lidocaine

g. Nitroglycerin

h. Epinephrine

i. Oxygen

j. Adenosine

k. Naloxone

Match the drug in Column I with its classification in Column II. Answers may be used more than once.

Column I

___ 12. Nitroprusside

___ 13. Epinephrine

___ 14. Lidocaine

___ 15. Norepinephrine

___ 16. Vasopressin

___ 17. Mannitol

___ 18. Diltiazem

___ 19. Albuterol

___ 20. Furosemide

Column II

a. Antidysrhythmic, class IB

b. Diuretic

c. Calcium channel blocker

d. Catecholamine

e. Beta-adrenergic agonist

f. Antihypertensive

g. Exogenous antidiuretic hormone

NCLEX Review Questions

Select the best response.

21. Sublingual nitroglycerin may be prescribed for chest pain. What is the most important vital sign to assess before giving this drug?
    a. Blood pressure
    b. Heart rate
    c. Respiratory rate
    d. Temperature

22. Following administration of IV morphine to treat chest pain associated with acute myocardial infarction, what is the most important aspect of patient monitoring?
    a. Assessment of respiratory status
    b. Documentation of neurologic function
    c. Measurement and strict recording of intake and output
    d. Measurement of central venous pressure

23. Which is an emergency drug indicated for the treatment of symptomatic bradycardia?
    a. Atropine
    b. Epinephrine
    c. Lidocaine
    d. Nitroglycerin

24. When monitoring a patient with a dobutamine infusion, the nurse must be alert to the development of adverse effects. Which one may require slowing or discontinuing drug administration?
    a. Bradycardia
    b. Confusion
    c. Diaphoresis
    d. Myocardial ischemia

25. In which category is the drug vasopressin?
    a. Beta blocker
    b. Calcium channel blocker
    c. Hormone
    d. Nitrate

26. Which is an endpoint of IV procainamide administration?
    a. Headache
    b. Hypotension
    c. Respiratory depression
    d. Vomiting

27. Which dysrhythmia(s) is amiodarone IV used to treat? *(Select all that apply.)*
    a. Asystole
    b. Atrial fibrillation
    c. Bradycardia
    d. Second-degree heart block
    e. Ventricular fibrillation

28. What is the best indication for sodium bicarbonate?
    a. Metabolic acidosis
    b. Metabolic alkalosis
    c. Respiratory acidosis
    d. Respiratory alkalosis

29. The patient is admitted to the critical care unit after sustaining a severe closed head injury in a motorcycle collision. Mannitol (Osmitrol) is ordered to decrease intracranial pressure. Through which mechanism does mannitol exert its pharmacologic effects?
    a. Cerebral vasoconstriction
    b. Loop diuresis
    c. Osmotic diuresis
    d. Peripheral vasodilation

30. The patient presents to the emergency department after eating soup at a wedding reception. She is allergic to shellfish, and it is discovered that the soup was lobster bisque. She has hives and is anxious. Her tongue and lips are swollen. Which medication would be appropriate to administer to this patient in this situation?
    a. Atropine
    b. Diltiazem
    c. Diphenhydramine
    d. Lidocaine

31. An unresponsive patient presents to the emergency department in respiratory distress. Her friends say that she has been "using a lot of those pain pills for her back." Her pupils are pinpoint and her respiratory rate is 4 breaths/min. Which medication will the nurse be prepared to administer?
    a. Diltiazem 0.25 mg/kg IV piggyback
    b. Flumazenil 2.5 mg IV push
    c. Naloxone 0.4 mg IV push
    d. Magnesium 2 g IV piggyback

32. For which type(s) of shock should dopamine be administered? *(Select all that apply.)*
    a. Cardiogenic shock
    b. Hypovolemic shock
    c. Insulin shock
    d. Neurogenic shock
    e. Septic shock

33. Through which mechanism does dobutamine elevate blood pressure?
    a. Increasing cardiac output
    b. Positive alpha effects
    c. Vasoconstriction
    b. Vasodilation

34. The patient has a diagnosis of septic shock. A norepinephrine drip is infusing through a central IV line. The bag of norepinephrine is almost empty. For which reason should the nurse make it a priority to prepare a new bag?
    a. Hypertensive crisis can result if the infusion is interrupted.
    b. Profound hypotension can occur if the infusion is abruptly discontinued.
    c. The patient is at high risk for bradycardia and heart block.
    d. The organisms responsible for septic shock will proliferate.

35. For which reason is dextrose 50% most commonly prescribed?
    a. As a maintenance infusion to keep a vein open
    b. To increase urine output
    c. To treat hyperglycemia
    d. To treat insulin-induced hypoglycemia

36. What is the proper method of administering adenosine?
    a. Slow IV push
    b. Diluted in 50 mL as IVPB
    c. Rapid IV push as a bolus
    d. Via a nebulizer

37. What is a priority nursing action after administration of a total IV lidocaine dose of 2 mg/kg to an adult and the arrhythmia has been suppressed?
    a. A continuous infusion of lidocaine must be initiated to maintain a therapeutic serum level.
    b. A therapeutic serum level will be achieved and maintained.
    c. Additional bolus doses must be administered to achieve a therapeutic serum level.
    d. It is recognized that a lidocaine overdose has occurred.

38. The nurse is preparing to administer epinephrine 0.3 mg IM to a patient with an allergic reaction. Which solution should the nurse select?
    a. 1:10,000 solution of epinephrine
    b. 1:1000 solution of epinephrine
    c. 1:100 solution of epinephrine
    d. 1:1 solution of epinephrine

39. The patient is in cardiac arrest. To administer epinephrine 1 mg for IV injection, which solution should the nurse select?
    a. 1:10,000 solution of epinephrine
    b. 1:1000 solution of epinephrine
    c. 1:100 solution of epinephrine
    d. 1:1 solution of epinephrine

40. The lowest adult dose of atropine for heart block or symptomatic bradycardia is 0.5 mg IV. What happens at lower dosages?
    a. Paradoxical bradycardia can occur.
    b. Miosis occurs.
    c. The patient is at high risk for tachycardia.
    d. Vagal activity is completely blocked.

41. Flumazenil is used to reverse the effects of which drug type?
    a. Antipsychotics
    b. Benzodiazepines
    c. Opioids
    d. Paralytic agents

42. Magnesium sulfate is indicated for treatment of which alteration(s)? *(Select all that apply.)*
    a. Atrial dysrhythmias
    b. Hypokalemia
    c. Hypomagnesemia
    d. Refractory ventricular tachycardia
    e. Torsades de pointes

43. Furosemide exerts its effects on pulmonary edema through which mechanisms?
    a. Bronchodilation and diuresis
    b. Bronchodilation and antiinflammatory actions
    c. Vasoconstriction and diuresis
    d. Venodilation and diuresis

44. Which statement(s) best describe(s) epinephrine? *(Select all that apply.)*
    a. Epinephrine is a catecholamine.
    b. Indications for epinephrine include asystole and ventricular fibrillation.
    c. Metabolic acidosis decreases the effectiveness of epinephrine.
    d. The action of epinephrine is enhanced if it is infused through alkaline solutions such as sodium bicarbonate.
    e. Patients cannot be allergic to epinephrine.

45. Which priority nursing intervention(s) should be implemented when caring for a patient with a nitroprusside (Nipride) infusion? *(Select all that apply.)*
    a. Always use nitroprusside with a blue or brown color to the solution.
    b. Monitor blood pressure continuously.
    c. Stop the nitroprusside abruptly if side effects are experienced.
    d. Protect the solution from light.
    e. Monitor thiocyanate levels.

46. Which clinical manifestation(s) is/are commonly associated with atropine administration? *(Select all that apply.)*
    a. Dry mouth
    b. Miosis
    c. Mydriasis
    d. Urinary retention
    e. Vomiting

Case Study

Read the scenario and answer the following questions on a separate sheet of paper.

M.E., 48 years old, calls emergency medical services (EMS) with complaints of chest pain and shortness of breath. He has a history of angina, asthma, and obesity. He states, "It just hit me hard. I think I'm going to die." He has taken three of his own nitroglycerin tablets, and he is given oxygen, an aspirin, and morphine en route to the hospital. On arrival at the hospital, an electrocardiogram is obtained. M.E. is not having a myocardial infarction but is diagnosed with unstable angina and is admitted to the coronary care unit. Vital signs on admission are temperature 37.2° C, heart rate 88 beats/min, respiratory rate 20 breaths/min, and blood pressure 214/118 mm Hg. A nitroglycerin drip is started.

1. How does nitroglycerin work to treat a patient with angina?

2. Why was the patient administered aspirin, oxygen, and morphine en route to the hospital? Why was the nitroglycerin drip started?

Answer Key

Crossword Puzzle

Across
1. pharmaceutic
5. pharmacogenetic
6. pharmacokinetic
7. tachyphylaxis
10. half life
11. protein binding

Down
1. pharmacodynamic
2. antagonist
3. toxicity
4. receptor
8. agonist
9. placebo

12. e
13. d
14. b
15. a
16. f
17. c
18. d
19. c
20. a
21. b
22. c
23. c
24. b
25. d
26. b
27. b, c, e. The gastrointestinal tract is not considered vital to a patient in shock and hypotensive, so blood is shunted away and drug absorption is slowed. Blood flow is also slowed due to pain and stress, resulting in prolonged emptying time of the stomach.

28. c
29. b
30. b
31. b
32. a. A medication that has a half-life of 24 to 30 hours will be taken once daily to maintain a steady state.
33. d
34. b. A creatinine clearance level of 30 mL/minute indicates renal dysfunction. Many medications, including trimethoprim, are eliminated through the kidneys. To prevent toxicity, the dose would need to be decreased.
35. a
36. b
37. c
38. b
39. a
40. a, b, d, e. The nurse must be completely familiar with any medication he or she is administering. Information needs to be obtained not only on the medication, but also on the specific patient's history. Drug reference books, drug pamphlets/inserts, or a pharmacist may be consulted with questions.
41. b
42. c
43. a, b, c
44. a, b, d, e. The nurse should assess the patient for side effects (both desirable and undesirable) when administering medications. This is especially important for medications that have nonselective actions. The nurse must be familiar with the medication, including its dose range, desired effects, side effects, and adverse effects prior to administration. This information can be obtained from a variety of sources including current reference books, drug inserts, and pharmacists. If the drug has a narrow therapeutic range or requires peak/trough levels, these should be evaluated prior to administration. The appearance of side effects may occur immediately or up to several days after a dose. There is no set time to wait to see if side effects disappear. The health care provider should be notified as soon as possible after the appearance of side effects, especially if they are undesirable.

Case Study

1. The receptor theory states that drugs bind to receptor sites to either produce (initiate) or inhibit (block) a response. Some receptor sites are specific to only one medication, while others may accommodate several different medications. However, some "fit better" and are more active. The drug binding sites are located on cell membranes and are primarily protein, glycoprotein, phospholipids, and enzymes in nature. The four receptor families are kinase-linked receptors (enzyme), ligand-gated ion channels, G protein-coupled receptor systems, and nuclear receptors.

   Verapamil is a calcium channel blocker. Ligand-gated ion channels stretch across the cell membrane. If the channel is open, ions (usually calcium and sodium) can flow across the membrane. A calcium channel *blocker* prevents the flow of calcium. In the case of verapamil, this causes a decreased force of contraction, less spasm, and ultimately less anginal chest pain.

2. As with any new medication, the patient should be taught about how to take the medication (with or without food, timing during the day), what effects to expect and how soon to expect to see results, any undesirable side effects or adverse effects, and what to report to the health care provider. It is important to stress that the medication must be taken "as prescribed" even if the patient is feeling better or not feeling any changes because some medications work immediately and some medications may take several weeks to build up to a therapeutic level.

Chapter 2—
The Drug Approval Process

Crossword Puzzle

Across

3. digitalis
6. misfeasance
8. nonfeasance
10. codeine
11. brand

Down

1. VIPPS
2. malfeasance
4. iron
5. heroin
7. generic
9. amphetamines

12. b
13. d
14. c
15. a
16. d
17. d
18. c
19. b
20. d
21. a
22. b
23. c
24. c
25. d
26. d
27. d
28. a
29. a
30. b
31. c
32. a, c, d, e. Differences in appearance, either in the medication or the packaging, can be an indication of a counterfeit medication. However, it is important to remember that pharmacies may change their pharmaceutical supplier, so the drug may appear to be a different color or shape than the patient is used to. This is an opportunity for the nurse and the pharmacist to work together to provide patient education.

Case Study

1. The Health Insurance Portability and Accountability Act (HIPAA) sets the standards for maintaining patient confidentiality and delineates how PHI (protected health information) can be used. As it specifically pertains to his prescriptions and medications, the nurse will tell L.L. that his personal information will be shared with the pharmacist as it pertains to his care. The pharmacist will be able to discuss the medication and treatment with the patient in a separate counseling area, away from other patients.

Chapter 3—
Cultural and Pharmacogenetic Considerations

1. e
2. f
3. b
4. a
5. d
6. c
7. a
8. d

9. b
10. c. It is important for the nurse to recognize that people of African descent, which many Jamaicans are, use home remedies that have been passed down through generations. Clay is high in minerals such as calcium, iron, copper, and magnesium. Eating clay (geographia) or dirt is also considered a home remedy for nausea and vomiting associated with pregnancy.
11. d. Since the patient has consulted with a traditional healer, the patient may be more compliant with the drug regimen if he or she can continue to follow the guidance of the healer. Studies have not shown that sabila will help control glucose.
12. a, b, c
13. a, c, d, e

Case Study

1. The first concern for the nurse is the dose of erythromycin. A standard dose of erythromycin for this patient would be 800 mg per day. Assuming that the bottle contains enough for 10 days, the bottle would contain a little over 8000 mg. If the bottle is almost half empty, the patient has ingested 4000 mg. This is an overdose and puts the patient at risk for liver dysfunction. The health care provider should be notified immediately.
2. The family and patient should be approached in a quiet and calm manner, using a quiet voice, and allowing periods of silence. Should a translator be required, a professional translator or language line should be utilized to obtain further history. Many non-native English speakers of Asian descent will simply nod when asked questions to avoid showing disrespect. The parents may not have understood the exact amount (teaspoon) of the medication required and the spoon used in the home may have been what they used as a "teaspoon." To prevent any further misunderstandings regarding dosing, a syringe or measured spoon should be given at discharge or directions to the pharmacist to provide the same.

Chapter 4—
Drug Interactions and Over-the-Counter Drugs

Crossword Puzzle

Across
3. amphetamines
6. absorption
8. distribution
9. excretion

Down
1. FDA
2. biotransform
4. two
5. synergistic
7. OTC

10. c
11. d
12. a
13. b
14. e
15. a
16. b
17. a, c, d, f
18. a, b
19. b
20. a, b, e. It can be safe to take over-the-counter (OTC) medications and prescription medications at the same time. The health care provider should be consulted prior to the addition of OTC medications to the regimen. It is very important for the parents not to add multiple medications without consultation because many medications may have the same drugs in differing combinations or dosages.
21. a. Carbamazepine is a hepatic enzyme inhibitor that increases drug metabolism, so a larger dose of warfarin may be needed to achieve therapeutic levels.
22. c. Vitamin K and warfarin essentially work against each other. The patient is taking warfarin to prevent clots that may occur due to atrial fibrillation, and vitamin K is required to help the blood clot.
23. b. The purpose of a laxative is to increase gastric motility and decrease transit time. There will be decreased absorption of the drug due to decreased time in the stomach for absorption.
24. a. Concurrent use of calcium-containing products may prevent the absorption of some fluoroquinolones like ciprofloxacin (Cipro).
25. a
26. a
27. d
28. b
29. d
30. b. Diuretics such as furosemide decrease the reabsorption of water, sodium, and potassium. Too great a loss of potassium (hypokalemia) can enhance the action of digitalis and lead to digitalis toxicity. Diuretics are to be taken on a regular basis and not only when the patient feels symptoms. Some studies have shown an interaction between digoxin and grapefruit juice, but not an interaction with cranberry juice.
31. d
32. b

33. c. To help prevent a drug-induced photosensitivity reaction, the patient should use sunscreen when outdoors. There is no need to remain indoors during daylight hours, and increasing vitamin C intake will not have an effect. Medication should be taken as prescribed by the health care provider.

34. a, b, c, d. A patient with a history of impaired renal function should avoid acetaminophen, aspirin, ibuprofen, and quinidine. Valproic acid should not be taken by patients with any hepatic disorders.

35. d

36. b. Propranolol can be used for migraines; however, it is not safe to use when the patient is also taking a calcium channel blocker. Bradycardia may result.

Chapter 5—
Drugs of Abuse

Crossword Puzzle

Across
2. drug addiction
6. relapse
7. cocaine
9. nicotine
11. cue-induced cravings

Down
1. drug misuse
2. drug abuse
3. detoxification
4. intoxication
5. tolerance
8. abstinence
10. bupropion

12. b
13. a
14. d
15. c
16. a
17. b. Cocaine-induced dysrhythmias are possible with the combination of tricyclic antidepressants. Dysrhythmias are also a concern in a patient taking digitalis or methyldopa (Aldomet).
18. c
19. a
20. a, c, e. A patient must be ready and motivated to quit any addictive substance or the likelihood of success is decreased. This is a difficult process that will require the patient's commitment. Certain triggers, like places where a person smokes or times that trigger the craving for a cigarette, should be identified and alternatives determined. There are a variety of aids, both prescription and nonpre-

scription, that can be utilized to help a patient quit smoking. Ideally, a quit date of two weeks should be set so the patient stays motivated. Tobacco in any form is still addictive, so chewing tobacco or smoking tobacco in a pipe instead of a cigarette are still abusing tobacco. Although it is difficult, some patients prefer to quit smoking "cold turkey" or without the use of aids.

21. b
22. d

Case Study

1. Even though the patient appears to be intoxicated, other causes of his unresponsiveness need to be evaluated. The patient's respiratory rate is insufficient and his respirations must be assisted. There is no antidote for alcohol intoxication other than supportive care. Should opiate abuse be suspected (evaluate for pinpoint pupils), a medication such as naloxone could be administered. If a benzodiazepine overdose is suspected, flumazenil (Romazicon) could be administered. It will be important for the nurse to assess the time of the patient's last drink, since alcohol withdrawal may start as early as 4 to 6 hours, peak at 24 to 36 hours, and last as long as 5 days.

2. Alcohol withdrawal is a serious medical concern and death can result. Seizures are possible and most frequently occur between 7 to 48 hours after the last drink. Delirium is also common. Withdrawal can be treated either with chlorodiazepoxide (Librium) or lorazepam (Ativan). Wernicke's encephalopathy may appear very similar to alcohol intoxication. It is imperative that the patient receive thiamine supplementation prior to administration of any dextrose to prevent the development of Wernicke's encephalopathy. Thiamine must also be continued at a dose of 100 mg/day until the patient is taking in adequate nutrition, either orally or enterally.

Chapter 6—
Herbal Therapies

Crossword Puzzle

Across
2. sage
7. saw palmetto
9. evening primrose
10. cranberry
11. garlic
12. milk thistle

Down

1. dong quai
3. valerian
4. ginger
5. bilberry
6. feverfew
8. peppermint

13. d
14. a
15. e
16. b
17. c
18. g
19. f

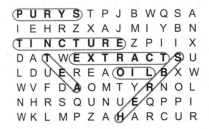

20. syrup
21. tea
22. tincture
23. extracts
24. oil
25. herbs
26. d
27. g
28. h
29. j
30. a
31. f
32. b
33. c
34. e
35. i
36. a
37. a
38. c
39. c
40. a. Kava may be used to promote sleep and relaxation; however, the FDA issued a consumer warning in 2002 about the risk of liver damage from kava use.
41. a, b, c, d
42. a, d. The nurse should assess for presence of edema and hypertonia as well as complaints of insomnia in a patient he or she suspects may have ginseng abuse syndrome.
43. b, d. Large quantities of any one herbal product can lead to an "overdosage" of that product. Since specific doses and quantities are not regulated in

this country, it is difficult to determine the correct amount. More is not necessarily better. Infants and children should not receive herbal preparations due to the lack of standardization and testing in a pediatric population.
44. a, b, e
45. a, b, c
46. a, b, d. The effects of antihypertensive medications may be decreased. Since licorice may have similar effects to aldosterone and corticosteroids, the effects of corticosteroid medications may be increased. Taking licorice with digitalis may increase the effects of digitalis and lead to digitalis toxicity.

Case Study

1. The most commonly utilized herbal preparation for migraine headaches is feverfew. It is believed that this preparation may inhibit platelet aggregation and act as a serotonin antagonist, which may help in vascular and migraine headaches. Feverfew may also help with nausea and vomiting. Ginger is another herbal preparation that may help in the treatment of migraine headaches and the associated nausea. Although researched, the mechanism of action is unclear. St. John's wort may be taken for mild depression and anxiety, but it is not effective in treating headaches. St. John's wort has not been shown to be effective in moderate or severe depression; in fact, when combined with an SSRI, there is a higher risk for suicide. The mechanism of action is unknown.

2. Ginger interacts with antiplatelet and anticoagulant medications. Feverfew also interacts with antiplatelet and anticoagulant medications. St. John's wort has interactions with many drugs, including central nervous system (CNS) depressants, selective serotonin reuptake inhibitors (SSRIs), and oral contraceptives.

3. As with any herb or medication, the patient should be encouraged to keep a list of her medications and dosages. Although many people believe herbs are automatically "safe" since they are natural, this is not always the case. Herbal preparations do not pass through an FDA approval process as medications do, so strength, amount of filler, and impurities may vary. Herbal preparations may also vary from one company to another, so the patient should be encouraged to continue to obtain it from the same reliable source or company.

Chapter 7—
Pediatric Pharmacology

1. fewer; lower
2. age; health status; weight; route of administration

3.   1; 3
4.   body fluid composition; tissue composition; protein-binding capability
5.   2 years; higher
6.   e
7.   d
8.   a
9.   b
10.   c
11.   a
12.   c. The dosage for a water-soluble medication may need to be increased in this age group because their bodies are about 70% water up until age 2 years. Therefore, there is more water in which the medication will be distributed.
13.   d
14.   a
15.   a, b, c, d
16.   a, b, c, e. In early adolescence, renal tubular function decreases, which may lead to impaired excretion and a higher risk for toxicity. Dehydration may also lead to toxicity. Since the patient is nauseated and vomiting, medications should not be administered orally. When providing care to any patient, developmental levels should be considered.
17.   b, c, d, f. If necessary, a child may be lightly restrained but should not be forcibly held down. The child should be praised for taking the medication. At no time should a child be threatened, forced, or made to view the medication as punishment. Depending on the developmental level of the child, explanations should be given to the child about what to expect, but the child should not be given the option of debating whether to take the medication. Herbal preparations are not usually given to children; however, cultural traditions should be respected as much as possible.

Case Study

1.   Preschoolers may respond to the use of hypnosis or creative imagery. They may also benefit from a familiar toy or stuffed animal as support. Allow the child to verbalize that she is scared or upset. Do not argue with the child or tell the child that she is being punished for falling from the tree. Tell the child what you are going to do before you do it. Do not just surprise the child.
2.   A topical anesthetic like eutectic mixture of local anesthetics (EMLA) or lidocaine, epinephrine, and tetracaine (LET) may be utilized to lessen the pain of establishing an IV. The downside to using these topical anesthetics is that they must be in place 60 to 90 minutes before the IV can be started for them to be effective.
3.   Caregivers may be involved in patient care (if they choose to be) by helping gently restrain the child.

They can also provide distraction ("What color sling would you like?" or "What should we have to eat tomorrow morning when we get up?"). Reassuring the preschooler that she is doing a good job holding still can also be beneficial.

Chapter 8— Geriatric Pharmacology

Crossword Puzzle

Across
2.   absorption
4.   distribution
6.   diuretics
8.   polypharmacy
10.   nonadherence

Down
1.   digoxin
3.   biotransformation
5.   kidneys
7.   laxatives
9.   adherence

11.   a
12.   b. Higher doses of certain antihypertensives like hydrochlorothiazide (HCTZ) can cause various electrolyte imbalances that may be life-threatening.
13.   b. Digoxin has a long half-life and may accumulate in the geriatric patient. Bradycardia (heart rate less than 60 beats/minute), nausea, vomiting, and visual changes may be an indication of digitalis toxicity.
14.   a. There is no reason that the patient cannot work outside if he is taking digitalis, and the patient's symptoms are not related to the digitalis. Diphenhydramine can be very sedating in the geriatric population, and there are substitutes that are equally effective with fewer side effects. Fluoxetine, an SSRI, is prescribed for depression. Patients of all ages should be advised not to take one another's medications.
15.   c. Drugs with a shorter half-life and less protein binding would have fewer side effects. There are fewer protein binding sites in older adults, resulting in more circulating drug. Because of less effective functioning of both hepatic and renal metabolism, drugs with a shorter half-life are safer.
16.   a, b
17.   d. Dizziness when going from a supine to a standing position is referred to as *orthostatic hypotension*. Although bradycardia may cause dizziness, this is not the most likely cause.

18.   a. Changing positions slowly should assist in decreasing the dizziness associated with hypotension related to changes in position. Taking a deep breath and checking his heart rate will not affect his dizziness. Having a chair close to the bed may be beneficial if the patient feels dizzy but may also pose a safety risk. If the patient faints, he may strike the chair as he falls.

19.   c. When a person has been hospitalized, a medicine reconciliation has been completed. Depending on the patient's response, medications may be added to or subtracted from the regimen and dose adjustments may be made. The patient should take only those medications that have been prescribed at discharge.

20.   b. The patient was discharged from the hospital with a new dosage of her medication. She should take digoxin 0.25 mg/day as prescribed. The pharmacist can be a resource; however, the medication should be taken as prescribed.

21.   a. Although a family member could assist with the daily medication regimen, the patient will be able to maintain more independence using a non-childproof cap. Using a non-childproof cap should make the container easier for the patient to grasp and open.

22.   b. Maintaining independence for as long as possible is crucial for a geriatric patient. A patient who has visual challenges can, with assistance, fill a medication-dispensing container for the upcoming week. The patient must have assistance in the setup to assure that the correct medications are in each separate compartment. Leaving the medication bottles on the counter could lead to a mix-up if they are displaced. Writing down which medications need to be taken is not beneficial if the patient has visual challenges. The patient does not forget what medications need to be taken, but is unable to clearly see which medication is to be taken at which time.

23.   b, e

24.   a, c, d, e. Of the listed factors, only height does not have a role in dosage adjustment. Older adults have more adipose tissue, so a greater amount of lipid-soluble medication would be absorbed. Protein is required for binding of some medications, so if a patient is malnourished there would be less protein available. Laboratory results, specifically those that assess renal and hepatic function, are important to trend, as well as those drug levels (digoxin, INR) needed to measure toxicity. As with any population, it is important to evaluate the patient for responsiveness to the medication.

25.   a, b, d, e. Older patients have less protein available for binding, so it is important to know if a drug is highly protein bound. Drugs with a short half-life

are less likely to cause problems for the patient. Certain drugs (some antibiotics, digoxin, warfarin) have very narrow therapeutic ranges, so they must be monitored closely. Vital signs may vary as a patient ages; therefore, it is important to obtain baseline vital signs to know the patient's norm.

Case Study

1.   Since both renal and hepatic function are important in drug metabolism and excretion, and both decrease with aging, the nurse would anticipate liver enzymes, BUN, creatinine, and creatinine clearance would be ordered. Since this patient also has diabetes, the patient's blood glucose will be evaluated.

2.   There are a variety of sleep aids besides triazolam (Halcion) that could be utilized. Since this patient is also taking a diuretic, it would be important to suggest the patient take her diuretic in the morning to prevent frequent awakenings during the night to go to the bathroom. Some nonpharmacologic measures include warm baths, decreasing stimulation in the evening, and eliminating caffeine late in the day. The patient also states that she likes chamomile tea, which may help induce sleep. A light bedtime snack will help maintain blood sugar throughout the night.

3.   The nurse should recognize and support the patient's desire to be compliant with her medication regimen; however, the patient does need further education about "doubling up" on medications. A variety of methods can be used to help the patient remember to take her medication. These can include commercial pill dispensers, making a list, keeping a calendar, or setting an alarm.

Chapter 9—
Collaboration in Community Settings

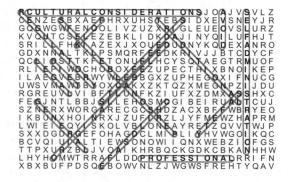

1.   professional; legal; regulatory
2.   avoid
3.   general; diet; self-administration; side effects; cultural considerations

4.   safety
5.   original-labeled; child-safe
6.   personal beliefs
7.   traditional; folk
8.   c. The nurse should provide contact information so that if any questions arise, they may be addressed. Waiting until the next appointment is a safety issue, and the patient must be reassured that it is important to call with questions.
9.   a. The medication regimen varies from patient to patient. Although some medication is only taken once per day and can be taken with other medications, the set dosing will be prescribed by the health care provider.
10.   a, b, c, e
11.   d. Patients who are allergic to any medications should wear some kind of Medic-Alert identification and carry a wallet card indicating the allergies. Receiving an annual flu shot is important for all patients, not just those on medications or with medication allergies.
12.   d
13.   c. Self-care centers are best suited to handle minor situations without the potential for a serious condition or for the patient to deteriorate.
14.   b
15.   a, b, c, e

Case Study

1.   The most common medications administered now to the school-age population are medications for asthma and attention deficit/hyperactivity disorder (ADHD), and OTC medications such as acetaminophen.
2.   The school nurse must have a legal, written prescription from the health care provider to administer the medication. The medication must be presented in a pharmacy-labeled bottle or sealed OTC bottle, and there must be written consent from the legal guardian to administer the medication. Safety is paramount when administering medications in a school setting. The nurse's actions will be governed by the nurse practice act for the state. There must be written policies, procedures, and guidelines to follow, and there must be a formal medication record. With regards to the medications themselves, they must be kept in a secured area accessible only to those staff members who are dispensing the medications. There must be a sharps container for any needles and biohazard bags for any contaminated materials.
3.   To ensure that culturally competent care is provided, respect should be shown to all involved. When offering a prescription, instructions, or pamphlets, use both hands to show respect. Recognize that traditional medicine must be respected as long as it does not conflict with the legal duties of the nurse in providing care to the student.

Chapter 10— The Role of the Nurse in Drug Research

1.   d
2.   a
3.   g
4.   b
5.   c
6.   f
7.   e
8.   i
9.   j
10.   h
11.   k
12.   e
13.   a
14.   g
15.   f
16.   d
17.   c
18.   b
19.   a
20.   c
21.   a
22.   c
23.   b
24.   c
25.   c
26.   a, b, d, e
27.   a, b, d. The role of the research nurse is to help protect the patient from harm. Answering questions that the patient may have about the process is part of informed consent. This is the role of the health care provider; however, the nurse is also responsible for ensuring that the patient's questions are answered and that the patient is not coerced into participating in a study. The patient is given a copy of the signed consent form along with the assurance that he or she may withdraw from the study at any time without prejudice. Some studies provide financial compensation, but this is not a requirement. A copy of the institutional review board (IRB) proposal is not given to the patient, but the purpose of the study is discussed. The results of the study may or may not be shared with participants at a later time.

Case Study

1.   A *double-blind* trial means that both the participant and the researcher are "blinded" to the treatment. Neither one knows whether the patient is receiv-

ing the drug or a placebo. Patients are either in the study group that receives the drug or in the control group. The control group is matched to the study group using several characteristics like gender, age, or weight. The double-blind study is designed to prevent bias.

2. There are many factors that might prevent a drug from moving from phase II to phase III. If the drug is found to be ineffective in treating patients with the disease or condition it is designed for, it would not move forward to phase III. If the drug is found to be harmful or dangerous in any phase, it would not move to the next phase. The fact that there have been several minor side effects does not mean that the drug will not move to phase IV.

Chapter 11—
The Nursing Process in Patient-Centered Pharmacotherapy

1. b
2. a
3. c
4. a
5. d
6. a
7. e
8. d
9. d
10. a
11. e
12. b
13. a
14. b
15. a
16. b
17. a
18. a
19. d
20. a
21. c
22. c
23. b
24. b
25. d
26. b
27. c
28. c

Case Study

1. The assessment phase of the nursing process for this patient would include not only subjective and objective data, such as a patient history and physical examination, but also reviewing current medications and allergies. Other items to assess include

the home environment and, most importantly, the patient's readiness to learn. If any laboratory tests are available, these should also be reviewed.

The next phase in the nursing process is the development of nursing diagnoses. These are based on actual concerns discovered in the assessment phase or potential problems due to risk factors that arise in the assessment. The patient's statements suggest several potential diagnoses, including those related to anxiety, knowledge deficit, and noncompliance.

In the planning phase, patient-centered, measurable goals are established in collaboration with the patient, family, and other members of the health care team. The goals must be realistic and measurable and occur in a certain time frame. A realistic goal for this patient could include something that addresses the need to prepare and administer insulin properly and accurately.

During the implementation phase, the nurse provides the education necessary for the patient to be able to achieve the goal. In this situation, the teaching needs to address several areas, including the psychomotor skill of preparing and administering an insulin injection. A demo-return demo scenario could be utilized. The nurse must also educate the patient and family about insulin and the side effects/adverse reactions to report. The importance of proper diet and the need to eat after taking insulin is a key safety point. The patient and family also must be educated on signs and symptoms of hypoglycemia. Adequate time for questions must be provided, as well as contact information for the health care provider. The nurse must ensure that the patient is ready to learn, the material is presented in an appropriate manner for learning to occur, and the materials are culturally appropriate.

The final step in the nursing process is evaluation. The goal must be evaluated and changes made if necessary. Was the patient able to demonstrate insulin administration? Did the patient have problems with anxiety surrounding the administration? Was the patient able to verbalize concerns to the health care provider? From a purely objective standpoint, were the patient's blood glucose levels within the prescribed range?

Chapter 12—
Safety and Quality in Pharmacotherapy

1. c
2. f
3. j
4. g

5. a
6. h
7. b
8. d
9. e
10. i
11. a
12. a
13. b
14. a
15. b
16. a
17. c
18. d
19. a
20. e
21. b
22. c. Antibiotics must be taken at regularly spaced intervals to maintain therapeutic blood levels.
23. b
24. c
25. c. A nurse must never administer a dose that seems large or out of range without rechecking the calculations. If there continues to be a question, another nurse could double-check the dose as well.
26. c, e
27. a. The nurse's first action is to document the refusal immediately. It is important to remember that the refusal to take a medication is the patient's right. The nurse should determine the patient's reasoning behind refusing to take a medication and stress the importance of the mediation regimen. The health care provider should be notified of the refusal.
28. b, c, d, e
29. b, d, e

Chapter 13—
Medication Administration

1. Enteric-coated; timed-release
2. fine-sized particle
3. semi- or high Fowler's
4. 50
5. 20
6. c
7. a
8. b
9. ventrogluteal
10. vastus lateralis
11. deltoid
12. gluteal
13. dorsogluteal
14. c
15. a
16. d

17. c
18. a. Over-the-counter medications and herbal preparations may interact with prescription medications. Patients must be encouraged to discuss the use of these preparations with their pharmacist or health care provider.
19. a, b, e
20. b. The patient should rinse out the mouth after administering a dose from a metered-dose inhaler. This will help prevent secondary infection and irritation.
21. b, d

Chapter 14—
Medications and Calculations

Section 14A

1. b
2. f
3. g
4. c
5. k
6. l
7. m
8. r
9. d
10. e
11. h
12. q
13. p
14. i
15. o
16. a
17. n
18. j
19. A. 1000 mg; B. 1000 mL; C. 1000 mcg
20. 3000 mg
21. 1500 mL
22. 100 mg
23. 2.5 L
24. 0.25 L
25. 0.5 g
26. 4 pints
27. 32 fl. oz
28. 48 fl. oz
29. 2 pints
30. 16 fluid drams
31. grams to milligrams
32. 1000 mg; 15 gr
33. 0.5 g; 7½ gr
34. 100 mg; 1½ gr
35. 60 or 64 mg
36. $\frac{1}{150}$ gr
37. 1 L; 1 qt
38. 8 fl. oz; 1 medium-sized glass

39.   1 fl oz; 2 T; 6 t
40.   1 t
41.   1½ fl oz; 9 t
42.   150 mL; 10 T

Section 14B
1.   d
2.   b
3.   a
4.   250 mg per 5 mL
5.   d
6.   A. d; B. b
7.   A. a; B. b
8.   A. d; B. b
9.   d
10.   b
11.   A. b; B. a
12.   b

Section 14C
1.   c
2.   b
3.   A. a; B. b
4.   a
5.   c
6.   A. a; B. a
7.   A. a; B. d
8.   A. c; B. c
9.   A. c; B. c
10.   d. This lithium level is too high, and adjustments need to be made. Withhold the dose and contact the health care provider.
11.   A. b; B. c
12.   A. a; B. a
13.   a
14.   b
15.   c
16.   c. The nurse should acknowledge the patient's concerns and provide an appropriate answer. The first two responses negate the patient's concerns, while the last response is incorrect.
17.   b
18.   b
19.   b
20.   e
21.   b
22.   a

Section 14D
1.   b, c, d, e
2.   c, d
3.   self-sealing rubber tops; reusable if properly stored
4.   a, b
5.   is not
6.   units
7.   a

8.   c
9.   b
10.   b
11.   c
12.   d
13.   A. a or b (as long as the dose is calculated accurately); B. c
14.   a
15.   c
16.   Withdraw 36 units of Humulin L insulin.
17.   A. First withdraw 8 units of Humulin R (regular) insulin and then 44 units of Humulin N (NPH) insulin. Total: 52 units of insulin. B. c; the regular insulin should be drawn up first.
18.   b
19.   A. a; B. a
20.   b
21.   A. c; B. c
22.   b
23.   c
24.   b
25.   A. 2.7, 500; B. c
26.   A. 1.8, 2; B. a
27.   d
28.   c
29.   A. 2, 2.6; B. b
30.   A. c; B. d; C. b
31.   b
32.   c

Section 14E
1.   a, b, c
2.   c
3.   10-20 gtt/mL; 60 gtt/mL
4.   microdrip set
5.   keep vein open; 250-mL IV bag
6. D_5W
7.   NSS or 0.9% NaCl
8. D_5½ NSS, 5%D/½ NSS, or 5%D/0.45% NaCl
9. D_5LR or 5%D/LR
10.   small; short
11.   calibrated cylinder with tubing; intermittent IV drug administration
12.   volumetric
13.   uniform concentration of the drug, patient control and ownership of the pain
14.   27-28 gtt/min
15.   31-32 gtt/min
16.   A. b; B. 83 gtt/min
17.   A. 1000 mL; B. 2500 mL; C. 100 mL/hr (104 mL/hr); D. macrodrip set; E. 16-17 gtt/min
18.   A. e; B. 27-28 gtt/min
19.   A. c; B. c
20.   A. 10 mL of sterile water; B. 1 g = 10 mL; C. b
21.   A. 6.6 mL; B. 2 g = 8 mL; C. b
22.   A. c; B. b

23. A. 4 mL of sterile water; B. 1 g = 4 mL; C. c; D. c
24. A. a; B. c
25. A. 7.5 mL; B. c
26. A. 1.6 mL; B. b
27. A. c; B. c
28. a
29. A. b; B. b
30. A. b; B. b

Section 14F

1. A. b; B. d
2. A. b; B. d
3. A. a; B. b
4. c
5. A. a; B. b
6. b
7. b
8. A. b; B. a; C. e
9. A. 0.87; B. c
10. A. a; B. a
11. A. b; B. b
12. A. b; B. b
13. A. b; B. b
14. A. 2 mL, 2 mL; B. b; C. b
15. A. a; B. b

Chapter 15—
Vitamin and Mineral Replacement

1. a
2. b
3. b
4. a
5. a
6. a
7. a
8. a
9. b
10. b
11. a
12. d
13. c
14. e
15. a
16. b
17. a, b, c, e, g
18. d
19. c. Newborns are vitamin K–deficient at birth and it is a common practice in the United States to administer a one-time dose of vitamin K to prevent hemorrhagic disease of the newborn, which can present up to 6 months after birth.
20. c
21. a. Folic acid (folate) is very important during the first trimester of pregnancy to prevent neural tube defects such as anencephaly or spina bifida. All women who may become pregnant should be encouraged to take folate 400 mcg/day, since frequently a woman does not know she is pregnant until well into the first trimester.
22. c
23. b. Vitamin B_1 is also known as *thiamine*. Thiamine deficiency is evident in Wernicke's encephalopathy, which, if left untreated, leads to Wernicke-Korsakoff syndrome and irreversible brain damage. Thiamine should be administered prior to any dextrose. Vitamin B_6 deficiency can also be seen in alcohol abusers, but does not necessarily create the above symptoms.
24. a
25. c
26. d
27. b. Vitamin A deficiency can be seen in patients with biliary and pancreatic disorders. Celiac disease damages the lining of the intestine and impairs absorption of vitamin A.
28. b
29. a, b, c, d. Any dose changes should be discussed with the health care provider prior to changes being made. Symptoms of hypervitaminosis A include nausea, vomiting, anorexia, lethargy, peeling skin, hair loss, and abdominal pain. Alcohol ingestion will decrease the absorption of vitamin A.
30. b. Pyridoxine or vitamin B_6 might be considered beneficial for a patient with neuritis from INH therapy. Signs and symptoms of neuritis include numbness, tingling, "pins and needles" feeling, and difficulty gripping an object.
31. d. Patients who are receiving parenteral nutrition are at risk for zinc deficiency. Zinc will also be crucial for this patient for wound repair and tissue healing.
32. c
33. d
34. d. Vitamin K is needed for synthesis of prothrombin and the clotting factors VII, IX, and X. Vitamin K_1 (phytonadione) is the only form that is available to treat an overdose of an oral anticoagulant.

Chapter 16—
Fluid and Electrolyte Replacement

1. d
2. f
3. b
4. e
5. a
6. c
7. c
8. a
9. d

10. e
11. b
12. a
13. d
14. c
15. a
16. a. Oral potassium supplements can be irritating to the stomach and should be taken with at least 6 ounces of fluid or with a meal.
17. d. IV potassium must be given using a rate-controlled device and cannot be allowed to run freely. In many hospitals, the nurse does not prepare this medication, and it is either mixed in the pharmacy or comes prepackaged from the manufacturer.
18. d. Potassium is very irritating to the vein. If the site has become reddened and swollen, the IV should be discontinued immediately and the health care provider should be contacted to establish central venous access.
19. b, c
20. d. Administering sodium bicarbonate IV (50 mEq/L) as a one-time dose may help temporarily by driving potassium back into the cell.
21. a, b, d, e. A patient who is taking a potassium supplement should be taught the signs and symptoms of both hypo- and hyperkalemia and when to notify the health care provider. Since there is a narrow range for potassium level, the patient should anticipate routine blood work to evaluate if the potassium is in the expected range. Because potassium is irritating, the supplement should be taken with a meal or full glass of liquid and the patient should remain upright for a minimum of 30 minutes to prevent esophagitis.
22. b
23. c
24. b
25. b
26. a
27. b
28. b
29. b
30. b
31. a
32. a
33. d. This patient is hypokalemic. Signs of hypokalemia may include anorexia, nausea, and vomiting. Muscle weakness is not usually apparent until after the potassium level is less than 2.5 mEq/L. Untreated hypokalemia can lead to cardiac arrest and death.
34. a
35. a. A potassium level of 3.2 mEq/L is considered hypokalemia and may require a supplement. Potassium supplements are taken over an extended peri-od of time and not just a few days. Hypokalemia is rarely caused by inadequate intake. This response is also accusatory and is not therapeutic. GI losses due to vomiting and diarrhea may lead to hypokalemia; constipation will not.
36. c. A sodium level of 150 mEq/L is considered hypernatremia. The normal range for serum sodium is 125-135 mEq/L.
37. a, d, e. GI disturbances; paresthesias of the face, hands, and feet; and arrhythmias are commonly seen with hyperkalemia.
38. c, d, e
39. a, b, e. This patient is hypocalcemic. Signs of hypocalcemia include anxiety, irritability, tetany, seizures, hyperactive deep tendon reflexes, and carpopedal spasms.

Case Study

1. D.M. is in hemorrhagic shock as indicated by his vital signs. Stab wounds to the chest and abdomen can penetrate vital organs, causing large blood loss and risk of death. The priority assessment for this patient, as with any patient, is airway assessment. Airway always comes first. After a systematic assessment of the patient, two large-bore IVs (14 or 16 gauge) should be established in large veins. Another option is to assist the health care provider in placing a central line for rapid fluid resuscitation with blood.
2. The patient needs to be resuscitated with blood and blood products.
3. Whole blood may be more beneficial because it contains all of the components (plasma, platelets); however, uncrossmatched packed red blood cells (PRBCs) may be easier to obtain in the emergent setting of trauma.

Chapter 17— Nutritional Support

Crossword Puzzle

Across
3. hypoglycemia
4. elemental
5. air embolism
6. infection
7. pneumothorax
9. polymeric

Down
1. hyperglycemia
2. hyperalimentation

3.   hypervolemia

8.   hydrothorax

10.

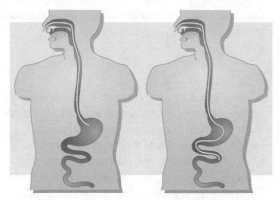

| Nasogastric | Nasoduodenal/nasojejunal |

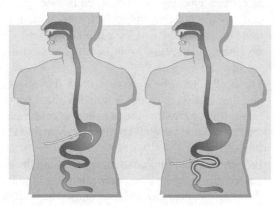

| Gastrostomy | Jejunostomy |

11.   d

12.   a

13.   b

14.   c

15.   a. The enteral nutrition of choice for a diabetic patient is Glucerna because it is low carbohydrate, high fat, and lactose-free.

16.   d. Respalor is a low-carbohydrate, high-fat formula used for patients requiring enteral nutrition who have respiratory conditions.

17.   c

18.   d

19.   b. Patients with burns have a higher calorie requirement than most other types of patients. In the acute phase, this is due to a hypermetabolic state. The patient requires nutritional support to assist in wound healing. Total parenteral nutrition (TPN) would be an option; however, there is an increased risk of infection. The best response is cyclic tube feeding in which the nutrition is administered over 8-16 hours, allowing the patient to be ambulatory and active during that time.

20.   d. Due to the tonicity of the fluid from the high glucose levels, TPN must be administered through a central venous line.

21.   d

22.   b

23.   b

24.   c. If a patient is receiving continuous parenteral nutrition, residuals should be checked every 2-4 hours. A residual greater than 50 mL indicates potential delay in gastric emptying. If residual is more than 50 mL, stop the infusion for 30 minutes to 1 hour and then recheck.

25.   a, c, d. Enteral nutrition is the preferred method if there is a functioning GI tract. It tends to be much less expensive than TPN and has a lower risk of infection, since TPN must be administered through central access. There is no risk of central line–associated bloodstream infection (CLABSI) from enteral feeding, because it is administered into the gastrointestinal tract.

26.   a, c, d

Case Study

1.   Transitioning a patient from TPN to enteral nutrition is common when a patient has a long-term need for nutritional support. Certain steps must be followed for a successful and safe transition. The first step is to see if a patient is ready for enteral feeding and how much he or she will tolerate. This is accomplished by giving small amounts of feeding at a slow rate. The usual start rate is 25-40 mL/hour. The next step is a gradual increase in rate by 25-40 mL/hour over an 8- to 24-hour period. During this transition, the TPN rate is reduced by the same amount. TPN can be discontinued when the patient is able to tolerate taking approximately 75% to 80% of their needs by the enteral method. It is important to remember that a critically ill patient may require between 3000 and 5000 calories/day.

2.   A patient who will require long-term enteral nutrition will likely require a gastrostomy tube. Prior to that time, the patient may have received nutrition via a nasogastric or orogastric tube. Aspiration is a serious risk for those patients receiving tube feedings and may lead to aspiration pneumonia. Elevating the head of the bed between 30 and 45 degrees when possible may be beneficial. This is not an option if there is a question of spinal cord injury. The nurse should aspirate to check for residual before administering the next feeding and every 4 hours between feedings.

Chapter 18—
Adrenergic Agonists and Adrenergic Blockers

1.   c

2.   d

3. b
4. e
5. a
6. smooth
7. adrenergic
8. sitting up
9. do
10. sympatholytics
11. phentolamine mesylate (Regitine)
12. reserpine
13. beta blocker
14. hypertension
15. asthma; COPD
16. antagonism (The two drugs could counteract each other—as *antagonists*—thus negating a therapeutic action.)
17. d
18. c, a
19. a
20. a
21. b
22. d
23. c
24. d
25. b
26. b. Although albuterol will increase the patient's heart rate, this may cause a feeling of nervousness and not an ease of breathing. It has no effect on urinary output. Albuterol causes smooth muscle dilation, not constriction or contraction. Bronchodilation and relaxation of smooth muscles will improve air flow into the lungs.
27. a. Assuring a patent airway is the first step in providing care to any patient. There is no indication at this time for an electrocardiogram. Although epinephrine is beneficial in allergic reactions, 1 mg of 1:1000 exceeds the subQ dosage. Establishing an IV would not be the first action to take.
28. d. Although all pieces of information are important, the nurse should ask the patient how many puffs of the inhaler were taken to determine that the patient did not overdose on the medication. Other side effects of albuterol, besides shaking and trembling, include sweating, nausea, headaches, blurred vision, and flushing.
29. b, c, e
30. b
31. a, b, c. Carvedilol (Coreg) is an adrenergic blocker. The other three medications are adrenergic medications. Adrenergic agonists are contraindicated in narrow-angle glaucoma.
32. b
33. b. Dopamine acts only on dopaminergic receptors and is located in renal, mesenteric, coronary, and cerebral arteries. These dopaminergic receptors can only be activated by dopamine.

34. c, e
35. a
36. b. The proper dosage for timolol (Blocadren) is initially 10 mg b.i.d., with a maximum dose of 60 mg/day. The above-ordered dose is 10 times the initial starting dose.
37. a

Case Study

1. An EpiPen contains epinephrine, which is a naturally occurring catecholamine useful in the treatment of allergic reactions and anaphylaxis. It acts on both alpha and beta receptors and promotes CNS and cardiac stimulation and bronchodilation. It also decreases mucus congestion by inhibiting histamine release. Although epinephrine can be used for a variety of processes, including cardiac arrest and hypotension, an EpiPen is used specifically for allergic and anaphylactic reactions and must be used at the first indication of difficulty breathing, hoarseness, hives, itching, or swelling of the lips and tongue.
2. The EpiPen must be stored in a cool, dark place, and the solution must be clear and without particles. It is crucial that the patient appreciate and understand that the EpiPen must be available at all times.
3. Proper use of an EpiPen includes pressing the device firmly against the outer thigh and holding the device in place for 5-10 seconds. The injection must be delivered into the subcutaneous tissue. Massage the area for 10 seconds to promote absorption and decrease vasoconstriction. Should the EpiPen be needed more than twice per week, the health care provider must be notified.

Chapter 19—
Cholinergic Agonists and Anticholinergics

1. c
2. e
3. d
4. h
5. a
6. b
7. f
8. g
9. d
10. a
11. b
12. c. Anticholinergic medications are contraindicated in a patient with glaucoma because they increase the intraocular pressure.
13. b

14. c
15. c
16. a, c
17. d. Bethanechol is used to treat urinary retention but will not be effective and should not be used in the case of a mechanical obstruction. If this patient was prescribed bethanechol for urinary retention and the urine output is decreasing, the health care provider should be notified to investigate another cause.
18. d. Bethanechol is a cholinergic agonist. The patient is experiencing an adverse response and the treatment of choice is atropine.
19. c
20. a, b. Atropine would be beneficial as a preoperative medication to help control oral secretions. It is also used for patients who are symptomatic with a heart rate fewer than 50 beats/minute.
21. d. Atropine-like drugs should not be administered to patients with narrow-angle glaucoma because they will increase the intraocular pressure.
22. c. Due to the decrease in gastrointestinal motility that can be associated with propantheline, the patient should be encouraged to eat foods that are high in fiber and drink adequate amounts of liquid to prevent constipation.
23. a, b, c, e. Hyoscyamine is an anticholinergic medication that will have similar side effects to the prototype drug atropine. Adequate fluid intake will help prevent constipation. Vision may be blurry, and the patient should be advised not to drive until aware of how the medication may affect vision. Sucking on hard candy or sugar-free ice pops, as well as increased fluid intake, may help with dry mouth. The patient should be educated as to baseline heart rate and advised to report tachycardia (rates above 100) to the health care provider. Increased sweating is not a common side effect.
24. a, c, d
25. d
26. b, c, d, e. Common side effects of anticholinergic drugs like benztropine may include dry mouth, constipation, and urinary retention. Dizziness and hallucinations should be reported to the health care provider as these may become dangerous to the patient. Because there is a decreased ability to perspire, life-threatening hyperthermia may develop. Palpitations may be due to tachycardia.

Case Study

1. Tolterodine tartrate blocks cholinergic receptors selectively in the bladder to decrease the incidence of incontinence.
2. The common side effects are those associated with other cholinergic medications and may include dizziness, vertigo, dry mouth, nausea, vomiting, weight gain, and urinary retention.
3. Tolterodine is contraindicated in patients with glaucoma or gastric or urinary retention and in women who are lactating.
4. Besides discussing side effects and adverse reactions with the patient, H.H. should be encouraged to take the medication on an empty stomach as absorption is delayed with food. Grapefruit juice should also be avoided since it decreases drug levels. Before taking any other medications, the health care provider should be consulted because this drug interacts with several other classes of drugs such as phenothiazines, macrolides, and antifungals.

Chapter 20—
Central Nervous System Stimulants

Crossword Puzzle

Across
4. dependence
6. ADHD
9. anorexiants
10. analeptics

Down
1. amphetamines
2. phenylpropanolamine
3. methylphenidate
5. narcolepsy
7. hyperkinesis
8. armodafinil

11. a, c, d
12. c
13. a, b, c, d
14. b
15. a, b, c, d, f
16. b
17. a. Methylphenidate and amitriptyline are not usually used together since methylphenidate increases serum levels of amitriptyline and may cause hypertension. There are other, safer alternatives to use in combination for prophylaxis in migraines.
18. d
19. b
20. a, b, e
21. c. Hemorrhagic stroke is the most likely diagnosis of those listed. There is a 16-fold greater risk in females for hemorrhagic stroke in those patients taking appetite suppressants or anorexiants. Pregnancy-induced hypertension is a possibility, but not

the most likely cause at this point. A pregnancy test should be obtained.

22. a, d, e. CNS stimulants are absolutely contraindicated in patients with coronary artery disease, hypertension, and liver failure. Cautious use is recommended for those patients with any degree of liver disease.

23. a

Case Study

1. Both of these medications are CNS stimulants that are used in conjunction with appropriate counseling for treatment of ADHD. The best time to give the medication is 30-45 minutes before meals, so the nurse will need to review the lunch schedules of the students and plan accordingly on how best to administer the drugs.

   Baseline height, weight, and vital signs should be obtained and monitored throughout the course of treatment. A record of the students' complete blood count, including a white blood cell count with differential and platelet count, should be on file. Routine vital signs should be assessed since both of these medications can cause an elevation in heart rate and blood pressure, especially if taken in conjunction with caffeine. Patients should also be monitored for an increase in hyperactivity.

   Health teaching is important for not only the student, but also the family and the teachers on staff. The goal of these medications is to increase focus and attention and decrease impulsiveness and hyperactivity. The student and family should be encouraged to eat three nutritious meals per day along with healthy snacks since anorexia may be a side effect. Dry mouth may also occur so, as possible within school policy, the student should be allowed to chew gum or suck on hard candy. The importance of avoidance of caffeinated beverages and foods, including chocolate, sodas, and energy drinks, must be stressed since high plasma levels of caffeine may be fatal.

   Medication administration at school must be handled with tact and ease. If possible, the school nurse's office should not be open and in the main hall where all other students can observe the comings and goings of the students requiring medication or care. Privacy is crucial.

Chapter 21—
Central Nervous System Depressants

Crossword Puzzle

Across

1. saddle block
2. nitrous oxide
3. hangover
5. insomnia
6. kava kava
7. benzodiazepines
8. local anesthetic
12. balanced anesthesia
13. barbiturates

Down

1. spinal block
4. epidural block
9. sedation
10. caudal block
11. flurazepam

14. sedative-hypnotics; general anesthetics; analgesics; opioid and nonopioid analgesics; anticonvulsants; antipsychotics; antidepressants
15. rapid eye movement; nonrapid eye movement
16. sedation
17. may
18. ultrashort-acting
19. central nervous; pain; consciousness
20. surgical; analgesia; excitement or delirium; medullary paralysis
21. spinal
22. respiratory distress or failure
23. saddle block
24. are
25. short
26. zolpidem tartrate (Ambien) (also eszopiclone [Lunesta], zaleplon [Sonata], and ramelteon [Rozerem])
27. flumazenil (Romazicon)
28. esters; amides
29. d
30. f
31. e
32. a
33. b
34. c

35. c
36. b
37. c, d. Maintaining the patient flat in bed for 24-48 hours and encouraging adequate oral fluid intake as tolerated may help prevent a spinal headache. The patient may also require IV fluids to supplement intake.
38. c. By explaining the reason for positioning (either seated with an arched back or fetal position), the patient will feel as if she has more control. The nurse can reassure the patient that he or she will assist her in maintaining the proper position.
39. d
40. d, e
41. a
42. a, b, c, e. Older patients may have more problems with Stage 3 and Stage 4 nonrapid eye movement (NREM) sleep and awaken frequently. Establishing a bedtime routine, maintaining a schedule of going to bed and arising in the morning, and avoiding caffeine and alcohol at bedtime may help. Although it sounds intuitive to take naps, they may actually hinder a patient getting a good night's sleep if they are longer than 20-30 minutes. Diuretics should be taken in the morning and fluids should be limited at bedtime to prevent frequent trips to the bathroom, which may interrupt sleep.
43. d, f

Case Study

1. Benzodiazepines are frequently prescribed prior to surgery. They increase the action of the inhibitory neurotransmitter gamma-aminobutyric acid (GABA) to the GABA receptors and reduce the excitability of the neurons. Medications such as alprazolam (Xanax) or lorazepam (Ativan) might be prescribed for anxiety.
2. Balanced anesthesia includes many parts leading up to surgery. By using a variety of agents, there tends to be fewer cardiovascular side effects, less nausea and vomiting, and a quicker recovery. This is also true of utilizing a laparoscopic approach instead of an "open" approach to this surgery.

    The night before the surgery, a medication such as zolpidem (Ambien) might be prescribed to ensure a good night's sleep. After the patient has arrived in the preoperative area and approximately 1 hour prior to surgery, a combination of an opioid or anxiolytic and an anticholinergic such as atropine would be given. The purpose of the anticholinergic is to decrease secretions, and therefore, the risk of aspiration. Once the patient is transferred to the operating room, a short-acting sedative such as pentothal, propofol, or etomidate may be given and the patient will be given inhaled anesthetics.

This procedure will require general anesthesia, so the patient will also receive a muscle relaxant to facilitate endotracheal intubation and maintain neuromuscular blockade.

Chapter 22— Anticonvulsants

Crossword Puzzle

Across
2. atonic
3. petit mal
4. myoclonic
7. convulsions
9. partial
11. teratogenic

Down
1. grand mal
2. anticonvulsants
5. clonic
6. anoxia
8. seizure
10. EEG

12. EEG
13. idiopathic
14. generalized; partial
15. preventing; do not
16. are not
17. phenytoin
18. over-the-counter
19. intramuscular
20. a
21. b. Although it is important to know the patient's medical history regarding seizures, the best response is asking about the medications that have been prescribed. Although no seizure medications for epilepsy are pregnancy category A or B, some category C medications may be utilized if the benefits outweigh the risks.
22. a, d
23. b
24. a, b, d. Valproic acid is taken in divided doses. Doses start at 10-15 mg/kg/day and increase to a maximum of 60/mg/kg/day until seizures are controlled. Increased fluid is not required with valproic acid. There are no food restrictions with valproic acid, as may be seen with other anticonvulsants.
25. b, c, d. An absolute contraindication is heart block and bradycardia. Cautious use is recommended for

patients with hypoglycemia and hypotension. Dilantin is excreted in small amounts in the urine.

26. d. Intravenous phenytoin is irritating to the tissue and it is recommended that a central line or peripherally inserted central catheter (PICC) line be utilized when possible. The health care provider does not need to be notified immediately to change the medication to oral form. Continuing the infusion, even with a saline flush, may cause sloughing of the tissue.

27. a. Although a variety of anticonvulsants may be utilized over a patient's lifetime, at this time, there is no cure for seizure disorders. The patient will need to take a medication for the duration of his life.

28. b

29. a, b, d, e. Documenting the type of movements (tonic/clonic), duration of seizure activity, and where the movements started and progressed are important pieces of gathering the history of the seizure event. It is important to know, if possible, what the patient had been doing prior to the event and if the patient reported any warning prior to the seizure. The patient is unable to stop true seizure activity voluntarily.

30. c. Nosebleeds and sore throats may be a sign of blood dyscrasias and should be reported to the health care provider. A reddish-pink discoloration of the urine may be expected. To prevent injury to the gums, a soft toothbrush should be utilized. Orthostatic hypotension is not associated with phenytoin use.

31. a

32. a. The first-line drug of choice for status epilepticus is either diazepam or lorazepam.

33. a, b, c

34. c

Case Study

1. Oxcarbazepine is taken by mouth with an initial dose of 300 mg b.i.d. One of the benefits of this medication is that there are fewer adverse effects than with carbamazepine and drug level monitoring is usually not necessary, which may be more convenient in the patient's role of elementary school teacher. This medication also is pregnancy category C, so it *may* be somewhat safer in the event of pregnancy.

Chapter 23—
Drugs for Neurologic Disorders: Parkinsonism and Alzheimer's Disease

1. c
2. a
3. d
4. e
5. b
6. dopamine; acetylcholine
7. dopamine
8. levodopa
9. carbidopa
10. tacrine (Cognex) [also donepezil (Aricept); rivastigmine (Exelon)]
11. enhance
12. selegiline
13. Stalevo (carbidopa, levodopa, entacapone)
14. trihexyphenidyl (Artane) [also benztropine (Cogentin) or biperiden (Akineton)]
15. a, c, d. A dose of carbidopa 10 mg/levodopa 100 mg t.i.d./q.i.d. is the correct dose if this is initial dosing. Carbidopa 25 mg/levodopa 250 mg t.i.d./q.i.d. is the correct as a maintenance dose.
16. a
17. b, c, d, e. Carbidopa-levodopa may make the patient's movements smoother, although at high doses, dyskinesia may be noted. Jaundice will not result from missing doses. Vitamin B_6 helps the body eliminate levodopa. Taking supplements would decrease the effectiveness of the medication. Nausea and vomiting are side effects, so taking the medication with meals may be beneficial. There is no indication that carbidopa-levodopa affects glucose levels.
18. a, b, e. Aged cheeses, chocolate, and yogurt are all foods that are high in tyramine. These foods should be avoided when taking selegiline to prevent a hypertensive crisis from occurring.
19. d. Tricyclic antidepressants decrease the effect of rivastigmine.
20. c. When taken with levodopa, COMT inhibitors like entacapone will increase the levodopa combination in the brain.
21. a, e. Glaucoma and angina are contraindications for the use of anticholinergic medications. Shingles and diabetes are not contraindications. A patient with a history of urinary retention, not frequency, should not take anticholinergic medications.
22. c

23. c. Memantine (Namenda) is prescribed for the treatment of mild to severe Alzheimer's disease. Increased wandering and hostility can indicate that the disease is progressing and an increase in the dose may be beneficial.

24. a. Sucking on hard candy or chewing sugarless gum may help with dry mouth associated with anticholinergic medications such as benztropine mesylate. This medication is initially taken at bedtime and twice per day in divided doses as a maintenance dose. The nurse should remind the patient that all medication adjustments need to be made by the health care provider. Urinary retention is a side effect of anticholinergic medications; however, the nurse should encourage the patient to urinate when he or she feels the urge and not on a set schedule.

Case Study

1. Alzheimer's disease has seven stages of cognitive decline, and the progression may occur over many years or decades. Stage 3 is considered mild, and the patient may start to show some signs of decreased ability to function in work or social settings and have problems with recall and memory. Anxiety may also be a component. Stages 4 and 5 require the patient to have more assistance with performing complex tasks (stage 4), leading to the need for a higher level of assistance as the patient needs reminders to bathe, lock doors, and turn off stoves, for example (stage 5). Disorientation becomes more noticeable and the patient may become tearful. Stage 5 is considered moderately severe and marks the beginning of early dementia. In stage 6, the patient needs assistance with activities of daily living and may have incontinence of urine and feces. Psychological disturbances such as paranoia, agitation, delusions, and violent behavior become more prominent. In stage 7 (late dementia), the patient is unable to care for him- or herself and may make only sounds or speak a few words. Patients will eventually become comatose.

2. Tacrine is an acetylcholinesterase inhibitor (AChE) that is used in the treatment of mild to moderate Alzheimer's disease. Tacrine increases cognitive function by preventing the breakdown of acetylcholinesterase, which allows for more acetylcholine to be available as a transmitter.

3. Safety is a primary concern for the grandmother as she moves into a new home with her family. As Alzheimer's disease progresses, the patient may begin to wander more and is at higher risk for falling. Removing obstacles from the patient's path may help prevent falls, as will eliminating loose rugs and quickly cleaning up spills. Assuring adequate locks on outside doors may prevent the patient from wandering outside unattended; how-ever, the patient should be able to have an escape route from the house as needed. Door alarms are also available. Covers may be placed over dials for the burners on a stove. These are similar to those utilized for preventing young children from adjusting the burners. The family will need additional resources and support, as caring for a patient with Alzheimer's is a full-time job. Organizations such as the Alzheimer's Association can provide direction.

Chapter 24—
Drugs for Neuromuscular Disorders: Myasthenia Gravis, Multiple Sclerosis, and Muscle Spasms

Crossword Puzzle

Across
1. acetylcholine
4. myasthenic crisis
5. edrophonium
8. hemiplegia
9. ptosis
10. fasciculations

Down
2. neostigmine
3. cholinergic crisis
4. miosis
6. myelin sheath
7. dantrium

11. b
12. b. Drooling, excessive tearing, sweating, and miosis are signs of a cholinergic crisis.
13. a
14. c
15. d. There is an increased toxicity when taken with tetracycline.
16. c. Imuran and Betaseron are biologic response modifiers and immunosuppressants. They are used to decrease the inflammatory process of the nerve fibers.
17. b
18. a, c
19. b. Diazepam is contraindicated in narrow-angle glaucoma.

Case Study

1. Patients with spinal cord injuries may have spasticity due to hyperexcitability of neurons caused by increased stimulation from the cerebral neurons or

lack of inhibition in the spinal cord or at the skeletal muscles.

2. Carisoprodol (Soma) is a centrally acting muscle relaxant and is utilized for muscle spasms. Baclofen is used specifically for muscle spasticity, either due to trauma or multiple sclerosis.

3. Side effects of these medications include drowsiness, dizziness, nausea, and hypotension. They should not be taken with other central nervous system depressants or alcohol. Baclofen can be used for an extended period of time without developing tolerance. It does not have abuse potential. Carisoprodol is now a Schedule IV drug and has the potential for abuse.

Chapter 25— Antiinflammatory Drugs

1. d
2. c
3. e
4. h
5. b
6. a
7. f
8. g
9. i
10. injury; infection
11. redness; swelling (edema); heat; pain; loss of function
12. delayed
13. does
14. higher (or increased)
15. 24
16. d
17. a, c, d, e. Heartburn can be a side effect of NSAIDs. Taking the medication with food may help decrease heartburn. Dark, tarry, or bloody bowel movements are an indication of GI bleeding, which is an adverse effect of NSAID use. The dosage range for NSAIDs varies from medication to medication, but large doses may cause erosive esophagitis, which would cause heartburn-type pain. There are many types of heartburn, including those associated with acute myocardial infarction. Not all heartburn is of GI origin due to a drug effect.
18. b
19. a. Warfarin is an anticoagulant that may be taken by patients with atrial fibrillation. Aspirin displaces warfarin from its protein-binding site. This increases the anticoagulant effect and may lead to excessive bleeding, which may initially be indicated by bruising. Although the other medications may have

drug-drug interactions, they do not cause increased anticoagulant effects, as evidenced by the bruising.
20. d
21. c. Ibuprofen can cause bronchospasms in a patient with asthma; therefore, its use is contraindicated.
22. a
23. b. Since ibuprofen is excreted in the urine, adequate fluid intake and urine output should be maintained. Ibuprofen is category C in early pregnancy and category D in the third trimester.
24. c
25. a
26. b
27. a
28. c
29. a, c, d. Corticosteroids may be used for a variety of disease processes including flare-ups of arthritic conditions. They have a long half-life and are usually taken once a day in a large prescribed dose and then the dose is tapered for 5-10 days. Corticosteroids are never simply stopped. They may be given in combination with other medications including prostaglandin inhibitors.
30. b, c, d, e. Fluid intake should be increased to promote uric acid excretion. Avoiding alcohol is important because alcohol causes an overproduction, as well as an underexcretion, of uric acid. Purine is required to synthesize uric acid. Taking the medication with food will help avoid GI upset. Some studies have shown that vitamin C may help increase uric acid elimination; however, large doses of supplemental vitamin C are not recommended and, since vitamin C is an acid, there is a higher risk of kidney stone formation.
31. d. Although side effects of infliximab may include headache, dizziness, cough, nausea, and vomiting, an adverse reaction to the medication is severe infection due to immunosuppression. A fever of 38.8° C in an adult who is taking infliximab needs to be evaluated.

Case Study

1. The normal therapeutic dosage is 325-650 mg q4h as needed, up to a maximum of 4 g/day. If the patient takes 975 mg every 4 hours as stated, this patient will be taking 5,850 mg/day, which exceeds the maximum daily dose.
2. Side effects may include anorexia, nausea, vomiting, dizziness, abdominal pain, and heartburn. Adverse reactions include tinnitus, GI bleeding, blood dyscrasias including thrombocytopenia and leukopenia, and liver failure.
3. The patient appears to be hypotensive, tachycardic, and tachypneic. These vital signs could be indicative of a hypovolemic state, potentially due to a GI bleed. Interpretation of the vital signs is com-

pounded due to the use of caffeine with the aspirin. Metabolic acidosis, as can be seen in aspirin overdose, can also cause tachypnea.

Chapter 26—
Nonopioid and Opioid Analgesics

1. central nervous system; peripheral nervous system
2. respiration; coughing
3. antitussive; antidiarrheal
4. head injury; respiratory depression (shock and hypotension are also acceptable answers)
5. side effect; health care provider
6. IV
7. a. Frequent monitoring of blood pressure is required since opioids will lower blood pressure.
8. c
9. b. Monitoring fluid intake is the least important. The nurse should monitor bowel sounds to identify constipation, a common side effect of opioids. The patient's pain should be frequently assessed. The nurse should assess vital signs, noting rate and depth of respirations for future comparisons; opioids commonly decrease respirations and systolic blood pressure.
10. b, c, d, e. There are no dietary restrictions associated with the use of hydrocodone. Adequate fluid intake and including fiber in the diet will assist with constipation.
11. d. Drugs with long half-lives are more beneficial to patients dealing with chronic pain, as they have a longer duration of action.
12. b
13. b
14. b
15. c
16. b, c. Adequate pain control is important for patients of all ages. Dose adjustments will be made in an older patient just as they would be in a pediatric patient. This may also be based on hepatic and renal function. By working together to stay on top of the pain, it may be easier to treat. The concept behind PCA is that it is *patient*-controlled analgesia. The family must be advised not to use the PCA device for the patient.
17. b, d, e. The best people to assess how a child is acting are those who are with the child the most. Ask the parents or other caregivers how the child usually acts when he is in pain or upset. Utilizing developmentally appropriate communication skills and pain scales should yield the best result for the nurse treating this patient's pain. Opioids are appropriate to utilize if nonopioid methods are ineffective.
18. b. Cholestyramine will decrease the effectiveness of acetaminophen. An alternative nonopioid would

be an option for the patient instead of stopping the cholestyramine.
19. b, c, f
20. b. It does not appear that the patient's pain is well controlled with the current medication or scheduling. The health care provider should be notified so adjustments can be made or other options can be explored.
21. c
22. c. Alcohol must be avoided while taking opioid pain medications. Vicoprofen contains ibuprofen so anything that also contains ibuprofen must be avoided.
23. c
24. a, b, d. Nonopioid pain medications are appropriate for minor injuries such as abrasions and minor aches and pains.

Case Study

1. Migraines are caused by dilation and inflammation of the blood vessels in the brain. The exact cause is unknown, but it may be due to deficiencies of 5-hydroxytryptamine (5HT), a neurotransmitter that causes vasoconstriction. If levels are low, there is vasodilation that leads to migraines.
2. A classic migraine is preceded by an aura. This may include flashing lights or certain smells or sounds. Each person may have an aura unique to him or her that occurs before the headache begins. Common migraines are not preceded by auras.
3. Treatment may include analgesics, ergotamine preparations, and selective serotonin$_1$ receptor agonists (triptans). The triptans (sumatriptan, naratriptan, zolmitriptan) should be taken as early as possible during a migraine to be effective. All triptans are contraindicated if the patient has uncontrolled hypertension. Nausea may be controlled with medications such as ondansetron. If the triptans are not effective, opioid medications may be necessary. Medications may also be prescribed to prevent future headaches. These include medications in the beta blocker, anticonvulsant, or tricyclic antidepressant classes.

Chapter 27—
Antipsychotics and Anxiolytics

1. e
2. d
3. f
4. g
5. a
6. h
7. b
8. c

9. thought processes; behaviors; dopamine
10. dihydroindolones; thioxanthenes; butyrophenones; dibenzoxazepines
11. drowsiness
12. pruritus; photosensitivity
13. decrease
14. are not
15. tolerance
16. sedative-hypnotics
17. c
18. a
19. a
20. b
21. b
22. c
23. c
24. b
25. b. Orthostatic hypotension may occur with phenothiazines and nonphenothiazine medications within this class. The patient should be encouraged to change positions slowly to prevent orthostatic hypotension.
26. d
27. a
28. b
29. c, d, e. Either hypo- or hypertension may be indications of an adverse reaction. Although it may be safe to take some herbal medications while taking fluphenazine, taking kava kava may increase dystonic reactions. There are numerous side effects associated with fluphenazine, including dizziness, headache, and nausea.
30. c. Because of less effective hepatic and renal function, doses of antipsychotics should be decreased by 25% to 50% in older patients.
31. d. The correct answer is always maintaining the airway. It does not matter what the suspected overdose or illness may be. Airway is always the top priority.
32. a
33. c
34. c
35. d
36. b. Hyperglycemia is a side effect of taking risperidone. Blood glucose levels should be obtained at baseline and monitored carefully.
37. b
38. a, b, e
39. b, c, d. Patients with liver damage, subcortical brain damage, and any kind of blood dyscrasia should not take fluphenazine.
40. a, b, d, e

Case Study

1. Clonazepam (Klonopin) is a benzodiazepine that is in the same family as diazepam and alprazolam. It is used for anxiety associated with depression and seizures.
2. Benzodiazepines enhance the action of GABA (gamma-aminobutyric acid), an inhibitory neurotransmitter. It has a fairly rapid action and is readily absorbed from the GI tract.
3. Side effects include drowsiness, dizziness, and coma if taken in large doses. The action of benzodiazepines is potentiated when taken with alcohol.
4. H.K. may have taken an overdose. A respiratory rate of 8 and an O_2 saturation of 78% require immediate action by the nurse. Maintaining an airway is the priority intervention. Oxygen should be administered, and an airway adjunct should be inserted. Her ventilations should be assisted with a bag-mask and high-flow oxygen until her airway can be secured. An IV will need to be established and flumazenil (Romazicon) administered. Flumazenil acts very quickly, but is only effective for benzodiazepine overdoses. An emetic is not an option for this patient as she is unresponsive. Gastric lavage is the intervention of choice. Blood pressure may need to be supported with IV vasopressors.

Chapter 28—Antidepressants and Mood Stabilizers

Crossword Puzzle

Across

4. St. John's wort
6. major
8. reactive
10. bipolar
11. bedtime
12. tyramine

Down

1. imipramine
2. lithium
3. ginseng
4. St. John's wort
5. imipramine
7. feverfew
9. two to four

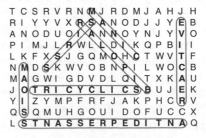

13. bipolar
14. SSRIs
15. MAOIs
16. manic
17. antidepressants
18. reactive
19. tricyclics
20. a
21. a
22. b
23. d
24. c
25. b
26. c
27. d
28. b. Orthostatic hypotension is a frequent side effect of tricyclic antidepressants (TCAs). The patient should be encouraged to change positions slowly to avoid this side effect.
29. a, b, e. Bananas, chocolate, and wine are contraindicated in a patient who is taking a monoamine oxidase inhibitor (MAOI). Any food that is high in tyramine such as aged cheeses, processed meats, and soybeans or soy products should also be avoided.
30. d. St. John's wort is a common herbal remedy for depression. St. John's wort, when taken in combination with selective serotonin reuptake inhibitor (SSRI) drugs, can precipitate serotonin syndrome, which presents as headache, sweating, and agitation.
31. c
32. c. Monitoring the patient is one of the most important roles of the nurse. Trending vital signs, weight, and lab work will be important to the patient's ongoing care. The patient needs to maintain a fluid intake of 2-3 L of fluid/day initially and must be especially vigilant to maintain an adequate intake in hot weather. Manic patients frequently stop taking their medication when they feel better. They must be advised to continue taking the medication even if they feel better.
33. a. Monitoring hepatic and renal function in a patient taking lithium should be completed with weekly blood work, which includes BUN and creatinine.
34. b. The patient's lithium level is still subtherapeutic, and he remains in a manic phase. Therapeutic levels for acute mania are 1-1.5 mEq/L, and a therapeutic range is usually reached in 1-2 weeks.
35. a. The patient needs further education requiring the purpose of the medication. Lithium may be used in bipolar disorder as a mood stabilizer, but its effect is on the manic phase.
36. d. Venlafaxine is a serotonin-norepinephrine reuptake inhibitor. Side effects of this medication may include drowsiness, insomnia, photosensitivity, and ejaculatory dysfunction, among others. Taking St. John's wort while taking venlafaxine may increase the risk of serotonin syndrome or neuroleptic malignant syndrome.
37. a. Some studies have linked lithium to a congenital anomaly involving the tricuspid valve of the heart if taken during the first trimester of pregnancy. Lithium is a pregnancy category D drug.

Case Study

1. SSRIs block the reuptake of the neurotransmitter serotonin at the nerve terminal. One of the possible causes of depression is a lack of circulating serotonin. By preventing the reuptake, more serotonin is available and depression is lessened. SSRIs may be effective in the treatment of depression in cases where the patient was nonresponsive to a TCA.
2. In the initial interview, the nurse should inquire about medical history, medications, allergies, and past coping behavior. The nurse should directly ask the patient about suicidal thoughts. The use of herbal agents should also be investigated. A thorough psychiatric history should be obtained with a specific focus on past episodes of depression and treatments. Vital signs should be obtained as well as weight. Baseline laboratory work should be reviewed, since this medication should be used with caution in patients with a history of renal or liver problems.
3. Discharge teaching should include recommendations for counseling, since studies have shown that medication and counseling together are more successful than either modality alone. Support groups have also shown benefit. The nurse should teach the patient to take the medication as prescribed and that it may take 2-4 weeks for the onset of action. Alcohol should be avoided while taking SSRIs. The medication should be taken with food. Dry mouth may be a side effect that can be relieved somewhat with sucking on hard candy or chewing gum. If the patient feels suicidal at any time, she should contact the health care provider, suicide hotline, or go to the emergency department immediately.

Chapter 29— Penicillins and Cephalosporins

Crossword Puzzle

Across
3. cross-resistance
6. bacteriostatic

7. methicillin
10. acquired resistance
11. immunoglobulins
12. natural resistance

Down

1. nosocomial infections
2. nephrotoxicity
3. culture and sensitivity
4. superinfection
5. antibacterial
8. penicillin
9. bactericidal

13. e
14. g
15. f
16. h
17. a
18. b
19. c
20. d
21. d
22. a
23. d
24. b
25. c. The correct dose is 30 mg/kg q6-8h. This child weighs approximately 17 kg. The correct dose would be 510 mg every 6 hours.
26. c
27. a. Anorexia, along with nausea and vomiting, are common side effects of ceftriaxone. It is possible the patient will begin to eat more and regain weight as her illness is cured; however, this is not the best answer.
28. b. Acidic fruits or juices may make dicloxacillin less effective. Abdominal pain is a possible side effect. The entire course of antibiotics must be completed to prevent resistance from developing. Rashes can be associated with dicloxacillin, but may also be an indication of allergic reaction. The patient would need to be evaluated for other indications of an allergic reaction, such as difficulty breathing or hives.
29. d
30. b
31. c. Antibiotics, especially penicillins, may make oral contraceptives less effective, so an alternate method of birth control should be utilized.
32. a, c, d. Ideally, culture and sensitivity should be obtained before starting antibiotics. Allergic reactions are a possibility with any antibiotics. Because cephalosporins are eliminated in the urine, monitoring for adequate urine output is important.
33. a
34. c. Amoxicillin is contraindicated in a patient with asthma. Use in pediatric patients and diabetics is

not contraindicated. Amoxicillin is pregnancy category B and is considered relatively safe in pregnant women to treat infections.
35. c. A dose of 750 mg every 8 hours would not provide the correct blood levels. The standard dose for adults is 250-500 mg q6h or 500 mg-1 g q12h. The maximum dose is 4 g/day.
36. c. Because this medication contains large amounts of sodium, it must be used carefully in patients with hypertension or heart failure. The medication is safe for all of the other patient populations listed.

Case Study

1. The mechanism of action for penicillins is to inhibit synthesis of the cell wall. Piperacillin-tazobactam (Zosyn) is a penicillin that is considered an extended-spectrum penicillin. By combining a broad-spectrum antibiotic like piperacillin with an enzyme that inhibits beta-lactamase (tazobactam), the resultant drug is able to work more effectively and longer against beta-lactamase–producing bacteria.
2. Signs of an allergic reaction would include hives, edema, stridor, and hypotension. Severe anaphylactic reactions leading to death are possible. Monitoring the patient during the first few doses is critical. A superinfection occurs when the normal body flora are altered due to antibiotic administration. Symptoms can include stomatitis, anal or genital itching, and oral infections such as thrush.
3. Piperacillin-tazobactam (Zosyn) is only administered parenterally. The nurse will share with the patient that they will be observing for allergic reactions to the medication as well as evaluating the IV site for patency.

Chapter 30— Macrolides, Tetracyclines, Aminoglycosides, and Fluoroquinolones

1. g
2. b
3. f
4. a
5. c
6. a
7. e
8. h
9. a
10. h
11. d
12. a. The correct dose of IV levofloxacin is 500 mg/day.

13. a
14. d
15. b, c, d, e. Doxycycline should be taken with meals for improved absorption. Products that contain milk will bind to the medication and prevent absorption. There are no restrictions regarding eggs.
16. a, b, c, e. Outdated medications of any kind should be discarded; however, tetracycline will break down into toxic byproducts so it must be assured it is discarded. Superinfections, which occur when normal bacteria are destroyed, are common with the use of antibiotics. Tetracycline should not be taken during first and third trimesters of pregnancy due to possible teratogenic effects. Tetracycline does not cause urinary urgency.
17. b, e. Ototoxicity is a serious adverse effect of gentamicin. Thrombocytopenia may be a life-threatening adverse effect. Nausea, headache, and photosensitivity may be side effects; however, they are usually not considered serious.
18. a, b, c, e. Iron, which is found in prenatal vitamins, and antacids prevent absorption of doxycycline. Studies have shown that the effects of warfarin (Coumadin) may be increased by taking doxycycline, placing the patient at higher risk for bleeding. Cautious use should be exercised in a patient taking doxycycline and a proton pump inhibitor like omeprazole (Prilosec).
19. b, c, d, e. Drugs in the tetracycline family should be stored away from light to prevent breakdown. Cautious use is recommended in patients with renal and/or liver disease. Baseline levels should be assessed and reevaluated as needed. Due to mutations within the strains of various sexually transmitted infections, a culture and sensitivity should be obtained prior to starting treatment. It is also possible that various sexually transmitted infections could be present at the same time, and it would be beneficial to the patient if the most effective antibiotic is prescribed for each. Tetracyclines may make oral contraceptives less effective, so additional contraceptive use is recommended.
20. b. Peak blood levels are drawn 45-60 minutes after a drug has been administered.
21. b. The correct trough level for gentamicin is 0.5-2.0 mcg/mL. The health care provider should be contacted prior to administering the dose because it is elevated.
22. c
23. c
24. c. Contact the health care provider. Vancomycin may be nephrotoxic, and a decrease in urine output may be an early indication of renal damage. Decreasing renal function is also a part of normal aging, putting this 70-year-old patient at higher risk for renal failure.

25. a, b, c. Amikacin may cause hepatotoxicity, so the patient needs to be monitored for signs of liver failure. Jaundice may be an indication of liver failure and is noticeable in the sclera of the eyes early in the course. The urine may also take on a dark hue in liver failure. Rising levels of liver enzymes AST/ALT are also an indication.
26. c. Conjunctivitis is a possible side effect of azithromycin. If this occurs, the patient should not wear contact lenses. Photosensitivity is not a side effect of this medication. Taking azithromycin with food may help prevent nausea. If a headache occurs as a side effect, medications such as ibuprofen or acetaminophen are not contraindicated.

Case Study

1. Levofloxacin is a fluoroquinolone that interferes with bacterial DNA synthesis.
2. The nurse should educate the patient on the side effects of nausea, vomiting, abdominal cramping, and diarrhea. Headache, blurred vision, dizziness, depression, and confusion may also occur.
3. Adverse effects may be life-threatening. Levofloxacin is both nephrotoxic and hepatotoxic and encephalopathy is possible. Depression may lead to suicidal ideation. Stevens-Johnson syndrome is another life-threatening adverse effect associated with levofloxacin.
4. A.B. has a history of both asthma and a seizure disorder. It will be important for the nurse to carefully review her medication history, since use of levofloxacin and theophylline preparations requires caution. Patients with seizure disorders also should be monitored carefully for worsening of seizure activity.

Chapter 31—Sulfonamides

```
W J Q I O K O N F A B U L H N R Q
W D P E N I C I L L I N O K R H K
B L R Y E D R M C P S D D O V P A
L K C O V N V E E A U L G Y Q N M
M C R C C E R M V F C L J M E C T
P A A N Y Y I U A I F U S Q X Y
V X B J D S C D C D F L S K K E
E Q A R G I N C R E A S E O N W S
B Q A R E N O T L Q V U Z D P D L
Y N C I T A T S O I R E T C A B E
R T R I M E T H O P R I M C J C F
```

1. folic acid
2. penicillin
3. trimethoprim
4. are not
5. is not
6. liver; kidneys

7. bacteriostatic
8. increases
9. b
10. b
11. a
12. d
13. a
14. b, c, d, e. TMP-SMZ is contraindicated in a nursing mother. It is possible that there is cross-sensitivity between sulfonamides, so it is important to determine if the patient is allergic to any other antibiotics. There are a variety of etiologies for kidney stones; however, crystallization of the urine may occur with sulfonamides and lead to kidney stone formation. Some patients are more prone to kidney stones than others. TMP-SMZ has a variety of interactions with several medications, including warfarin, oral hypoglycemic agents, ACE inhibitors, digoxin, phenytoin, and potassium-sparing diuretics.
15. a, b, c, d. To prevent crystallization in the urine, fluids should be encouraged. Urine output should be carefully monitored since this medication is excreted in the urine. Adverse reactions are possible and include abdominal pain, nausea, vomiting, diarrhea, and anorexia. A desired effect of TMP-SMZ will be resolution of the bronchitis as evidenced by decreasing coughing and clear lung sounds.
16. b
17. c
18. d
19. a

Case Study

1. Bactrim is a sulfonamide that is bacteriostatic. It inhibits the bacterial synthesis of folic acid, which is required for bacterial growth. The standard IV dosage range is 8-10 mg/kg/day given in 2-4 divided doses. For this patient, the appropriate dose would be 560-700 mg/day, administered in 2-4 divided doses over 60-90 minutes each.
2. Patient and family teaching will include the need for IV access and adequate fluid intake to maintain a urine output of more than 600 mL/d. The patient will have his intake and output monitored, so the family must be taught to either record, or let the nurse know, what additional fluids are taken by the patient. The nurse will advise the patient of the potential side effects of anorexia, nausea, vomiting, diarrhea, and abdominal pain. Other side effects include headache, fatigue, vertigo, and insomnia. The patient should be advised to ask for help when getting out of bed or ambulating due to the potential for vertigo and risk of falling.
3. The nurse will need to be aware of the potential for increased effects of anticoagulation, such as bruising and bleeding, due to the interaction between warfarin and Bactrim. There is also a potential for increased hypoglycemic effects of glyburide. The nurse will need to carefully monitor lab work, including BUN and creatinine for renal function as well as liver panel (AST, ALT, ALP). The nurse will also need to monitor for life-threatening adverse effects, including electrolyte imbalances (hyperkalemia, hyponatremia, hypoglycemia), seizures, angioedema, anemias, leukopenia, pseudomembranous colitis, and Stevens-Johnson syndrome (erythema multiforme major). Stevens-Johnson syndrome is characterized by fever, feeling ill, joint pain, and skin lesions. Severe cases can be life-threatening and may require intensive care hospitalization and the use of immunoglobulins.

Chapter 32—Antituberculars, Antifungals, Peptides, and Metronidazole

Crossword Puzzle

Across
1. first-line drugs
4. rifabutin
7. amphotericin B
9. vagina
10. gram-positive
11. hepatotoxicity

Down
2. lungs
3. streptomycin
5. fluconazole
6. bactericidal
8. IV

12. a
13. a
14. b
15. a
16. a
17. b
18. b
19. b
20. a
21. b
22. b. Alcoholism is a contraindication to prophylactic treatment for tuberculosis with isoniazid. Alcohol ingestion with this drug can increase the incidence of peripheral neuropathy.

23. c
24. b, c, d, e. All of the foods listed except apples are high in vitamin B$_6$, which is important in preventing peripheral neuropathy.
25. a. Taking a combination of echinacea and ketoconazole can promote hepatotoxicity.
26. b, c, e. It will be important to obtain a history of medications taken and drug allergies prior to starting treatment. A history of tuberculosis (TB) exposure and the results and dates of most recent purified protein derivative (PPD) and chest x-rays will also be important information. A history of IV drug abuse, although important overall, is not specific to this disease process.
27. b
28. c
29. c. Antacids should not be taken at the same time as INH. Antacids decrease the absorption of INH.
30. a, b. Vitamin B$_6$ supplements or increased intake may be necessary to prevent peripheral neuropathy. Alcohol should be avoided since INH can be hepatotoxic. Rifampin, not INH, may turn body fluids brownish-orange.
31. b
32. b
33. b. The standard dose range is 0.3-1 mg/kg/day. This is mixed in 500 mL of D$_5$W and infused over 2-6 hours. The maximum dose is 1.5 mg/kg/day. Because this medication is highly toxic, the initial dose would be as low as possible.
34. c. Amphotericin B is only given intravenously and side effects include flushing, nausea, vomiting, hypotension, and chills. The patient does not need to be NPO prior to receiving a dose of amphotericin B, and it may in fact be beneficial to have a light, nongreasy meal or even some crackers to help decrease the nausea. Amphotericin B is nephrotoxic, so any changes in urination should be reported immediately to the health care provider.
35. a, c, d, e. There are no contraindications or documented interactions between amphotericin B and alcohol.
36. a
37. c
38. a, b, c
39. b
40. a, b, c. Laboratory values that assess hepatic and renal function should be obtained at baseline and trended. PT may be altered if the patient is taking warfarin.

Case Study

1. The nurse must complete a thorough assessment including questions regarding medications currently taken, allergies, and vital signs. Specific questions regarding vaginal or anal itching should also be asked.
2. Frequent use of antibiotics can destroy the normal flora in the body and cause a superinfection to occur. This infection is likely thrush, which is caused by *Candida* spp.
3. To correctly take this medication, the patient should put 1-2 tsp (5-10 mL) in her mouth and swish it around. The medication should then be swallowed.

Chapter 33—
Antivirals, Antimalarials, and Anthelmintics

1. c
2. e
3. a
4. b
5. d
6. d
7. b
8. b. 400 mg taken t.i.d. or three times per day will yield 1200 mg total in a 24-hour period.
9. c. Gentamicin is an aminoglycoside. Taking an aminoglycoside and acyclovir together may increase the risk for nephrotoxicity.
10. c. Famcyclovir 125 mg b.i.d for 5 days is a treatment option for HSV-1. There are also other dosing regimens available, including 1000 mg b.i.d. for 1 day or as a 1500-mg one-time dose. HSV-1 is spread in the saliva, so the paramedic may or may not be able to work while there is an active lesion. It is not true that he would never be able to work as a paramedic again.
11. a, c. It is crucial to have an evaluation of baseline renal function, since ganciclovir is excreted in the urine and it can be nephrotoxic. Ganciclovir can also cause hyperbilirubinemia.
12. c
13. b
14. c, d, e, f. With the use of chloroquine, red blood cell count, hemoglobin, and hematocrit may be lowered. Liver enzymes such as AST may be elevated. Baseline laboratory values should be obtained and monitored.
15. b. Chloroquine is taken for 2 weeks before and 6-8 weeks after exposure to potentially infected mosquitoes to prevent growth of the parasites. Abdominal cramping, nausea, and vomiting are among the expected side effects. Ringing in the ears may be an indication of ototoxicity and needs to be reported immediately. Taking either antacids or laxatives may decrease the effectiveness of chloroquine.

16. b. Artemether/lumefantrine (Coartem) is a combination drug that has a high success rate and may be used if other drugs have failed due to resistance. It is especially useful in patients with high fevers.

17. b, d, e. Proper hygiene for a patient who has worms includes frequent handwashing, especially after using the toilet and before eating. Since the worms may live on a variety of materials, all clothing, towels, and bedding should be changed on a daily basis and washed in hot water. The patient should shower instead of sitting in a bathtub and should not swim in pools or use hot tubs while infected. To prevent trichinosis, caused by *Trichinella spiralis,* all pork and pork-containing products must be thoroughly cooked to destroy the larvae.

18. c, d, e

19. b

Case Study

1. "The flu" is a viral disease that is spread by droplets. Three antigen types, A, B, and C, are the causative agents. Type C is not as common in humans as types A and B, and type B occurs only in humans. Type A is responsible for most of the outbreaks annually.

2. The flu can be diagnosed by obtaining a nasal swab, a throat swab, or nasal aspiration, depending on the test. It is a quick test that can be completed in the health care provider's office. Since the flu is a virus, antibiotics will not be effective for treatment. There are several antiviral medications that can be used in the treatment of the flu. Amantadine and rimantadine may be used. These are older medications and, since the influenza virus mutates frequently, do not appear to be as effective as zanamivir and oseltamivir phosphate. The newer medications impair virus replication but are only effective if taken early in the course of the illness. The best "treatment" is rest, fluids, and limited contact with others to prevent the spread of the disease.

Chapter 34—
Drugs for Urinary Tract Disorders

Crossword Puzzle

Across

1. acute pyelonephritis
4. urinary stimulants
7. bacteriostatic
8. acute cystitis

Down

2. cranberry
3. *Pseudomonas aeruginosa*

5. nitrofurantoin
6. bactericidal
9. c
10. b. Cranberry juice will help lower the pH and make the urine more acidic. Whole milk may make urine more alkaline and increase the pH. Although increased fluid intake is important when a patient has a urinary tract infection (UTI), simply increasing the amount of water alone will not decrease the urine pH.
11. b
12. b, c, d. Photosensitivity may occur and extra protection should be taken when outside or exposed to sunlight. Increasing fluid intake is important because medications in this class are eliminated in the urine. Drowsiness may occur when taking nalidixic acid, so operating machinery and driving should be avoided. Orange discoloration of the urine is not associated with nalidixic acid, and absorption is improved if taken with food.
13. c, d, e
14. a, c, e
15. d. Swelling around the eyes and lips are classic indications of angioedema, which is an adverse effect associated with nitrofurantoin and needs to be evaluated immediately. Brown- or rust-colored urine and diarrhea can be side effects of nitrofurantoin (Macrodantin), but they do not need to be immediately reported to the provider. Frequency in urination is common with UTIs.
16. a, b, e
17. c
18. d. Bright reddish-orange urine is to be expected when taking phenazopyridine (Pyridium). This can be very startling to the patient if she is not told in advance to anticipate the change. Undergarments can also be stained orange while taking this medication.
19. b
20. a, c, e. Bethanechol is a urinary stimulant and would not benefit this patient. Nitrofurantoin is an antiinfective and, unless this patient has a UTI, there is no need for it. Tolterodine tartrate, although beneficial to patients with overactive bladder, is contraindicated in patients with narrow-angle glaucoma.
21. a. Chest pain and difficulty breathing could be indicative of an allergic reaction. To prevent GI upset, the majority of the fluoroquinolones can be taken with food. Headaches, dizziness, and photosensitivity may occur.
22. b. Bethanechol chloride (Urecholine) is a urinary stimulant that increases bladder tone. It is prescribed when bladder function is lost due to spinal cord injuries with paralysis.

Case Study

1. Oxybutynin chloride (Ditropan) is a urinary antispasmodic that has direct action on the smooth muscles of the urinary tract. By relaxing these muscles, the spasms are decreased.
2. Patients who have urinary or GI obstruction as well as those with narrow-angle glaucoma should not take this medication. Oxybutynin blocks acetylcholine receptors that mediate parasympathetic function. Should the patient experience severe abdominal pain, constipation, or urinary retention, the health care provider should be contacted immediately.
3. Common side effects may include dry mouth, drowsiness, and blurred vision. The patient should be encouraged not to participate in any activities where dizziness could be an issue (climbing, skateboarding, etc.). Adult patients should be encouraged not to drive until they know how the medication will affect them.
4. No, the dosage range for adults is 5 mg b.i.d./t.i.d., with a maximum adult range of 20 mg/day. The range for children over 5 years old is 5 mg b.i.d., with a maximum of 15 mg/day.

Chapter 35—
HIV- and AIDS-Related Drugs

Crossword Puzzle

Across
3. cell-mediated
6. nucleoside analogues
7. efavirenz
8. nonnucleoside analogues
10. innate
11. viral load

Down
1. reverse transcription
2. tenofovir
4. acquired
5. budding
9. adherence

12. b
13. a, c, e
14. b, c, e
15. c
16. c
17. d
18. b
19. b
20. b

21. a, b, c. Hepatic and renal function will be monitored at baseline and throughout treatment. A CBC with differential will be followed to watch for indications of infections.
22. a, b, c, d. Seizures would be an adverse reaction, not a side effect.
23. c
24. d
25. d
26. a, c. Most of the side effects associated with efavirenz are CNS side effects such as dizziness, insomnia, agitation, and hallucinations. Gastrointestinal side effects include nausea and diarrhea.
27. a, c, d. Efavirenz has effects on the liver and the potential for liver failure. Alcohol should not be consumed while taking this medication. The patient should discuss the use of any herbal preparations with the health care provider. St. John's wort should not be taken with efavirenz.
28. d
29. c, d. Monitoring of liver enzymes and triglycerides is important while taking tenofovir. Some studies have shown that this medication may also have an effect on cholesterol, but the link is unclear.
30. a, b, d. St. John's wort should not be taken with any antiretrovirals, as it may change the levels in the blood. A benefit of tenofovir is that it may be taken with or without food. This is important because nausea, vomiting, diarrhea, and flatulence are potential GI side effects. The patient may have to work with the health care provider to make adjustments with regards to timing, diet, and side effects. Dizziness may be a side effect also, so the patient may wish to wait to drive until after he or she knows the medication's effects; however, a patient will be able to drive while taking tenofovir.
31. a
32. b, c. This medication has few side effects. They include rash, cough, and nausea.
33. a, b, d, e. Anything that will help the patient keep track of timing on medication and increase compliance will be of benefit. This can be in the form of pill organizers, timers to remind the patient of medication schedule, and wall calendars or charts where the medication can be crossed off after it has been taken.

Case Study

1. Although occurring less frequently than in years past, health care provider exposure still occurs. The first step the nurse should take is to completely wash the exposed area with soap and water.
2. Policies vary from institution to institution; however, postexposure prophylaxis (PEP) should start within hours of exposure and continue for 4 weeks.

Both the basic and expanded versions of PEP include combinations of medications.

3. The potential side effects of therapy include nausea, malaise, and fatigue. These occur in between 17% and 47% of all providers taking the prophylactic treatment and may be a cause of noncompliance.

Chapter 36— Vaccines

Crossword Puzzle

Across
3. seroconversion
5. anaphylaxis
7. passive
8. pathogen

Down
1. attenuated viruses
2. recombinant
4. vaccine
6. antibodies

9. d
10. b, c, e. Acquired passive immunity is provided through administration of antibodies pooled from another source. Newborns receive immunity through maternal antibodies at birth. Pregnant women should not receive immunizations, with a few exceptions such as the seasonal flu vaccine.
11. c
12. d
13. d
14. a
15. a
16. a
17. a
18. c
19. d
20. a
21. c
22. c
23. c
24. d
25. d. Influenza vaccine is not given until at least 6 months. Hepatitis B is not due again until 6 months.
26. a. Redness and tenderness are common side effects.
27. b
28. a, b, c, e. Parents should be given a copy of the immunization record as well as an appointment card with a contact phone number for the clinic at the time of discharge. A Vaccine Information Statement should be given to any patient, not just children, when they receive any immunizations.
29. a
30. c. Although diphenhydramine is used for allergic reactions, in the case of an anaphylactic reaction, epinephrine should be readily available.

Case Study
1. A concern for a patient who has sustained a puncture wound is the potential for tetanus.
2. Signs and symptoms of tetanus include headache, irritability, muscle spasms that usually begin in the jaw ("lockjaw"), fever, and drooling. If not treated, tetanus can be fatal.
3. The patient should receive a Td vaccine. Other vaccinations could include zoster, pneumonia, and, if in contact with infants or young children, pertussis.

Chapter 37— Anticancer Drugs

1. h
2. j
3. a
4. d
5. i
6. c
7. g
8. b
9. f
10. e
11. a. Combination chemotherapy is used as a treatment across all (or most) phases of cell life; therefore, it tends to be more effective.
12. d
13. c
14. a. The goal of palliative chemotherapy is not to cure but to help improve the patient's quality of life by treating symptoms such as pain or shortness of breath that may be associated with advanced disease.
15. a. White blood cells are used to fight infection. If the white blood cell count is decreased, the patient is at higher risk for an infection. Temperature changes, even if slight, may be an indication of a developing illness.
16. a. Chemotherapy causes myelosuppression, involving red cells, white cells, and platelets. Platelets are involved with clotting and healing injured tissue. If the platelet count is low, the patient is more prone to occult bleeding (GI tract, for example) and may be unable to effectively clot wounds (like IV sites).

17. d. Caffeine may have a laxative effect, so it should be limited in patients with diarrhea.

18. b. When both drugs are given orally, cyclophosphamide decreases digoxin levels by impairing GI absorption.

19. d. Metronidazole may increase the toxicity of 5-FU by inhibiting elimination.

20. a. Adriamycin has serious cardiac side effects. Cardiac function should be assessed prior to and during treatment with this medication. Cardiac ejection fraction should be obtained prior to commencing treatment. Depending on studies, a drop in the ejection fraction between 5% and 10% can be an early indication of cardiotoxicity.

21. c. Doxorubicin (Adriamycin) may cause congestive heart failure. Shortness of breath and crackles could be an indication of early heart failure.

22. c

23. c. When the blood count is at its lowest is when the patient is at the highest risk for infection.

24. c. Hemorrhagic cystitis is a result of severe bladder inflammation, which may occur with cyclophosphamide. Adequate hydration while giving this medication is important to potentially prevent this complication.

25. a. Hydration should be started before treatment and maintained throughout. Antiemetics should be given 30-60 minutes prior to beginning treatment prophylactically.

26. d. Pregnancy should be prevented during chemotherapy treatment, including use of cyclophosphamide, due to the effects on the fetus.

27. c. Hyperpigmentation can occur along the vein where 5-FU was administered. This may not be reversible. Oral hygiene is very important, and the mouth should be rinsed every 2 hours.

28. c. Nausea, vomiting, and diarrhea associated with chemotherapy can place the patient at risk for altered nutrition. Adequate nutrition is required for healing. Small, frequent meals and snacks may be better tolerated than three large meals per day.

29. d. Doxorubicin may change the urine to a pink or reddish color. This is due to bladder irritation.

30. c. Adriamycin has both cardiac and pulmonary side effects. These should be reported to the health care provider.

31. a

32. b. Chemotherapeutic agents suppress the bone marrow. Laboratory work should be monitored for abnormalities. The nadir for many chemotherapeutic agents occurs between 7 and 10 days.

33. d. Disposable powder-free gloves (nitrile, polyurethane, neoprene) should be worn when preparing chemotherapy and disposed of after administering the medication or if they become punctured or contaminated.

34. b. The patient and his family will need to be alert for signs of infection due to the effects of chemotherapy. Assessing his temperature will need to become a part of his routine.

35. a. Antiemetics should be administered prophylactically before chemotherapy is initiated.

36. c. Petechiae, ecchymoses, and bleeding gums are an indication of bleeding.

37. a

38. d. Vincristine lowers the effects of phenytoin, so the patient must be carefully observed for an increase in seizure activity.

39. a, c, d. Each of these herbals has shown some effect when taken with vincristine. A daily multivitamin may be beneficial in patients undergoing chemotherapy. There is no contraindication for taking valerian.

40. c. An alcohol-based mouthwash will be very uncomfortable for a patient with mucositis. Also, if the skin barrier is broken, using an alcohol-based mouthwash will potentially cause further irritation.

41. c. Neutropenia, or a lowered white blood cell count, puts the patient at risk for infection.

Case Study

1. Cyclophosphamide (Cytoxan) is an alkylating agent. It works by causing the DNA strand to cross-link, strands to break, and abnormal base pairing. This prevents the cancer cells from dividing. Cyclophosphamide is also a CCNS (cell cycle–nonspecific) drug that kills cells across the lifespan.

2. Some major side effects of cyclophosphamide include nausea and vomiting, anemia, risk for infection, and bleeding. Some side effects specific to this medication include the potential for hemorrhagic cystitis, discoloration of the nails, cardiomyopathy, and syndrome of inappropriate antidiuretic hormone (SIADH) secretion.

3. A thorough nursing history and physical assessment are crucial for this patient throughout the course of therapy. A baseline assessment of laboratory values, x-rays, and vital signs is very important. A psychosocial assessment should also be completed. Careful monitoring of the patient's temperature on a daily basis is crucial to watch for early signs of infection.

4. The patient should be taught that adequate fluid intake (both oral and IV) will be very important to prevent hemorrhagic cystitis. Even if the patient is nauseated, small sips of water at frequent intervals may be beneficial. The goal for fluid intake is 2-3 L/day. The patient should be advised not to become pregnant while undergoing treatment. Cyclophosphamide is pregnancy category D. Also, before using any OTC medications or herbal preparations, the patient should confer with her health care pro-

vider since there are several herbs (ginseng, garlic, kava kava, echinacea, ginkgo, St. John's wort) that may have interactions with chemotherapy. If the patient has a desire for complementary therapy, it should be respected as much as possible.

Chapter 38—
Targeted Therapies to Treat Cancer

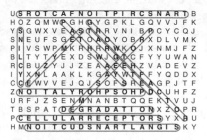

1. growth factor
2. Signal transduction
3. phosphorylation
4. Transcription factors
5. Cyclins
6. proteasome; degradation
7. Targeted; cellular receptors; enzymes; pathways
8. d. Shortness of breath and itching could be an indication of an anaphylactic reaction. The infusion must be stopped immediately and the reaction treated.
9. c
10. b
11. a
12. b
13. c. Patients who have preexisting respiratory problems should not take erlotinib, as pulmonary fibrosis may occur.
14. a. Imatinib (Gleevec) may cause thrombocytopenia and increase risk for bleeding. This may be initially apparent with bleeding gums, bruising, and petechiae.
15. a, c, d, e. Gastrointestinal and integumentary symptoms are associated with this medication.
16. a, b, d, e. The cardiovascular system is not affected by imatinib (Gleevec).

Case Study

1. For metastatic breast cancer, bevacizumab is administered 10 mg/kg every 2 weeks in combination with paclitaxel. It is always mixed in normal saline and infused over 60-90 minutes depending on how it is tolerated. The first dose is given over 90 minutes.
2. Bevacizumab binds to vascular endothelial growth factor (VEGF) and prevents the binding of VEGF with its receptors. It blocks angiogenesis, and the goal is to slow the disease spread.
3. Bevacizumab has a black box warning for GI perforations, wound dehiscence, impaired wound healing, hemorrhage, and fistula formation after surgery. Other side effects include proteinuria, hypertension, increased risk for deep vein thrombosis, and hematopoietic suppression. Although there are many side effects, this medication is used for those patients with metastatic disease where the benefits outweigh the risks.

Chapter 39—
Biologic Response Modifiers

Crossword Puzzle

Across

2. oprelvekin
4. nadir
5. absolute neutrophil count
6. interleukin
8. pegylation
9. interferon
10. tumoricidal
11. sargramostim
12. myelosuppression
13. hybridoma technology

Down

1. colony stimulating
3. erythropoietin
7. thrombocytopenia

14. b
15. c
16. a
17. d
18. e
19. a, b, d
20. a. Bone pain is the only consistently observed reaction attributed to G-CSF. This is due to expansion of the bone marrow.
21. d. Granulocytes may become sequestered in the pulmonary system and cause dyspnea. This will cause an additional stress on the already compromised patient. Special attention should be paid to complaints of difficulty breathing.
22. a, b, c, d. Single-dose vials are for a single use only. They do not contain preservatives and must be disposed of immediately. Multidose vials do have preservatives, but they must be discarded 21 days after being opened. Hemoglobin should be obtained at baseline and then throughout treatment

and levels should not exceed 12 mg/dL. Aranesp should be protected from light.

23. b
24. a
25. a
26. a
27. a, c, d, e
28. a, b, c, e. The patient and her significant others should be educated regarding side effects, adverse effects, and how to administer the medication. The side effects from BRM administration usually disappear 72-96 hours after discontinuation of therapy.
29. b, c. GM-CSF should be administered to both allogenic and autologous BMT recipients. It is not recommended for Kaposi's sarcoma. GM-CSF is used for an ANC < 1500/mm³, and it should not be used within 24 hours of chemotherapy.

Case Study

1. G-CSF is not a chemotherapeutic agent, but is used in conjunction with myelosuppressive chemotherapy to increase production of neutrophils and enhance phagocytosis to help fight infection. It is an adjunct to chemotherapy, and some initial effects may be seen within 1-2 days.
2. Side effects of this medication are similar to those of other BRMs (nausea, vomiting, fatigue, etc.); however, bone pain is consistently reported with G-CSF because of the action on the bone marrow. Bone pain occurs more frequently in patients receiving higher IV doses (20-100 mcg/kg/day) than in patients receiving lower subcutaneous doses (3-10 mcg/kg/day).
3. Priority teaching instructions include the use of nonopioid pain medication to help relieve bone pain. Should the patient become pregnant, she should notify her health care provider immediately, as caution should be used in administering this medication to pregnant patients. The patient should also report any abdominal pain, including pain referred to the left shoulder, as well as chest pain or hematuria.

Chapter 40—
Drugs for Upper Respiratory Disorders

1. c
2. a
3. d
4. b
5. b
6. a

7. d
8. a
9. d
10. a
11. c
12. a, b, d, e
13. d
14. c
15. a, b, c, e. The common cold is spread by droplets, so good hand hygiene and covering the nose and mouth when sneezing are important to prevent the spread of the illness. Adequate fluids and rest are also important. The use of any herbal preparations should be discussed with the health care provider prior to implementing them. Nasal sprays are only used every 4-6 hours for a set period. If used longer than 5-7 days, rebound congestion may develop.
16. a, b, c, d
17. a, b, c, d. Decongestants are not contraindicated in obesity unless the patient also has any of the other diagnoses.
18. c, d. Antihistamines may cause drowsiness. Diphenhydramine is a common ingredient in OTC sleeping preparations. Should the patient choose to take any OTC medications, he or she should be instructed to read the label carefully to check for interactions. The best option, however, is to check with the health care provider or pharmacist. Decongestants taken at bedtime may cause insomnia or jitteriness. Antibiotics are ineffective against a virus.

Case Study

1. Oxymetazoline is a decongestant nasal spray that is used to help constrict the vessels within the nasal cavity. The nasal mucous membranes shrink, and it is easier for the patient to exchange air through the nose.
2. The correct dose for this patient would be 2 puffs in each nostril, morning and night. It should not be used for longer than 3-5 days due to the potential for rebound congestion.
3. Rebound congestion occurs due to irritation of the nasal mucosa leading to vasodilation instead of vasoconstriction. Use of nasal decongestants can also lead to nasal dryness and, if overused, epistaxis. Some brands of oxymetazoline are listed as moisturizing. Another option is to use saline nasal drops, although this will only moisturize and not serve as a decongestant. Oral decongestants such as phenylephrine or pseudoephedrine may also be used. Also important with this patient is to determine the cause of the nasal congestion. Allergies may be treated with intranasal glucocorticoids and first- or second-generation antihistamines. A common cold will not be treated with glucocorticoids.

Chapter 41—
Drugs for Lower Respiratory Disorders

1. d
2. e
3. b
4. c
5. a, b
6. b
7. cyclic adenosine monophosphate (cAMP)
8. epinephrine
9. beta$_2$-adrenergic agonists
10. nonselective
11. cAMP
12. increases
13. synergistic
14. shorter
15. methylxanthine (xanthine); asthma
16. glucocorticoids
17. prophylactic; histamine
18. rebound bronchospasm
19. beta$_2$
20. montelukast (Singulair)
21. evening
22. 10 mg/day; 5 mg/day
23. mucolytics
24. antibiotic
25. c. The inhaler should be shaken well before each use. Inhalers do not require refrigeration. By testing the inhaler each time to see if the spray works, the patient is losing a dose of the medication.
26. a, b, d, e. Inhaled doses of medications for asthma have a more rapid onset and fewer side effects than oral medications. They are shorter-acting. Some inhaled medications and oral medications can be taken together.
27. b
28. a
29. a, c
30. b
31. c, d
32. d. Taking theophylline and ephedra together may increase the risk of theophylline toxicity. Hyperglycemia is a sign of theophylline toxicity.
33. a, b, c, d. It is not necessary to wait 5 minutes between inhalations.
34. d, e
35. a, b, c, e. Beta blockers increase the half-life of theophylline. Theophylline increases the risk of digitalis toxicity and decreases the effects of lithium. Phenytoin decreases theophylline levels.
36. a, c, d, e
37. b. Cromolyn sodium is used as a prophylactic medication to prevent asthma attacks by preventing the release of histamine and suppressing inflammation in the bronchioles. It will not stop an attack once it has started and is not a bronchodilator.
38. c. The therapeutic range for theophylline is 10-20 mcg/mL.

Case Study
1. Albuterol is a selective beta$_2$ agonist. It can be used on an as-needed basis during an asthma attack because it is fast-acting and provides bronchodilation. Since it is a selective beta$_2$ agonist, there are fewer side effects than with other medications. Montelukast sodium (Singulair) is a leukotriene modifier. Leukotrienes are chemical mediators that cause airway edema and increased mucus production. Leukotriene modifiers like Singulair decrease inflammation. They must be taken daily and are not effective to treat an asthma attack. Advair Diskus 100/50 is a glucocorticoid combination drug that contains fluticasone propionate 100 mcg and salmeterol 50 mcg. Glucocorticoids have antiinflammatory properties, and they work synergistically with beta$_2$ agonists.
2. H.K. should be encouraged to keep all appointments as scheduled and to contact her health care provider before taking any over-the-counter medications. If she smokes, she should be given information on smoking cessation programs and advised to notify her health care provider if she is contemplating pregnancy. Patients with asthma should be encouraged to stay hydrated and report any increased use of "rescue inhalers" like albuterol. A patient with asthma should also be encouraged to wear a medical identification bracelet or necklace to indicate the medications he or she is taking.

Chapter 42—
Cardiac Glycosides, Antianginals, and Antidysrhythmics

Crossword Puzzle

Across
1. hypercapnia
2. preload
3. antianginal
6. repolarization
8. depolarization
10. hypokalemia
11. afterload
12. bradycardia
13. antidysrhythmics

Down

1. hypoxia
4. nitrates
5. ischemia
7. glycoside
9. tachycardia

14. weakens; enlarges
15. increase
16. pump or cardiac
17. digitalis glycosides
18. increase; decrease
19. positive inotropic action (increases heart contraction); negative chronotropic action (decreases heart rate); negative dromotropic action (decreases conduction of the heart cells); and increased stroke volume
20. decrease
21. it undergoes first-pass metabolism by the liver
22. 1-3; 3
23. headache
24. beta blockers
25. verapamil (Calan)
26. reflex tachycardia; pain
27. stressed (or exerted)
28. at frequent times daily with increasing severity
29. is at rest
30. spasm
31. reduction of venous tone or coronary vasodilator
32. hypoxia; hypercapnia
33. fast sodium channel blockers; beta blockers; calcium channel blockers; also drugs that prolong repolarization
34. alcohol; cigarettes
35. b
36. a
37. b
38. a
39. c
40. d
41. b
42. c
43. c
44. d
45. d
46. a
47. a, b
48. d
49. a, c. Constipation is a side effect of verapamil, and it is taken three times per day. Verapamil may cause hypotension, not hypertension.
50. c
51. d. Calcium channel blockers may have an effect on kidney and liver function, so baseline liver enzymes should be obtained and trended.
52. c

53. d. Normal values are less than 100 pg/mL. Greater than 100 pg/mL is considered elevated. Older women tend to run higher than older men; however, a level of 420 pg/mL is markedly elevated and is of concern for heart failure.
54. a
55. a
56. b
57. d. Nausea, vomiting, dizziness, headache, and bradycardia are signs of digitalis toxicity. The patient cannot wait until his next appointment to be seen. Digoxin levels will need to be evaluated and an antidote may need to be given.
58. b
59. a, b, c. Cortisone, furosemide, and hydrochlorothiazide all promote loss of potassium, which increases the effect of digitalis and can lead to digitalis toxicity.
60. a
61. a. A heart rate of less than 60 beats/min or irregular is concerning. A heart rate of less than 60 *and* irregular is the most concerning.
62. c. There are not any specific drug-food contraindications for digoxin. The patient should be encouraged to eat foods high in potassium such as fruits and vegetables (including potatoes). A patient with heart failure should avoid hot dogs due to high sodium content.
63. a, b, c, d, e
64. b
65. a, b. Nitroglycerin tablets should not be chewed but should be placed under the tongue. If chest pain persists after one tablet, the health care provider should be notified. There are no dietary restrictions when taking nitroglycerin. Tablets must be stored in a cool, dark place and preferably in the original bottle to prevent decomposition. A very dry mouth will hinder absorption, so sips of water may be taken.
66. c
67. b
68. c
69. c
70. a. Abruptly stopping acebutolol can lead to palpitations.
71. a, b, d, e
72. a, d, e
73. a, b, e. Electrolyte imbalances, especially potassium, calcium, and magnesium, can lead to cardiac dysrhythmias. Excessive catecholamines may lead to rapid atrial or ventricular rates as well as ectopy. Hypoxia and *hyper*capnia may also cause arrhythmias (dysrhythmias).

Case Study

1. The three different types of angina are classic, unstable, and variant. Classic angina is fairly predictable and occurs with stress or exertion. Unstable angina is also known as *preinfarction angina*. It is unpredictable and increases in frequency. Unstable angina may or may not be related to stress. Variant angina is also known as *vasospastic* or *Prinzmetal's angina*. It occurs at rest. Patients frequently have a combination of both classic and variant angina. Classic angina is caused by an actual narrowing of the coronary arteries, whereas variant angina is caused by vessel spasms.

2. Since stress plays a part in angina attacks, getting adequate rest and using relaxation techniques may be beneficial nonpharmacologic methods to treat vasospastic angina. Smoking cessation is very important to overall cardiac health.

3. Nitrates such as nitroglycerin or calcium channel blockers such as diltiazem or verapamil are used to treat variant angina. Beta blockers are not effective for variant angina, but are effective for classic or stable angina. Nitrates help dilate the coronary vessels and calcium channel blockers relax spasms.

4. Nitrates cause vasodilation and reduce both preload, and indirectly, afterload, leading to a drop in blood pressure.

Chapter 43—Diuretics

Crossword Puzzle

Across

3. natriuresis
6. osmolality
7. mannitol
8. hyperkalemia
9. diuresis
10. hypertension
11. hyperkalemia
12. oliguria

Down

1. carbonic anhydrase inhibitor
2. furosemide
4. aldosterone
5. hyperglycemia
13. hypokalemia
14. hypomagnesemia
15. hypercalcemia
16. hypochloremia
17. minimal bicarbonate loss

18. hyperuricemia
19. hyperglycemia
20. hyperlipidemia
21. b, d, e
22. d
23. b
24. b
25. a
26. c. Spironolactone (Aldactone) blocks the action of aldosterone and inhibits the sodium-potassium pump, so potassium is retained. This is important in maintaining a regular cardiac rhythm. It is frequently prescribed by cardiologists and is not contraindicated in patients who have had a myocardial infarction. Sodium is excreted with this medication. Patients should be advised not to overindulge in foods rich in potassium such as bananas, as this could cause above-normal levels (hyperkalemia).
27. d. To prevent hearing loss, furosemide must be administered slow IV push over at least 1-2 minutes. It does not need to be diluted and does not require a central line for administration. Cardiac monitoring is not essential, as furosemide does not cause arrhythmias.
28. a, b, d. Hypokalemia, or low serum potassium, is a risk for patients taking thiazides. This could be a life-threatening condition. Sodium is also lost, causing hyponatremia. Calcium is elevated since thiazides block calcium excretion. There is minimal effect on bicarbonate levels. Cautious use in hepatic failure patients is recommended, but trending of AST/ALT is not always indicated. Baseline values may be beneficial.
29. a. The normal range for serum potassium is 3.5-5.3 mEq/L. A level of 5.8 mEq/L is considered hyperkalemia, which may be life-threatening. The dose of spironolactone should be decreased, and the patient should decrease intake of potassium-rich foods such as bananas, apricots, leafy greens, and salmon.
30. a. Acetazolamide is recommended for patients with open-angle glaucoma.
31. a. Acetazolamide is a carbonic anhydrase inhibitor. It blocks the action of carbonic anhydrase, which is an enzyme that affects hydrogen ion balance. If the action is blocked, more bicarbonate will be excreted, leading to metabolic acidosis.
32. d. Because the onset of action is 2 hours, it may be best to take the medication when the patient will be awake for several hours so sleep is not disturbed. Hydrochlorothiazide can be taken with food to prevent GI upset. The medication needs to be taken consistently, even if the patient is not having symptoms.

33. a. Furosemide will cause an increased loss of potassium when given with amiodarone, which may predispose the patient to ventricular arrhythmias.

34. c. Muscle weakness, abdominal distention, severe leg cramping, and cardiac arrhythmias are indications of hypokalemia (lowered potassium levels). Lowered potassium may occur with the use of loop diuretics.

35. b

36. a, b

37. b

38. c. The combination of furosemide and alcohol can increase orthostatic hypotension.

39. a. Loop diuretics are contraindicated in patients with anuria. Giving diuretics to a patient without any urine output will not force urine production.

40. a, c, d. Raisins, baked potatoes, and tomatoes are high in potassium, which is beneficial since loop diuretics cause a loss of potassium. Rice and white bread are low in potassium.

41. d. Daily weights and vital signs need to be trended at home on a daily basis. The patient and family should be educated on how to take these measurements or arrangements should be made for home health services to assess, at least initially. The onset of action for hydrochlorothiazide is 2 hours. Hyperglycemia is a side effect of hydrochlorothiazide, so blood sugar should be monitored. This medication can be taken with food to prevent nausea.

Case Study

1. Mannitol is an osmotic diuretic that is used for patients with increased intracranial pressure and increased intraocular pressure. Osmotic diuretics increase osmolality and sodium reabsorption. Sodium, chloride, potassium, and water are excreted. This shift in fluid will cause, at least temporarily, a decrease in intracranial pressure.

2. The standard dosage range in adults for mannitol is 1-2 g/kg, followed by 0.25 mg to 1 g/kg of a 15% to 25% solution infused over 30-90 minutes. Mannitol crystallizes easily, so it must be warmed prior to administration. It is suggested that it be given through a filtered needle.

3. For this patient, the correct dose would be 80-160 g, followed by 20-80 g over 30-90 minutes.

Chapter 44— Antihypertensives

1. beta-adrenergic blockers; centrally acting alpha₂ agonists; alpha-adrenergic blockers

2. calcium channel blockers; ACE inhibitors; also diuretics

3. prehypertension; stage 1; stage 2

4. beta blockers; ACE inhibitors; also angiotensin II receptor blockers, potassium-sparing diuretics

5. diuretics

6. stage 2

7. diminished; lowered

8. cardioselective

9. decrease very–low-density lipoprotein (VLDL) and LDL; increase HDL

10. c

11. d

12. b

13. e

14. f

15. g

16. b. According to the guidelines, the patient falls in the category of prehypertension with a reading of 136/82 mm Hg, since prehypertension is defined as systolic blood pressure of 120-139 and diastolic blood pressure of 80-89.

17. d

18. b. Nonselective alpha-adrenergic blockers are used for severe hypertension associated with catecholamine-secreting tumors of the adrenal medulla (pheochromocytomas).

19. d

20. d. Diuretics are frequently given with a variety of antihypertensive agents to decrease fluid retention and peripheral edema.

21. a, b, c

22. b

23. a

24. d. African Americans are not as responsive to ACE inhibitors given as monotherapy, but may respond better if an ACE inhibitor is combined with a thiazide diuretic.

25. c. Calcium channel blockers and alpha₁ blockers may be more effective in the African-American patient population for treating hypertension.

26. a

27. a

28. c

29. a

30. d. Captopril has low protein-binding power, so there will be no drug displacement.

31. b

32. e. The only group that should absolutely not take valsartan are pregnant women in their third trimester due to decrease in placental blood flow.

33. b. Because of the action of ACE inhibitors such as captopril, potassium-sparing diuretics should not be used.

34. b. Compliance with the medication regimen can be very frustrating to a patient who "feels better." Stopping an antihypertensive abruptly can lead to rebound hypertension.

35. c

36. a
37. a, d
38. d
39. d
40. b. Ankle edema may occur with calcium channel blockers such as amlodipine. There are other options that may be utilized to treat the patient's hypertension.
41. b
42. b
43. d, e. Cardioselective beta blockers will help maintain renal blood flow and have fewer hypoglycemic effects than those associated with noncardioselective beta blockers. Rebound symptoms are a possibility if the medication is stopped abruptly. Cardioselectivity does not confer absolute protection from bronchoconstriction.
44. a, b, c
45. b

Case Study

1. Combipres (chlorthalidone with clonidine) combines a thiazide diuretic with a centrally acting alpha$_2$ agonist. Centrally acting alpha$_2$ agonists decrease the sympathetic response from the brainstem to the peripheral vessels. The result is decreased peripheral vascular resistance and increased vasodilation, thereby reducing blood pressure. Because clonidine can cause fluid retention, a diuretic is frequently prescribed, which accounts for the combination of clonidine with chlorthalidone.

2. *Hypertensive emergencies* are defined as a systolic blood pressure greater than or equal to 180 mm Hg and a diastolic greater than or equal to 120 mm Hg with acute impairment of one or more systems (cardiovascular, renal, neurologic). If left untreated, permanent damage may occur. J.H. is showing signs of neurologic dysfunction (headache and dizziness). Epistaxis may also be seen in hypertensive patients.

   The blood pressure needs to be lowered quickly, but in a controlled setting. Options include immediate-release nifedipine and sodium nitroprusside. Sodium nitroprusside (Nipride) is administered intravenously in a critical care unit and is the drug of choice for hypertensive emergencies. The patient must be monitored closely in a critical care unit during administration.

3. Priority teaching instructions at discharge for this patient include the importance of taking the medication as prescribed. Determining why the patient skips doses is important, and priority teaching instructions may be directed toward the cause. If the patient remains on a similar medication that is combined with a diuretic, the nurse should suggest the patient take the medication during waking hours so sleep is not interrupted. Decreasing stress, increasing exercise, and evaluating the diet are important pieces of the entire care plan for a patient with hypertension.

Chapter 45— Anticoagulants, Antiplatelets, and Thrombolytics

```
J B S J A G G R E G A T I O N U O
V M L K I N W P O F L W Y W W I L
A S S Y L O N R B I F Q H E D
D V T N G M X L U S P C G X Z T U
Q F S R B W A R L K C Q U U H S S
B T L K O H B P V D G H Z I H I E
Q S R A P K V W D Q C G F S Q A
W T P N Q F B J W G L V D M O U
T A N T I C O A G U L A N T D U
Q F Y X K C P Y M K H H H B A W
J F U C I T Y L O B M O R H T G Y
```

1. aggregation
2. anticoagulant
3. fibrinolysis
4. ischemia
5. thrombolytic
6. stroke
7. INR
8. LMWH
9. DVT
10. PT

11. artery; vein
12. clot formation
13. do not have
14. venous thrombus that may lead to pulmonary embolism
15. subcutaneously; intravenously
16. standard heparin; lower the risk of bleeding
17. warfarin
18. decrease
19. 4
20. plasminogen; plasmin
21. hemorrhage
22. fondaparinux (Arixtra)
23. c
24. d
25. a
26. a
27. e
28. d
29. f
30. b
31. f
32. c
33. a, b, c. Patients on warfarin therapy are maintained at an International Normalized Ratio (INR) of 2-3.
34. c
35. b

36. a. Abciximab (ReoPro) is an antiplatelet medication in the glycoprotein (GP) IIb/IIIa receptor antagonist family. It is used primarily for acute coronary syndromes and for preventing reocclusion of coronary arteries following PTCA.

37. a. The correct dose for continuous infusion is 0.125 mcg/kg/min. This patient weighs 76 kg (168 pounds ÷ 2.2 = 76 kg). 76 kg × 0.125 mcg/kg/min = 9.5 mcg/min.

38. d

39. a. Various laboratory values will be monitored while a patient is taking warfarin (Coumadin). The most important levels to trend will be PT, aPTT, and INR. The INR and PT are closely related, and the patient will have the aPTT evaluated prior to changing to warfarin completely.

40. b

41. d. Vitamin K is the antidote for warfarin poisoning or overdose. Protamine sulfate is the antidote for heparin poisoning.

42. a

43. b. There is the potential for drug displacement of warfarin, leading to higher free drug levels in the blood. This can result in bleeding.

44. a. Bleeding is considered an adverse reaction to fondaparinux.

45. a

46. a, b, c, d

47. b. Used after bleeding during cardiovascular surgery, aminocaproic acid may also be used to help with bleeding from thrombolytics.

48. a, c, e. Vital signs should be continually assessed while a patient is receiving thrombolytics. Cardiac monitoring should be performed to observe for reperfusion arrhythmias. The nurse should also monitor for signs and symptoms of bleeding.

49. a, b, d. Anticoagulants would be beneficial for patients with a history of deep vein thrombosis and those who have received an artificial heart valve. They are also beneficial in patients who have had major orthopedic surgeries, such as hip or knee replacements, to prevent pulmonary emboli.

Case Study

1. Heparin combines with antithrombin III, which accelerates the anticoagulant cascade of reactions that prevents thrombus formation. By inhibiting the action of thrombin, conversion of fibrinogen to fibrin does not occur and the formation of a fibrin clot is prevented. Heparin will not dissolve a clot like a thrombolytic, but it prevents the formation of further clots. Prior to discharge home, a patient must be transitioned to either a low–molecular-weight heparin (LMWH) like enoxaparin sodium, which is administered subcutaneously, or an oral medication such as warfarin (Coumadin).

2. Warfarin inhibits hepatic synthesis of vitamin K, thus affecting clotting factors II, VII, IX, and X. If the blood cannot clot as well, the likelihood of another pulmonary embolus forming is lower.

3. Priority teaching for this patient prior to discharge includes information regarding compliance with lab testing (INR) and communication with the health care provider before taking any medications, herbals, or OTC preparations. Dietary restrictions include limiting the amount of green leafy vegetables in the diet, as well as careful consumption of vitamin C. Green leafy vegetables are high in vitamin K. Herbals such as St. John's wort, ginkgo, kava, and ginseng also decrease the effectiveness of warfarin. The nurse should also advise the patient that aspirin should be avoided; acetaminophen may be used as a substitute as needed.

Safety precautions should also be taken to prevent anything that would lead to a risk of bleeding. The patient should be advised to use a toothbrush with soft bristles and only shave with an electric razor. If the patient does sustain an injury, bleeding should be able to be controlled with direct pressure for 5-10 minutes with a sterile dressing. If this is not effective, the patient should notify the health care provider. Any indications of bleeding such as epistaxis, hematemesis, or blood in the stool should be reported to the health care provider as well.

Chapter 46—
Antihyperlipidemics and Peripheral Vasodilators

1. b
2. c
3. a
4. a
5. b
6. d
7. c
8. d. Rhabdomyolysis is a severe side effect associated with atorvastatin. This occurs when muscle tissue breaks down.
9. b
10. c
11. c
12. d
13. d
14. a. An HDL level of 22 mg/dL puts the patient in the high-risk category for cardiovascular disease. A value less than 35 mg/dL is considered high risk.
15. b
16. c. Diet, exercise, weight loss, and medication all play a vital role in decreasing cholesterol. Diet continues to play a vital role, no matter what antihyperlipidemic medication is taken.

17. a

18. b, d, e. Cilostazol (Pletal) should be taken 30 minutes before or 2 hours after meals. Grapefruit juice will increase the levels of cilostazol, so it should be avoided. There is no contraindication for the use of acetaminophen. Headache and abdominal pain are both side effects of cilostazol. Blood pressure should be monitored frequently and the patient should be encouraged to change positions slowly to prevent a precipitous drop in blood pressure.

19. a, d, f

20. a

Case Study

1. Atorvastatin (Lipitor) is an HMG-CoA reductase inhibitor, or a "statin" drug. By inhibiting cholesterol synthesis in the liver, atorvastatin decreases LDL cholesterol ("bad") and slightly increases HDL ("good") cholesterol. It also decreases triglycerides between 20% and 50% based on the dosage.

2. Atorvastatin is pregnancy category X. Medications in this category have been shown to have a harmful effect on the fetus, and the benefits to the mother do not outweigh the risks to the fetus. Pregnancy is a contraindication to the use of statins.

3. Monitoring the patient for the desired effect is an obvious priority, although it is important for the nurse to advise the patient that changes in lipid profiles may take up to 3 months to become apparent. Liver enzymes should also be drawn at baseline and monitored throughout therapy. Vision should be tested at least yearly, as there have been some studies to indicate an increased risk of cataracts in patients taking statins. This risk is higher in patients with diabetes.

4. The nurse should emphasize that treatment of hyperlipidemia is a lifelong commitment. Making dietary changes, exercising, and using pharmacologic therapy will help decrease LDL levels, and therefore, potentially decrease the risk of coronary heart disease. Other important points in the health teaching plan for S.S. include the importance of keeping follow-up appointments with health care providers, taking the medication as scheduled even if she does not feel she is making any progress, and reporting any muscle pain or tenderness immediately, as this can be an indication of the life-threatening adverse effect of rhabdomyolysis.

Chapter 47— Drugs for Gastrointestinal Tract Disorders

1. f
2. d
3. e

4. b

5. g

6. c

7. a

8. a, e

9. a, b, c, e

10. b

11. a, b, c, d. Drinking weak tea and sodas that have gone flat may help with nausea. Open a can or bottle of soda and let it sit for several hours to get rid of the carbonation. Unsweetened gelatin may also be helpful. Crackers and dry toast may provide something to stay in the stomach. Relaxed breathing may help with the feeling of nausea, but it is usually more beneficial to breathe in through the nose and out through the mouth as is used in relaxation techniques.

12. c

13. c, d. Nonpharmacologic measures are now recommended for morning sickness. Some prescription antiemetics can be taken during pregnancy, but they are classified as pregnancy category C. Hydroxyzine (Vistaril) is classified as pregnancy category X. OTC antiemetics are no longer considered safe. Telling the patient it will just go away in a few months, while this may or may not be true, negates the patient's feelings.

14. b

15. d

16. b. Nausea, vomiting, and vertigo are classic signs of Ménière's disease. Diphenidol is used to treat these symptoms.

17. a

18. a, b, c

19. a, b, e

20. a, c, e

21. c

22. b, d, e

23. a

24. b

25. d. Patients with heart failure are not candidates for the use of saline cathartics. Saline cathartics pull fluid into the system, potentially making the heart failure worse.

26. c

27. b. Mineral oil absorbs the fat-soluble vitamins so the body cannot absorb them. This can lead to vitamin deficiency.

28. a, b, c, d. Stimulant laxatives like bisacodyl can cause diarrhea, leading to electrolyte imbalance. By increasing fluid and fiber intake in the diet, constipation can be prevented or lessened. Adequate amounts of regular exercise can prevent constipation. Laxatives that contain senna, cascara, and phenolphthalein can discolor the urine, turning it brown.

29. b
30. d. Patients with any kind of bowel obstruction or severe abdominal pain should not take laxatives.
31. a, c, d, e
32. a, c, d. Nonpharmacologic methods such as weak tea, broth, or flat soda, as well as crackers or toast, may help with nausea. These methods may also be used in conjunction with the antiemetic. Prochlorperazine may be sedating so driving, making serious decisions, and drinking alcohol should be avoided while taking the drug. Alcohol will intensify the sedative effect of prochlorperazine and should be avoided.
33. a
34. b
35. d. Certain antidiarrheals, including those containing diphenoxylate, difenoxin, or loperamide, are contraindicated in patients with severe hepatic disease.
36. a, b, c, d. Severe diarrhea can lead to electrolyte imbalance and hypovolemic shock. The patient should be carefully monitored for any arrhythmias associated with potassium loss. Frequent vital signs and assessment of bowel sounds are priorities.
37. c, d, e. A patient with diarrhea should avoid "heavy" fried foods, milk products, and raw vegetables. For the first 48 hours, fluid intake and replacing electrolytes are priority interventions.
38. a, b, d, e. Fresh fruits and vegetables, adequate water intake, and ingestion of whole grains may help prevent or treat constipation.

Case Study

1. Constipation has a variety of causes, including decreased fluid intake, poor diet, lack of exercise, fecal impaction, and current medications. Lack of appetite is a frequent complaint among the elderly. Poor dentition may lead to inability to eat raw fruits and vegetables. The opioid L.B. is taking for her postoperative hip pain, as well as the potential for decreased mobility and lack of exercise, may also lead to constipation.
2. Bisacodyl is a stimulant laxative that promotes defecation by irritating sensory nerve endings in the intestinal mucosa.
3. Omeprazole and other proton pump inhibitors will decrease the effect of bisacodyl, so dosage adjustments may need to be made. There are no interactions with either digoxin or calcium supplements.
4. It will be important for the nurse to encourage L.B. to eat well and exercise as possible. Including bran and whole grain in the diet may be beneficial. Bulk-forming laxatives can provide the fiber that she may not be getting in a regular diet. When possible, the patient should discontinue use of the opioid pain reliever. The nurse should also advise L.B.

that the medication should be taken whole, with a glass of water. Milk should be avoided around the time of administration, since milk also reduces the effectiveness of the laxative.

Chapter 48— Antiulcer Drugs

1. h
2. i
3. f
4. c
5. g
6. d
7. j
8. b
9. a
10. e
11. c
12. d
13. a
14. d
15. c
16. e
17. b
18. d
19. b
20. a
21. a, b, c, d, f
22. c, e
23. a, b, d, e. There are various nonpharmacologic methods to help prevent the discomfort associated with gastroesophageal reflux disease (GERD). Nicotine relaxes the lower esophageal sphincter so acid can reflux back into the esophagus. Elevating the head of the bed will allow the body to work with gravity instead of against it to keep acid in the stomach. NSAIDs are acids that will decrease the pH even further. Spicy foods are irritating to the lining of the esophagus.
24. d
25. a, b, e
26. a, b, c. Nizatidine should not be taken with meals, as it will delay absorption. The abdominal pain should have improved with 1-2 weeks, depending on the cause. Healing of the ulcer may take 4-8 weeks.
27. a
28. a, b, d, e
29. a, b, c. There are no documented interactions between esomeprazole and either lisinopril or propranolol. Esomeprazole interferes with the absorption of ampicillin, digoxin, and ketoconazole.
30. c. Hyperglycemia is an adverse reaction to sucralfate. Although the normal range for blood glucose

may vary, a blood glucose of 185 mg/dL is considered elevated.

Case Study

1. There are seven groups of antiulcer drugs: tranquilizers, anticholinergics, histamine$_2$ blockers, proton pump inhibitors, the pepsin inhibitor sucralfate, the prostaglandin E$_1$ analogue misoprostol, and antacids.

2. Aluminum hydroxide is an antacid. Antacids, as their name implies, neutralize acids that destroy the gastric mucosal barrier. They may be taken alone or in combination with other medications for ulcers.

3. The normal dose for aluminum hydroxide is 5-15 mL, 1 hour after meals and at bedtime. This patient is taking double the recommended dose.

4. The priority teaching right now for this patient is in regards to the proper dose. The patient should be advised to drink 2-4 ounces of water with the aluminum hydroxide and to decrease or eliminate consumption of alcohol and caffeinated beverages. There are many predisposing factors for ulcers, including environmental factors such as a high-stress job. Learning to utilize relaxation techniques and decrease stress may help the patient's discomfort. The patient should also be advised of the potential side effects, including anorexia and constipation.

Chapter 49—
Drugs for Eye and Ear Disorders

```
C X C P I  A I R U N A  L K L W G Z C G M G P A A U N D Z Q Z F R
L N F E A I S X L A G O G D K K Y X P K V N P V S O P R Z D R I
S R O T I  B I  H N I  E S A R D Y H N A C I  N O B R A C L T E M Z
U E A S M S T V R P Z P D S D E U E I X X W A N E T L Q Q H L W
A Y D L F O N J C W D U S Z V H B Z T D N Y E M M J V L B Y N Y
K R E N M X N T E A R S B Q U P T E P C P R T G L G O L K D S P
L R S I E C T C I N C R E A S E T O B Z D V P B T O Q K D R N O
T S F L S I R M S V A M O C U A L G V L E T C J S U I J G A Q M
S B K U A I A J H C I Y O B B L J Z I J O Z H M I L W F X T Y T
N T J W E J O T W Z I  D Y K T M H F D O Q O C C V Y P C I H K
I U X A R Z C W Y R D T C O B H C F D S S T D V Z W H Y U O S U
Q W V A C C U T O I S V E N B U N C E I S E S T C X A M N B H
N J Z V N Z L M I N B C V R U N N R S C C J B J U C L E P C P P
R D V Y U D A M A S W W E W U J G W S H C R H M K G C N F F Y I
L N P O E P R Y V E V X P D R J R O W F B I E R S P J O S
X L T Q S S B R R J A Q P I P K D O E I F O H A P X K R I D R O
E E B T B M F X G K L S E V S Y W E C R E Y W U S X Z T G Y D Q
Z C L R T W I P Z Q E A Y J R D J R Q W F B I X E R S P J O S
O B U L Q L B Z V N B D T U Y X D A Q Z Y B V X P L W G I Y V W
L Q X E W H C E A C Y C L O P L E G I C S K T O N U W I X W T F
```

1. foreign body
2. tears
3. intraocular
4. diuretics; (open-angle) glaucoma
5. decrease
6. anuria; dehydration
7. cycloplegics
8. children
9. increase
10. conjunctivitis
11. carbonic anhydrase inhibitors
12. osmotic

13. e
14. d
15. f
16. a
17. b
18. c
19. c
20. c
21. c
22. a, b, c, d. Small pupils or miosis is not a side effect of this medication.
23. d
24. b. Carbamide peroxide (Auro Ear Drops, Debrox) is an OTC medication that helps break up cerumen so it can be washed away.
25. a, c
26. c, d, e
27. a
28. a, d
29. e
30. a, b, c, d. Olopatadine has both antihistamine and mast cell–stabilizer effects. Tetracaine is a topical anesthetic. The other medications listed are decongestants to help with the eye irritation.

Case Study

1. Open-angle glaucoma occurs when there is too much aqueous humor that causes pressure and damages the optic nerve, which leads to decreased vision. As aqueous humor is formed, excess fluid drains though the trabecular meshwork structure of the eye. In open-angle glaucoma, the trabecular network is clogged and the excess fluid cannot drain. Primary open-angle glaucoma occurs gradually and the cause is unknown.

2. There are several different classes of medications that are used to treat glaucoma. Timolol is a beta blocker. Beta blockers are usually the first-line drug in glaucoma treatment. Beta blockers work by decreasing the production of aqueous humor.

3. The patient should wash her hands prior to administration of the drug and be very careful not to touch the tip of the bottle to the eye. The head should be tipped back and one drop instilled in the conjunctival sac of the lower lid. The patient should not rub her eyes after the medication is instilled. A tissue can be used to dab at the extra. Eyedrops should be instilled before any eye ointment.

4. This dose is too high. The standard dose is 1 gtt of 0.25%-0.5% solution b.i.d. initially, then decrease to 1 gtt/day as the condition stabilizes. The patient must be carefully observed for bradycardia, bronchospasm, and indications of developing or worsening heart failure, since this medication may cause systemic effects.

Chapter 50—
Drugs for Dermatologic Disorders

1. c
2. d
3. b
4. a
5. e
6. f
7. a, b, c, d
8. a, c, d
9. b
10. a
11. b
12. b, c, e
13. b
14. d
15. a, b, d. The patient should be encouraged to report to the health care provider if she is pregnant or plans on becoming pregnant since tetracycline has possible teratogenic effects. Harsh cleansers may be irritating to the skin that may already be sensitive. Tetracycline taken in combination with isotretinoin will increase the potential for adverse effects. Sunscreens with SPF 15 are recommended for all adults.
16. c
17. d
18. a, b, c
19. a, e

Case Study

1. Full-thickness burns extend down and include the epidermis, dermis, and the subcutaneous tissue in some cases. They have also been referred to as *third-degree burns*. Full-thickness burns may appear red, black, or white and are not painful because the nerve endings have been destroyed. Partial-thickness burns do not extend as deep; there may be blistering. Partial-thickness burns are very painful. Frequently partial-thickness (second-degree burns) surround a full-thickness burn.

2. Mafenide acetate is a broad-spectrum antibiotic that is applied topically (1/16-inch b.i.d.) to the burned area. Mafenide is a sulfonamide derivative, and it interferes with bacterial cell-wall synthesis and metabolism.

3. Another treatment option is silver sulfadiazine (Silvadene). It is also applied topically to the burned surface. Silver sulfadiazine acts on the cell membrane and cell wall. It is less likely to cause metabolic acidosis than mafenide.

4. Priority nursing interventions for this patient are pain control, adequate fluid resuscitation, and prevention of infection by providing sterile dressing changes. It will be easier for this patient to receive

skin grafting when appropriate if there have been fewer to no infections.

Chapter 51—
Endocrine Drugs: Pituitary, Thyroid, Parathyroid, and Adrenal Disorders

1. f
2. i
3. j
4. a
5. n
6. h
7. b
8. m
9. o
10. c
11. g
12. d
13. k
14. l
15. e
16. b
17. b
18. a
19. b
20. a
21. b
22. b
23. a
24. b
25. b
26. a
27. d
28. e
29. h
30. c
31. b
32. f
33. g
34. c. The normal dose is 25-50 mcg/day initially, with a maintenance dose of 50-200 mcg/day.
35. d
36. a, c, d
37. b, c, e. Strawberries, radishes, and peas inhibit thyroid secretions, and therefore must be avoided.
38. a
39. a, e. Over-the-counter drugs are generally contraindicated in patients with hypothyroidism. Patients with thyroid disorders should be encouraged to wear Medic-Alert–type identification. Medications for hypothyroidism should be taken on an empty stomach. Numbness and tingling of the hands occurs with hypoparathyroidism, not hypothyroidism.
40. b

41. d. Serum potassium levels could drop to <3.5 mEq/L, which could lead to arrhythmias.
42. b
43. b, c, d, e
44. c, d, e. Obtaining a medication history is important prior to starting a patient on prednisone, as there are many drug interactions possible with glucocorticoids. Vital signs and daily weights should be monitored. Weight gain is a side effect of prednisone.
45. b. Glucocorticoids can lead to fluid retention. Adequate fluid intake should be ensured but not forced.
46. b
47. b
48. a
49. a, b, c, d. Fresh fruit is not as high in potassium as dried fruit; although there are fresh fruit options, such as bananas and kiwi, that do provide a source of potassium.
50. a, b, e
51. b, c, d, e

Case Study

1. Signs and symptoms of adrenal insufficiency include muscle wasting, apathy, nausea, vomiting, electrolyte imbalances, hypovolemia, anemia, and cardiovascular collapse. An Addisonian crisis is a true emergency.
2. Hydrocortisone 20-240 mg/d in 3-4 divided doses can be given orally. This medication can also be administered IV or by suppository. The IV route is the fastest.
3. Priority teaching for this patient would include monitoring vital signs and weight. It is extremely important that the patient comply with the medication regimen and does not stop taking a glucocorticoid abruptly. The patient should be taught to watch for the signs of overdose or Cushing's syndrome (moon face, weight gain, puffy eyelids, edema). Laboratory values will be monitored closely to watch for hypoglycemia, hyponatremia, hyperkalemia, and anemia. The patient should be encouraged to carry Medic-Alert identification and a current list of medications. Herbal preparations should be avoided unless discussed with the health care provider or pharmacist.

Chapter 52— Antidiabetics

1. f
2. h
3. k
4. j
5. b
6. e
7. i
8. g
9. a
10. c
11. d
12. c
13. e
14. a
15. b
16. f
17. g
18. d
19. b
20. a
21. c
22. e
23. f
24. a, b, e
25. a, b, d
26. b
27. d
28. b, c, d, e
29. b, c, d, e, f
30. d. Tolazamide is a first-generation intermediate-acting oral antidiabetic agent. Oral medications in this class should not be used by patients with type 1 diabetes.
31. a, c, d, e, f. Insulin dose should be based on glucose testing and not how a patient is feeling. Compliance with regimen is crucial.
32. a, b, c, d. Oral antidiabetic medications should be taken on a regular, prescribed basis and not adjusted by glucose testing results.
33. a
34. a
35. c
36. c. When giving both NPH and regular insulin at the same time, the regular insulin is drawn into the syringe first.
37. d. U100 syringes are used for U100 insulin.
38. a, c, e
39. a. Regular insulin is short-acting, with an onset of 30 minutes to 1 hour.
40. c
41. b, d, e
42. c
43. c
44. a
45. b
46. a, c
47. b
48. d
49. b
50. b

51. d. Liver enzymes should be evaluated at baseline and monitored throughout treatment with thiazolidinediones.
52. b
53. b, c, d
54. b, c, d, e. Aspirin, oral anticoagulants, and sulfonamides can increase the action of sulfonylureas, especially the first-generation ones, by binding to plasma proteins and displacing sulfonylureas. The action of sulfonylureas may be decreased by taking several different types of medications, including anticonvulsants such as phenytoin (Dilantin).
55. a, b, c, d. Oral antidiabetic agents are only used for patients with type 2 diabetes because there have to be some beta cells functioning. Breastfeeding and pregnancy are contraindications. Severe infections, trauma, or physical stress can make blood sugar extremely difficult to control, so oral antidiabetic agents are not used. Because of the pharmacokinetics associated with oral antidiabetic agents, patients with renal or hepatic dysfunction should be treated with alternatives.

Case Study

1. Although there are a variety of causes for these symptoms, when a diabetic patient presents with a headache, confusion, slurred speech, and a glucometer reading of "low," a hypoglycemic reaction should be suspected. Although readings may vary depending on brand of glucometer, a reading of "low" may be in the 20 mg/dL range. This is an emergency that must be treated quickly.
2. As long as there is a gag reflex present and the patient is conscious, hard candy, glucose tablets, or glucose paste may be given. Other options include fruit juice or peanut butter crackers.
3. Once the patient becomes unconscious and loses the gag reflex, other options must be explored. The ABCs of patient care are top priority. After the ABCs are evaluated and treatment started, the patient may either receive glucagon (which stimulates glycogenolysis) or 50% dextrose IV. A benefit of giving glucagon is that it may be administered IM, IV, or subQ.

    This patient may or may not require admission to the hospital depending on his response; however, at discharge, priority education for this patient includes recognizing signs of hypoglycemic reactions, treatments at home (hard candy, etc.), and the importance of maintaining a routine with regards to monitoring and insulin administration.

Chapter 53— Female Reproductive Cycle I: Pregnancy and Preterm Labor Drugs

1. g
2. f
3. j
4. i
5. a
6. b
7. d
8. e
9. h
10. c
11. a, b, c, d
12. d
13. c
14. c
15. g
16. e
17. f
18. h
19. a
20. d, e
21. a
22. a, b, d
23. b, d
24. b
25. b
26. b, d, e
27. a, c, d
28. c
29. b. Acetaminophen is generally considered safe in pregnancy. Combination cold medications, especially those that contain aspirin or ibuprofen, are not recommended. Megadoses of vitamins and any herbal preparations are not considered to be safe.
30. a, b. It is important to provide culturally competent care to all patients. All patients should receive information in the language in which they are most comfortable. Either obtaining a translator or using a service like a language line is crucial to show your respect for the patient and her culture. Family members should not be used to translate in the health care setting if at all possible. Allow the patient and family adequate time to ask questions and do not hurry as time frame of reference is different in Hispanic culture.
31. a, c, d, e. Fluids should not necessarily be avoided before arising. Sometimes small sips of flat soda or apple juice may be beneficial.
32. a, b, c, e. Avoidance of spicy foods or foods known to cause heartburn is a mainstay in the nonpharmacologic treatment of heartburn. This includes citrus fruits and juices and tomato-based products. Smaller meals lead to less reflux of gastric con-

tents, as does keeping the head slightly raised for a period of time after eating. Many pregnant women late in their third trimester find it more comfortable to sleep in a recliner to prevent reflux.

33. a, b, d. The patient should be instructed to lie on her left side to prevent supine hypotensive syndrome. Maintaining an adequate diet with proper amounts of fluids, protein, and sodium is important for the well-being of both mother and baby. Recording daily weights and looking for trends, as well as keeping track of symptoms such as headache, nausea, and extremity swelling, are important for the patient with gestational hypertension.

34. b, c, e. Iron supplements should be taken 2 hours before or 4 hours after antacids so the medication can be absorbed. Although best taken on an empty stomach, iron can be taken with food if necessary. Jaundice should be reported immediately to the health care provider. Liver is an excellent source of iron.

35. a

36. b

37. a

38. a. Breath sounds should be auscultated every 4 hours and assessed for the presence of wheezes, rales, or coughing. Myocardial ischemia and pulmonary edema can be an adverse effect in patients taking beta-sympathomimetic agents.

39. b, d, e. The loading dose of magnesium sulfate 6 g is given over 20-30 minutes as an IVPB. It is administered via a pump. Too-rapid administration of magnesium sulfate can lead to cardiac arrest. Patients receiving magnesium sulfate are on bedrest while receiving therapy.

40. a, d

41. d

42. a, b, c

43. a, b, d

44. d

45. b, d, e. Diuretics such as furosemide and ACE inhibitors such as lisinopril are contraindicated in pregnancy.

Case Study

1. Some priority questions to ask include if K.R. has been receiving regular prenatal care and the date of her last visit. The nurse should inquire if there are any known complications with this pregnancy such as gestational diabetes, gestational hypertension, or hyperemesis. It will also be important to ask if she has been told she is starting to dilate or efface. K.R. should also be questioned regarding membrane rupture and if there has been any bleeding or changes in fetal movement.

2. K.R. is at high risk due to her age, history of miscarriage, and previous PTL.

3. Nonpharmacologic measures that the nurse can suggest while K.R. is waiting to hear back from the health care provider include lying down on her left side, or if that is not possible, at least sitting down and putting her feet up. Dehydration may lead to PTL, so K.R. should drink several glasses of water. Having an empty bladder may also help, so the patient should be advised to void. If nonpharmacologic measures are not effective, the patient may require tocolytics. These drugs include beta sympathomimetics (terbutaline), magnesium sulfate, or prostaglandin inhibitors. Terbutaline has come under scrutiny within the last 5 years and must be used cautiously. Magnesium sulfate is more commonly used. One of the major goals in tocolytic therapy is to interrupt or inhibit uterine contractions to create additional time for fetal maturation in utero.

4. Although the survival rate of a fetus at 33 weeks is fairly high, the baby will be small and will require a stay in the neonatal intensive care unit. The mother should also receive steroids, either betamethasone or dexamethasone, to accelerate fetal lung maturity and development of surfactant in the event her labor cannot be halted. Studies have shown that this will decrease the incidence of respiratory distress syndrome in preterm infants.

Chapter 54—
Female Reproductive Cycle II: Labor, Delivery, and Preterm Neonatal Drugs

Crossword Puzzle

Across
1. somatic
4. regional
5. kappa
7. ripening
8. Bishop score
9. meperidine
10. contraction
11. visceral

Down
1. surfactant
2. intratracheal
3. Pitocin
6. uterine inertia

12. a

13. d. Postdural headaches are caused by leakage of cerebrospinal fluid through a puncture site. The

decrease in pressure exerted by the CSF causes the headache.

14. a, b, c, d
15. a
16. d. Butorphanol tartrate, a narcotic agonist-antagonist, is absolutely contraindicated in this patient since it may precipitate withdrawal symptoms.
17. d
18. a
19. a. A fluid bolus of 500-1000 mL should be given to prevent hypotension that frequently accompanies an epidural.
20. d. Patients with hypotension are positioned on their left side to facilitate placental perfusion.
21. c
22. d
23. a. Patients with hypertension should not receive methylergonovine. When this medication is given IV, dramatic increases in blood pressure can occur.
24. b. Naloxone is a narcotic antagonist and will reverse the effects of meperidine, leading to an increase in pain.
25. d. The choice of pain control is very individual. Each woman has an expectation of what she wants with regards to the labor experience.
26. d
27. a, b, d, e. The time of delivery cannot be predicted, whether analgesics are utilized or not.
28. c. The patient should be placed flat immediately to ensure that the local anesthetic disperses evenly. The nurse must assess that the anesthetic is even. If this is not the case, the anesthesia provider should be made aware and the patient turned to the opposite side.
29. c
30. a, c
31. b, c, d, e. Deep tendon reflexes are usually assessed on a patient receiving magnesium sulfate, not oxytocin. A type and crossmatch should be obtained in the event that the patient will need an emergent cesarean section. The fetus may become hypoxic and there is an increased risk for uterine rupture.
32. a, c, e
33. b, d, e
34. a, b, c, d. Urinary retention is not a concern in the neonate of a mother who has received a sedative-hypnotic and antiemetic.
35. c, d
36. b, c, e
37. d

Case Study

1. Inductions are based on several factors, including intrauterine growth retardation. At 38 weeks gestation, K.E. is considered full-term. There are several options to induce labor. Prior to delivery, the cervix must efface, or thin, and dilate. A mechanical device such as a Foley catheter can be placed through the cervical os, and then 30 mL of sterile saline instilled into the balloon. This will act similarly to manual stripping of the membranes to start labor. Another method is to place prostaglandin E2 (PGE2) either intracervically or intravaginally. It is usually left in place for approximately 12 hours and then synthetic oxytocin (Pitocin) is started intravenously to augment labor. Once the cervix has dilated to approximately 5 cm, an amniotomy ("breaking the bag") may be performed under sterile conditions. Labor will tend to get into an established pattern within a few hours of the amniotic sac being broken.

2. Priority teaching for this patient includes advising her to communicate her needs and wants to the health care team regarding analgesia and delivery. Ideally a "birth plan" will have been developed by the patient and her partner in advance. This plan is usually submitted to the health care provider and is brought with the patient to the hospital. As much as is possible and safe, the patient should be able to control her delivery.

3. Analgesia may be provided by intravenous narcotic agonists, mixed agonist-antagonists, and regional anesthesia (epidurals, blocks). The patient should also have the option of refraining from the use of analgesics if she desires ("natural childbirth").

Chapter 55—
Postpartum and Newborn Drugs

Crossword Puzzle

Across
1. puerperium
2. erythromycin
4. congenital rubella
6. urticaria
7. folliculitis
8. episiotomy

Down
1. phytonadione
3. benzocaine
5. lactation

9. a, d, e
10. a
11. b
12. a, b
13. a, b, c. Drinking sage tea as well as applying ice or cold compresses to the breasts may aid in suppress-

ing lactation. Wearing a tight bra continuously for the first 10-14 days after delivery will also suppress milk production.

14. b
15. a
16. a, d, e
17. b, c, d
18. b
19. a. The swelling should decrease and disappear within 24-48 hours after administration of ophthalmic medications.

Case Study

1. The nurse's best response initially is to listen to J.G. and let her know that what she is feeling is all right. Pain control may be a first priority with regards to feeling sore and breast pain. Some non-pharmacologic methods to relieve her discomfort include warm or cool sitz baths, sitting on "donuts" or specially designed cushions, and gently washing the perineal area. NSAIDs may help with afterbirth pain. Narcotic analgesia may also be beneficial in the short-term, although this may pass to the infant while breastfeeding. Cool compresses with witch hazel, either homemade or commercially prepared, may be utilized. Benzocaine sprays may also be used judiciously. Discomfort from engorgement can be relieved by warm compresses or taking a warm shower and hand-expressing. Applying cabbage leaves to the breast tissue and areola may help with engorgement. Hand-expressing some milk and rubbing it on the nipple to ensure a good "latch" will also decrease breast tenderness.

Chapter 56— Drugs for Women's Reproductive Health and Menopause

Crossword Puzzle

Across

5. venous thromboembolism
10. progestin
13. menorrhagia
15. dysmenorrhea
17. osteoporosis
18. oophorectomy
19. methotrexate
20. mittelschmerz

Down

1. oligomenorrhea
2. dyspareunia
3. morning after

4. chloasma
6. ethinyl estradiol
7. menopause
8. mifepristone
9. menarche
11. the minipill
12. candida
14. amenorrhea
16. misoprostol

21. a, b, c, d. Oral contraceptives must be taken at the same time every day or within a few hours. The best choices for this patient, assuming there are no contraindications, would be medications that are injected, implanted, inserted, or applied topically. They stay in place or provide contraceptive coverage for a prolonged period of time. These would be more convenient for the patient.
22. b, c, d
23. a, b, d. Oral contraceptives can be expensive and may or may not be covered by insurance. Although not likely, patients can be allergic to oral contraceptives. This may be due to the fact that they are synthesized or it may be part of the packaging process (dye or filler).
24. c. A woman with breast cancer should not take oral contraceptives because the hormones could accelerate tumor growth.
25. a, b, c. There are no contraindications for using combined hormone contraceptives (CHCs) in epilepsy, but other medications that the patient takes must be evaluated. There is no contraindication for a patient with depression taking CHCs. The 45-year-old patient is, in all likelihood, perimenopausal, so there may not be a need for CHCs, but they are not absolutely contraindicated.
26. c. If only one dose has been missed, the patient should take the dose as soon as possible then get back on the regular schedule with the next dose.
27. b, c, d, e
28. d, e. Barbiturates like phenobarbital and topiramate, which can be used either for seizures or migraines, are contraindicated in patients taking oral contraceptives. All women of childbearing age should take folic acid.
29. c. Potassium levels should be monitored closely. Yasmin causes the body to retain potassium. Hyperkalemia is possible, especially in patients with undiagnosed kidney disease.
30. c. If the ring has been out less than 3 hours, it can be reinserted.
31. b. As part of the ACHES mnemonic [*A*bdominal pain (severe), *C*hest pain or shortness of breath, *H*eadache (severe), *E*ye disorders, *S*evere leg pain], severe headaches could be indicative of cardiovascular side effects and should be reported to the health care provider immediately.

32. b, c, d, e
33. c
34. a
35. b, e
36. c, d

Case Study

1. With these presenting symptoms and at her age, the patient is likely menopausal. Dyspareunia, frequency, urgency, thinning vaginal epithelium, and decreased elasticity on speculum exam are due to estrogen deficit. Frequency and urgency can also be associated with a urinary tract infection (UTI), so a urinalysis should be obtained; however, a UTI would not account for the findings on speculum exam. By definition, a lack of menstruation for 1 year is defined as menopause. Other symptoms associated with menopause may include hot flashes and night sweats.

2. Treatment may be symptomatic and include cool baths, using a fan, and sleeping in light clothing. Herbal options include chasteberry, red clover, black cohosh, and soy, although the research is equivocal. Bioidentical hormone therapy is made by a compounding pharmacist and matched to the individual. Bioidentical hormones are made with plants including soy and Mexican yams. The final option is hormone therapy (HT). HT should be administered at the lowest doses and for the shortest amount of time possible. HT improves vasomotor symptoms such as hot flashes, and it also improves vaginal dryness and irritation. It does, however, come with increased risks of cardiovascular events such as DVT, stroke, and MI and certain cancers (breast, ovarian, and lung). The health care provider should discuss the risk-to-benefit ratio with the patient to help her decide on the best option for her.

3. HT also decreases the risk of osteoporosis. C.W. is thin and Caucasian, which are two risk factors for osteoporosis. Using HT, increasing vitamin D and calcium intake, and exercise such as walking may help prevent bone loss. The use of medications for osteoporosis includes bisphosphonates and SERMs. These medications help prevent the breakdown of bone.

Chapter 57—
Drugs for Men's Health and Reproductive Disorders

1. g
2. h
3. j
4. f

5. e
6. i
7. b
8. c
9. a
10. d
11. d. Sildenafil is contraindicated in patients with significant cardiac disease.
12. d
13. c. The use of hormones to "bulk up" or improve performance occurs at all levels of sports competition. Side/adverse effects from the use of excessive intake of anabolic steroids include increased low-density lipoprotein cholesterol, decreased high-density lipoprotein cholesterol, acne, high blood pressure, liver damage, and dangerous changes in the left ventricle of the heart.
14. a. Blood glucose levels may be decreased in patients with diabetes when taking androgens. The patient should be instructed to carefully monitor blood sugar for changes so the insulin dose can be adjusted.
15. a, c
16. a, b, d
17. a, c, e

Case Study

1. Erectile dysfunction can occur in men at any stage of life. It occurs due to lack of sufficient blood flow to the penis. It may be seen in men with diabetes, and some studies indicate that up to half of all diabetic men will have erectile dysfunction at one time or another. Some of the medications used to treat hypertension, such as diuretics and beta blockers, may also cause erectile dysfunction.

2. One class of medications that the patient may be referring to is the phosphodiesterase (PDE-5) inhibitors, which includes sildenafil, tadalafil, and vardenafil. They work by increasing blood flow to the penis so the patient can maintain an erection.

3. Side effects may include upset stomach, blurred vision, flushing, and headache. The most serious side effect is a sustained erection (priapism) that lasts over 4 hours. Priapism is an emergency because a thrombosis may form in the corpora cavernosa, which can lead to permanent loss of function.

4. The nurse should teach the patient not to use any herbal preparations without discussing with his health care provider. The patient should also be advised to not use any nitroglycerin or nitrate-containing drugs while taking PDE-5 inhibitors because the combination can cause marked hypotension. PDE-5 inhibitors should also not be taken with grapefruit or grapefruit juice because it increases the amount of PDE-5 available.

Chapter 58—
Drugs for Disorders in Women's Health, Infertility, and Sexually Transmitted Infections

Crossword Puzzle

Across
2.   acanthosis nigricans
9.   leiomyomata
12. menorrhagia
13. peanut oil
14. anovulatory
16. progestational
20. amenorrhea
22. gonorrhea

Down
1.   endometriosis
2.   acyclovir
3.   hepatitis B
4.   St. John's wort
5.   syphilis
6.   insulin
7.   dysmenorrhea
8.   boxer shorts
10. infertility
11. Lupron Depot
15. danazol
17. penicillin
18. progestin
19. chasteberry
21. abstinence

23. c
24. a. Abstaining from sexual activity is the safest in preventing any further transmission; however, if that is not an option, all partners should wear a condom during sex.
25. a
26. d. If the patient wants to participate in sexual activity, using a condom is the safest.
27. a
28. b. Fluoroquinolones are contraindicated in pregnant women.
29. d
30. a, b, d
31. b, d, e. HIV cannot be cured. Early detection would promote earlier treatment. There is no legal requirement for an individual with STIs to be tested for HIV; it is the patient's choice.
32. d
33. c
34. a, b, c, e. Fibroids, depression, pregnancy, and ovarian failure are all contraindications. Gastro-

esophageal reflux disease (GERD) is not a contraindication for therapy with clomiphene.
35. b
36. c. Precise guidelines must be followed when taking Synarel. One spray is administered into one nostril in the morning and the other nostril in the evening.
37. b, c, e

Case Study
1. Premenstrual syndrome (PMS) occurs in up to 40% of all women at one time or another. Symptoms are classified as physical, emotional, or behavioral. If severe mood swings are present, the diagnosis of premenstrual dysphoric disorder (PMDD) may be applied. The patient's symptoms increase during the luteal phase (days 15-28) of the menstrual cycle.
2. Some nonpharmacologic methods for helping a patient with PMS may include allowing the patient to ventilate and express her feelings. Exercise will release endorphins, which will ease feelings of tension and anxiety. Dietary changes, including decreasing salty foods and caffeine, and eating frequent low-fat, high-carbohydrate meals may also help. Ensuring adequate amounts of vitamin B$_6$ may be helpful.
3. Although not regulated by the FDA, there are some herbal preparations that some patients find helpful. The supportive science is lacking to date. The herbal supplements may include St. John's wort, evening primrose, and chasteberry. If symptoms persist despite less aggressive methods, SSRIs and anxiolytics may be prescribed. Some patients also benefit from the use of hormone therapy to decrease the number of periods per year.

Chapter 59—
Adult and Pediatric Emergency Drugs

1.   h
2.   g
3.   k
4.   e
5.   i
6.   a
7.   f
8.   b
9.   d
10. c
11. j
12. f
13. d
14. a
15. d

16. g
17. b
18. c
19. e
20. b
21. a. Nitroglycerin can cause a rapid drop in blood pressure, especially in first-time users.
22. a. Morphine can cause respiratory depression so the patient's respiratory status must be monitored closely. Naloxone can be used to reverse respiratory depression if needed.
23. a
24. d. Myocardial ischemia can occur when a patient is receiving dobutamine. The nurse must monitor carefully for signs of myocardial ischemia, including chest pain and arrhythmias.
25. c
26. b
27. b, e
28. a
29. c
30. c. This patient is exhibiting signs of an allergic reaction. Besides receiving epinephrine, the patient will receive diphenhydramine (Benadryl). Diphenhydramine is an agent that reduces histamine-induced swelling and itching in allergic reactions.
31. c. Naloxone 0.4 mg IVP should be administered. If this is an opioid overdose, the medication should reverse fairly rapidly, and the patient will become responsive. If this is not an opioid overdose, there will be no response. Benzodiazepines, such as diazepam, are also used for back spasms, but they do not produce pinpoint pupils.
32. a, d, e. Dopamine may be used to treat hypotension in cardiogenic, neurogenic, and septic shock, although norepinephrine may be preferred in neurogenic shock. Hypovolemic shock should be treated with fluids, either crystalloids or blood. *Insulin shock* is actually misnamed and refers to a hypoglycemic reaction. It should be treated with glucose, not vasopressors.
33. a
34. b
35. d
36. c
37. a. Once the arrhythmia has been suppressed, as long as a total of 3 mg/kg has not been exceeded, a maintenance drip of lidocaine at a rate of 1-4 mg/min is started.

38. b. The correct solution to utilize for IM injection is 1:1000 solution.
39. a. The standard concentration of 1 mg of 1:10,000 epinephrine is used in cardiac arrest.
40. a
41. b
42. c, d, e
43. d
44. a, b, c, e
45. b, d, e. Blue or brown color indicates the solution has degraded and should not be used. The bottle should be protected from light. Because this medication is a potent antihypertensive, the patient will need to be monitored continuously in the critical care unit. As nitroprusside breaks down, the by-products include thiocyanate or cyanide; therefore, levels must be monitored closely and the drug should be used for the shortest amount of time necessary.
46. a, c, d

Case Study

1. M.E. took three of his own nitroglycerin tablets prior to calling EMS. Nitroglycerin (NTG), either in tablet form or as a spray, works to dilate the coronary arteries to provide blood flow and oxygen to the ischemic myocardium. It is the ischemic myocardium that causes angina.

2. An aspirin is given to patients having chest pain to decrease platelet aggregation in acute coronary syndrome and for acute myocardial infarction (AMI). It is not known if this patient is having an AMI, so the aspirin is given. Oxygen will be given to provide adequate supply to the heart. It can be administered either by nasal cannula, nonrebreather mask, simple mask, or by endotracheal intubation to maintain the oxygen saturation at >94%. This patient does not, at this point, require endotracheal intubation. Morphine is used to relieve pain, dilate venous vessels, and reduce the workload of the heart. IV nitroglycerin is reserved for patients with unstable angina or an AMI. A nitroglycerin drip is usually initiated at a rate of 10-20 mcg/min and increased by 5-10 mcg/min every 5-10 minutes, based on chest pain and blood pressure response. Nitroglycerin drips are not administered for prolonged periods of time. They are a temporizing measure.